Decision Making Series

Berman: *Pediatric Decision Making*
Bucholz, Lippert and Wenger: *Orthopaedic Decision Making*
Dubovsky and Feiger: *Decision Making in Psychiatry*
Friedman: *Gynecological Decision Making*
Goldstone: *Decision Making in Vascular Surgery*
Holt, Mattox and Gates: *Decision Making in Otolaryngology*
Korones: *Neonatal Decision Making*

Series Editor: Ben Eiseman, M.D.

Obstetrical Decision Making

By the Staff of the Beth Israel Hospital, Boston

Edited by

EMANUEL A. FRIEDMAN, M.D., Sc.D.

Professor of Obstetrics and Gynecology
Harvard Medical School
Obstetrician-Gynecologist-in-Chief
Beth Israel Hospital
Boston, Massachusetts

1982

B.C. Decker Inc. • Trenton, New Jersey
The C.V. Mosby Company • Saint Louis • Toronto • London

Publisher: **B.C. Decker Inc.**
3 Belmont Circle
Trenton, NJ 08618

U.S.A. and worldwide sales and distribution by:
The C.V. Mosby Company
11830 Westline Industrial Drive
Saint Louis, Missouri 63141

in Canada: **The C.V. Mosby Company, Ltd.**
120 Melford Drive
Toronto, Ontario M1B2X5

Obstetrical Decision Making ISBN 0-941158-01-2

Library of Congress catalog card number: 82-70759

Last digit is print number: 10 9 8 7 6 5 4 3 2

CONTRIBUTORS

BALMOOKOOT BALGOBIN, M.D.

Coordinator, Ambulatory Care Program, Beth Israel Hospital; Instructor in Obstetrics and Gynecology, Harvard Medical School

MAX BORTEN, M.D.

Coordinator, Residency Education, Chief, Section on Fertility Control, Beth Israel Hospital; Assistant Professor of Obstetrics and Gynecology, Harvard Medical School.

LOUIS BURKE, M.D.

Associate Director, Chief of Colposcopy Unit, Beth Israel Hospital; Associate Professor of Obstetrics and Gynecology, Harvard Medical School

WILLIAM D. COCHRAN, M.D.

Chief, Joint Program in Neonatology, Beth Israel Hospital; Assistant Clinical Professor of Pediatrics, Harvard Medical School

WAYNE R. COHEN, M.D.

Chief, Section on Fetologic Research, Beth Israel Hospital; Assistant Professor of Obstetrics and Gynecology, Harvard Medical School

EMANUEL A. FRIEDMAN, M.D., Sc.D.

Obstetrician-Gynecologist-in-Chief, Beth Israel Hospital; Professor of Obstetrics and Gynecology, Harvard Medical School

CATHERINE A. KEANEY, R.N., B.S.N., M.S.

Parent Education Coordinator, Beth Israel Hospital

HENRY KLAPHOLZ, M.D.

Director, Obstetrics Service, Section on Clinical Fetology, Beth Israel Hospital; Assistant Professor of Obstetrics and Gynecology, Harvard Medical School

CAROL S. LONDON, R.N., M.S.

Clinical Specialist in Sexually Transmitted Diseases, Beth Israel Hospital; Assistant Clinical Instructor, Boston College School of Nursing

WAYNE A. MILLER, M.D.

Director, Perinatal Diagnostic Laboratory, Assistant in Gynecology and Pediatrics, Massachusetts General Hospital; Assistant in Obstetrics and Gynecology, Beth Israel Hospital; Instructor in Pediatrics, Harvard Medical School

JOHN F. MODLIN, M.D.

Assistant in Medicine, Childrens Hospital and Medical Center; Assistant Professor of Pediatrics, Harvard Medical School

SELWYN P. OSKOWITZ, M.B., Ch.B.

Assistant in Obstetrics and Gynecology, Beth Israel Hospital; Instructor in Obstetrics and Gynecology, Harvard Medical School

JOHANNA F. PERLMUTTER, M.D.

Chief, Section on Human Sexuality, Adolescent Obstetrics Unit, Beth Israel Hospital; Assistant Professor of Obstetrics and Gynecology, Harvard Medical School

HAROLD RUBIN, M.D.

Obstetrician-Gynecologist, Beth Israel Hospital; Assistant Professor of Obstetrics and Gynecology, emeritus, Harvard Medical School

MACHELLE SEIBEL, M.D.

Chief, Gynecologic Endocrinology Laboratories, Beth Israel Hospital; Assistant Professor of Obstetrics and Gynecology, Harvard Medical School

LENARD R. SIMON, M.D.

Director, Gynecologic Service, Section on Gynecologic Oncology, Beth Israel Hospital; Instructor in Obstetrics and Gynecology, Harvard Medical School

DAVID J. SNYDER, M.D.

Head, Section on Obstetric Anaesthesiology, Beth Israel Hospital; Instructor in Anaesthesia, Harvard Medical School

AUSTIN WERTHEIMER, M.D.

Assistant in Obstetrics and Gynecology, Beth Israel Hospital; Instructor in Obstetrics and Gynecology, Harvard Medical School

PREFACE

The genesis of this book of decision trees is the oft-stated need perceived and expressed by generalist, obstetrical practitioners, and potential practitioners in training (that is, medical students and residents). Individually and collectively, our faculty is regularly besieged with requests for instruction and guidance in resolving diagnostic and therapeutic problems. Responding to such requests lucidly is a fitting role for those of us who consider ourselves to be both teacher and clinician. Indeed, our academic competence is sometimes challenged and the limits of our knowledge bared in the attempt to comply. Nonetheless, we continue to try to think logically so as to evolve a systematic sequence of interrelated steps leading to an end result that is appropriate vis-à-vis the correct diagnosis and the proper management regimen.

Our desire is not to replace the dogma of the past, which we eschew, with new dogma. Nonetheless, we recognize that much of what we consider today to be accepted and acceptable practice, even when based on apparently substantive scientific data, will be replaced in due course by modified practice as new data are developed.

In formulating this material, we have tried to be imaginative without being speculative; we have also tried to be comprehensive without being exhaustive or tautologous and, at the same time, to be concise without being superficial. In an effort to accomplish this, the editor has been merciless. I offer apologies to those authors whose work may have thereby been distorted, perhaps beyond recognition. Moreover, I accept full responsibility for the damage done, if any, and for errors that may have inadvertently been introduced. To all contributors, I extend special thanks for a difficult job well done. They have the added reward of an unexpected lesson well learned, namely that the simplicity of a decision tree is a delusion. Creating one that is meaningful is no small chore. Anyone who has ever tried will attest to the fact that the exercise forces one to think logically and systematically, a practice many of us are not accustomed to at all, even in the rarified atmosphere of academia.

Our collective aim in offering this material in its present form is to permit rapid dissemination and acquisition of information about specific obstetrical problems. We have deliberately kept comments to a minimum, somewhat more than telegraphic but much less than a full discourse on the subject at hand. Our intention was to provide the elements of the rationale for selecting from among the options that go to make the decision choice. Standard obstetrical textbooks are available and selected references are cited for the reader who wishes to (and should, of course) pursue the subject in greater depth.

We feel this material will prove especially useful to all who care for pregnant women, from midwife to obstetrician specialist, from student to seasoned practitioner. It will provide them with a framework, practical and conceptual at the same time, upon which they can build. The gratifying outcome results for mothers and offspring at our institution serve to justify our management recommendations.

Thus, this collection of decision trees should be more than a "how to" book (or more relevantly, a "how we do it" book), although it is a ready resource for such information. It is not intended to concretize clinical activities. Rather, we mean it to foster logical thinking about problems, to provide a necessary first step toward formal decision analysis, and above all, to help improve obstetrical practices.

Emanuel A. Friedman, M.D., Sc.D.
Boston

CONTENTS

FETAL STATUS EVALUATION

PREGNANCY-RELATED DISORDERS

INTERCURRENT PROBLEMS

LABOR AND DELIVERY COMPLICATIONS

POSTPARTUM MANAGEMENT

OPERATIVE PROCEDURES

FERTILITY CONTROL

INTRODUCTION

In the practice of medicine, decision making is commonplace. Almost every patient encounter involves one or more decisions. Some of these are pedestrian, others critical and challenging intellectual exercises. They range from simple matters of routine care to complex sequences of diagnostic and therapeutic steps. Inherent in some of the decisions we make is the logic of the basic tenets of medical science. Too many, however, derive from empiricism, dogma, rote, and intuition. Yet every decision should weigh benefits against risks or, more often, the risks of one option against the greater or lesser risks of another. To this end, a burgeoning scientific discipline of decision analysis is developing to quantitate the relative costs (principally monetary) of alternative options. Our collective efforts in this book have not directly addressed this sophisticated approach — which is still in its infancy with regard to technical development and practical application. Nonetheless, it is an objective toward which we should strive.

We recognize that the fine art of decision making can neither be taught simplistically nor learned easily. It is a skill that is acquired only by considerable effort after years of experience. It is a skill that needs continual sharpening and cultivation. Nonetheless, we felt we might facilitate the learning process somewhat by offering a spectrum of decision trees (algorithms or paradigms) reflecting the current practices at our institution. We do not consider any of them immutable. The central theme of each should serve the reader well as a practical guide to most of the decisions we are called upon to make for our obstetrical patients. Modifications, embellishments and tangents can be appended as needed, of course. Some of the more important "subroutines" are presented. These include approaches for assessing gestational age, cephalopelvic relationships, fetal growth, maturity, and well-being. We make repeated references to them wherever it is clear that the information they provide will help to make a logical decision. To avoid unnecessary complexity, we have chosen merely to cite cross references rather than to repeat them at each occasion. Whereas this means that some of the paradigms are incomplete entities that cannot stand alone, they have the advantage of being somewhat simpler as a consequence.

One may enter upon and find one's way in the forest of these trees — to maintain metaphorical consistency — by a variety of direct and circuitous routes. Choice can be addressed by a symptom (vaginal bleeding, shock, petechiae, pain), by an observed manifestation (hypertension, excessive uterine size, arrested labor, tetanic contraction, abdominal mass), by a laboratory finding (low hemoglobin, high alpha-fetoprotein, bacteriuria, glycosuria), by some historical information (renal or heart disease, hereditary hemorrhagic condition, exposure to infection) or by a known special attribute (teenager, addict, diabetic). One's objective may offer guidance to selection as well (desire to assess gestational age, to advise on and evaluate maternal nutrition, to screen for fetal genetic disorder, to provide pain relief in labor). Alternatively, the approach can be by way of an already established diagnosis (septic abortion, ectopic pregnancy, hydatidiform mole, hydramnios) or a suspected one (placenta previa, coagulopathy, amnionitis, fetal malpresentation), or even an anticipated interventive procedure (cervical cerclage, labor induction, fetal monitoring, forceps operation). Thus, access should not be difficult. Once a pathway has been selected, the direction one travels will depend on one's logical responses to considerations suggested by the sequence of road markers.

PREGNANCY VERIFICATION

Austin Wertheimer, M.D.

COMMENTS

A. Urine slide or tube pregnancy tests are usually positive by 26 days after ovulation. The newer tube tests may be positive at or before the missed period. A negative test, therefore, may merely reflect having obtained the test too early.

B. False-positive urine tests may occur if the following are present: proteinuria, hematuria, bacteriuria, detergents, LH peak, drug ingestion. If a positive pregnancy test is associated with an adnexal mass or with tenderness, consider ectopic pregnancy (see p. 34).

C. The beta-subunit of human chorionic gonadotropin (hCG) radioimmunoassay determination may be positive as early as 9 days following ovulation. Rare cases of hCG production from nongestational tumors have been reported. If this sensitive test is unavailable, repeat the urine test in 1–2 weeks when the level of circulating hCG may be high enough to be detectable.

D. Fetal heart (FH) tones may be detected as early as 13 weeks by Doppler ultrasound reflection techniques.

E. Fetal cardiac motion seen by real-time scanning gives clear-cut verification of pregnancy and fetal life. Uterine enlargement from a pathologic process, such as fibroids, hydatidiform mole, or missed abortion, will also be elucidated by this technique.

REFERENCE

Derman R, Corson SL, Horwitz CAL, Lau HL, Soderstrom R: Early diagnosis of pregnancy: A symposium. J Reprod Med 26:149, 1981

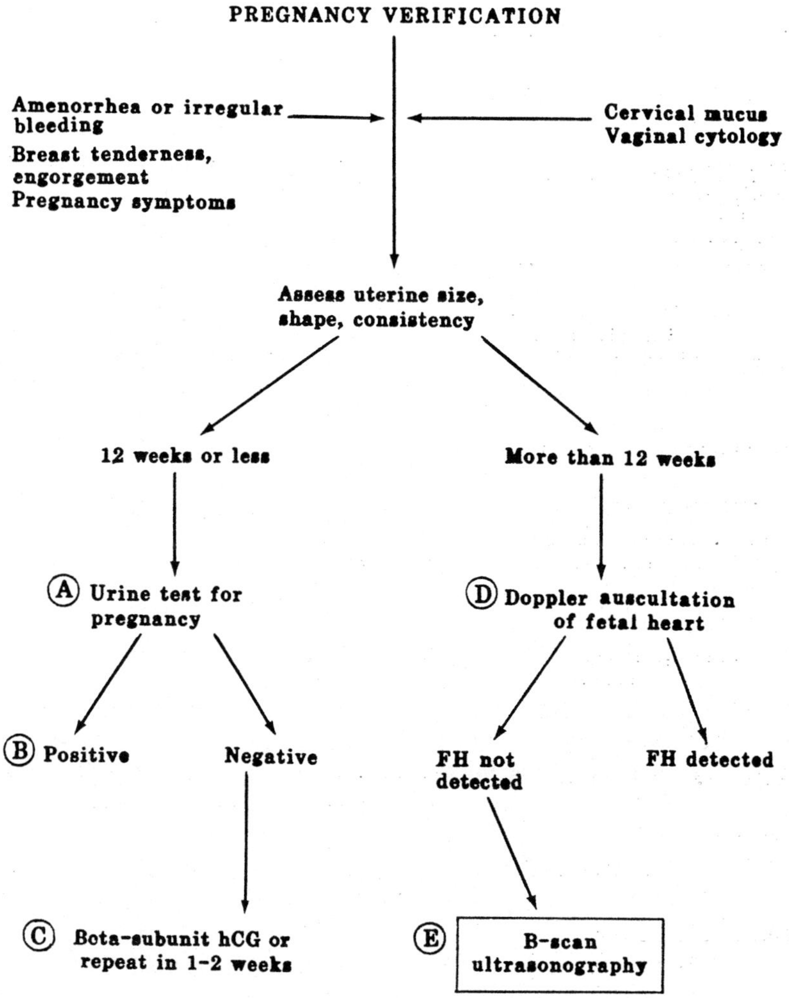
PREGNANCY VERIFICATION
Amenorrhea or irregular bleeding
Breast tenderness, engorgement
Pregnancy symptoms
Cervical mucus
Vaginal cytology
Assess uterine size, shape, consistency
12 weeks or less
More than 12 weeks
(A) Urine test for pregnancy
(D) Doppler auscultation of fetal heart
(B) Positive
Negative
FH not detected
FH detected
(C) Beta-subunit hCG or repeat in 1-2 weeks
(E) B-scan ultrasonography

FETAL DEATH

Emanuel A. Friedman, M.D.

COMMENTS

A. Subjective cessation of fetal movements is not a reliable sign but deserves to be evaluated. It is especially useful, however, for signaling problems with fetal well-being in patients at risk for chronic placental insufficiency (see p. 52). The principal predisposing factors include chronic hypertension, malnutrition, diabetes mellitus, and renal or other debilitating disease.

B. Definitive diagnosis of fetal death can be made with sophisticated ultrasound techniques, particularly the M-mode (time-motion cardiac imaging) and real-time scanning (using an array of transducers to produce a dynamic assessment of motion for visualizing fetal heart action).

C. If imaging ultrasonography is unavailable, one may have to wait 1–2 weeks to ascertain if the fetus is alive and the uterus is continuing to grow. Fetal heart tones may be heard again when the fetus moves into a more favorable position with its back up against the anterior uterine wall. Even if the FH is heard, one must still consider placental insufficiency in cases in which uterine growth is slowed or in which the uterine size is too small for the dates.

D. Prostaglandin (PG) induction with PGE_2 vaginal suppositories is an especially recommended method for concluding a pregnancy complicated by intrauterine fetal death. Its success rate is very high, although there may be need for an evacuation procedure for retained placenta following delivery of the fetus. Suppositories of 20 mg PGE_2 are inserted every 3–5 hours. Intramuscular 15-methyl-$PGF_{2\alpha}$ can be substituted in 250 μg doses every 1½–3½ hours if the membranes rupture or the suppositories prove ineffectual.

E. If PGs are unavailable, one awaits the spontaneous onset of labor. A potential risk of this delay is the development of coagulopathy. Weekly assessment of the patient's coagulation profile is, therefore, important. If the fibrinogen begins to fall, one can arrest the process of intravascular coagulation by using heparin in therapeutically anticoagulating doses. Once the coagulopathy is under control, delivery should be expedited by PG or oxytocin. Since the advent of PGs, cesarean section is almost never indicated here any longer.

REFERENCES

Southern EM, Gutknecht GD: The use of prostaglandins for the therapeutic termination of pregnancy. J Reprod Med 13:63, 1974

Lauersen NH, Secher NJ, Wilson KH: Mid-trimester abortion induced by intravaginal administration of prostaglandin E_2 suppositories. Am J Obstet Gynecol 122:947, 1975

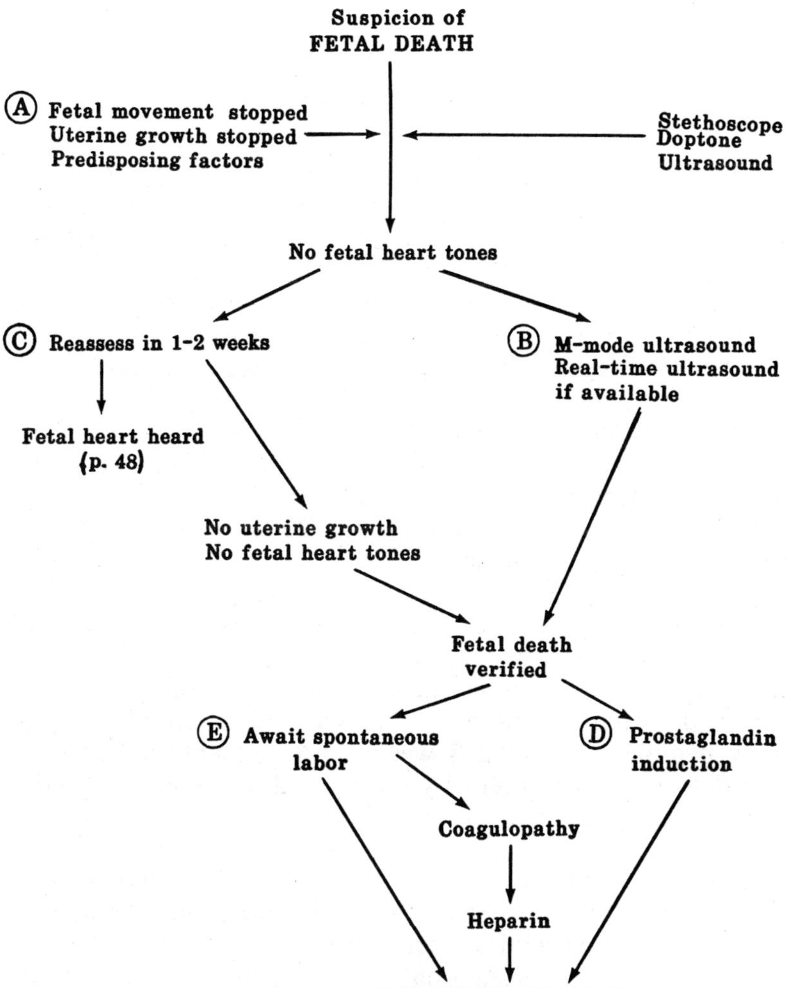
Suspicion of
FETAL DEATH
(A) Fetal movement stopped
Uterine growth stopped
Predisposing factors
Stethoscope
Doptone
Ultrasound
No fetal heart tones
(C) Reassess in 1-2 weeks
(B) M-mode ultrasound
Real-time ultrasound
if available
Fetal heart heard
(p. 48)
No uterine growth
No fetal heart tones
Fetal death
verified
(E) Await spontaneous
labor
(D) Prostaglandin
induction
Coagulopathy
Heparin
VAGINAL DELIVERY

GESTATIONAL DURATION

Emanuel A. Friedman, M.D.

COMMENTS

A. Naegele's rule calculates the expected data of confinement (EDC) by adding 9 months and 7 days to the first day of the last menstrual period (LMP). It assumes a gestational duration of 266 days from ovulation and fertilization plus 14 days from LMP to ovulation. It applies only to women whose menstrual cycles are rather regular and at 28-day intervals. Even among them, however, it is only accurate to within 2 weeks. Ovulation generally occurs about 12 days prior to the next period regardless of the interval between periods.

B. Irregular periods interdict use of Naegele's rule because ovulation cannot be predicted. The same tends to apply for women whose periods are spaced far apart. If ovulation symptoms are recognizable in them (e.g., mittelschmerz), EDC can be calculated by adding 8 months and 23 days (266 days) with a comparable degree of accuracy as for Naegele's rule.

C. If conception occurred following a single coital exposure, timing tends to be reliable. Other information may also be helpful, such as when the pregnancy test first became positive (usually about 3 weeks or more after conception for tube or slide tests), when the patient first experienced breast tenderness and nausea (usually beginning about 2–3 weeks past conception), when the fetal heart was first detected (8–10 weeks by ultrasound, 16 weeks by stethoscope), and when quickening occurred (16–18 weeks).

D. B-scan ultrasonography is reliable for determining gestational duration from crown-rump fetal length in the first trimester and biparietal diameter from 12 to about 30 weeks. The biparietal diameter measurements beyond 30 weeks are less accurate for determining gestational duration, but they are often helpful nonetheless. They are decidedly better than estimates based on uterine size observations by physical examination.

REFERENCES

Campbell S: Fetal growth. Clin Obstet Gynecol 1:41, 1974

Campogrande M, Todras T, Brizzolara M: Prediction of birth weight by ultrasound measurements of the fetus. Brit J Obstet Gynaecol 84:175, 1977

Robinson HD: Sonar measurement of fetal crown-rump length as a means for assessing maturity in first trimester pregnancy. Brit Med J 4:28, 1973

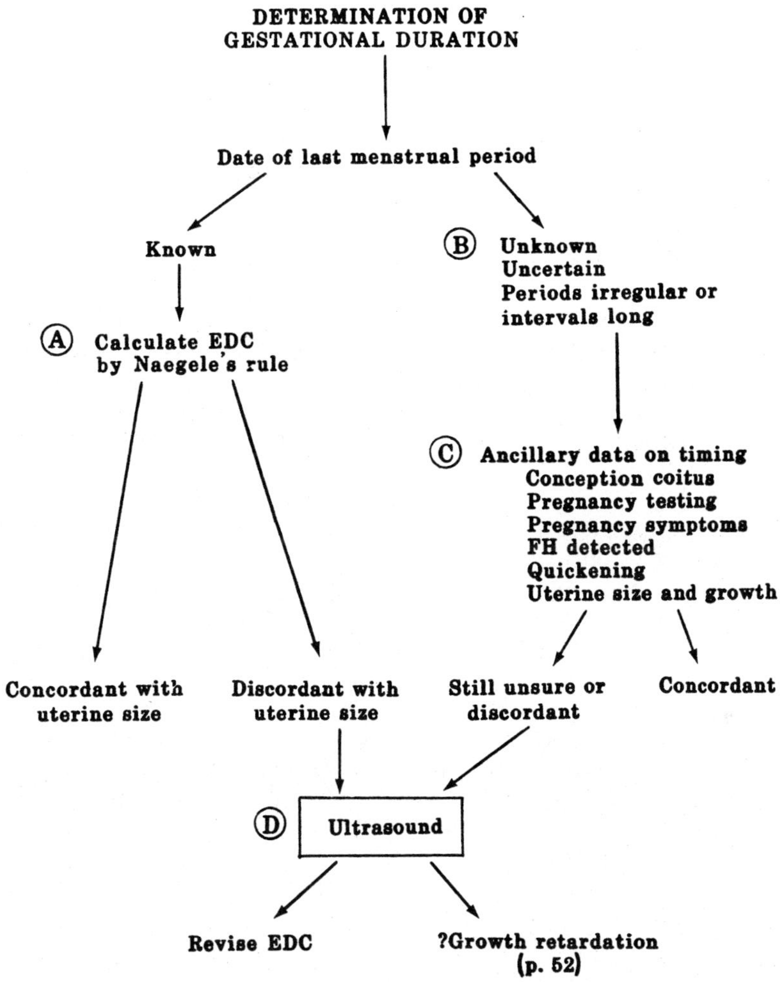
DETERMINATION OF GESTATIONAL DURATION
Date of last menstrual period
Known
Ⓐ Calculate EDC by Naegele's rule
Ⓑ Unknown
Uncertain
Periods irregular or intervals long
Ⓒ Ancillary data on timing
Conception coitus
Pregnancy testing
Pregnancy symptoms
FH detected
Quickening
Uterine size and growth
Concordant with uterine size
Discordant with uterine size
Still unsure or discordant
Concordant
Ⓓ Ultrasound
Revise EDC
?Growth retardation (p. 52)

ANTEPARTUM ASSESSMENT

Henry Klapholz, M.D.

COMMENTS

A. Thorough investigation into each patient's family, social, medical, and obstetric history is important. Of significance are multiple gestation, diabetes mellitus, hypertension, genetic disease, and exposure to cats and raw meat, as this pertains to toxoplasmosis prevention (see p. 104). A history of prior genital herpes genitalis infection will require cultures near term (see p. 114). Seek information on the use of alcohol, caffeine, and cigarette smoking.

B. The physical examination should focus on cardiopulmonary and orthopedic disorders, noting pelvic architecture and capacity (see p. 18), and obesity. Assess the nutritional state (see p. 10), gestational age (see p. 6), and uterine size concordance (see p. 52).

C. Laboratory survey should include CBC, serology (see p. 106), rubella titer (see p. 102), toxoplasmosis titer (see p. 104), herpes titer (see p. 114), Papanicolaou smear (see p. 116), urinalysis, urine culture (see p. 118), blood group and Rh factor. Alpha-fetoprotein (see p. 44) may detect open neural tube defects in the fetus. Routine gonococcal cultures are obtained in some areas (see p. 108).

D. Specific disease states uncovered require appropriate management in pregnancy. These include diabetes mellitus (see p. 68), chronic hypertension (see p. 70), renal disease (see p. 72), and cardiac disease (see p. 74). Proteinuria must be evaluated (see p. 58), as does glycosuria (see p. 68), anemia (see p. 82) and a positive serologic test for syphilis (see p. 106). Baseline toxoplasmosis titer is helpful for later use.

E. At each subsequent antepartum visit (monthly until 32 weeks, biweekly until 36 weeks, and weekly thereafter, unless more frequent visits are needed), urinalysis is repeated to detect albuminuria (see p. 58) and glycosuria (see p. 68). Hematocrit should be repeated at 20, 28, and 36 weeks (see p. 82). Rh antibody titer is done, when indicated, at similar intervals (see p. 54). Repeat serology for syphilis and gonococcal cultures is also valuable near term.

F. At each visit, the blood pressure must be checked (see p. 58). Uterine size (se p. 52) and weight gain (see p 10) are evaluated. The fetal heart is checked as well. Hyperreflexia and edema are noted, if present (see p. 58). Critical manifestations of potentially serious problems are searched for, such as decreased fetal movement (see p. 48), persistent headache or visual disturbance (see p. 58), venous and circulatory symptoms, vaginal bleeding (see p. 22), abdominal pain or cramping, and leaking vaginal fluid (see p. 120)

REFERENCES

Bowman JM: The management of Rh-isoimmunization. Obstet Gynecol 52:1, 1978

Gabbe SG, Quilligan EJ: General obstetric management of the diabetic pregnancy. Clin Obstet Gynecol 24:9, 1981

Harris R: Maternal serum alphafetoprotein in pregnancy and the prevention of birth defect. Brit Med J 280:1199, 1980

Kibrick S, Loria RM: Rubella and cytomegalovirus: Current concepts of congenital and acquired infection. Pediat Clin North Am 21:513, 1974

Krick JA, Remington JS: Toxoplasmosis in the adult: An overview. New Engl J Med 289:550, 1978

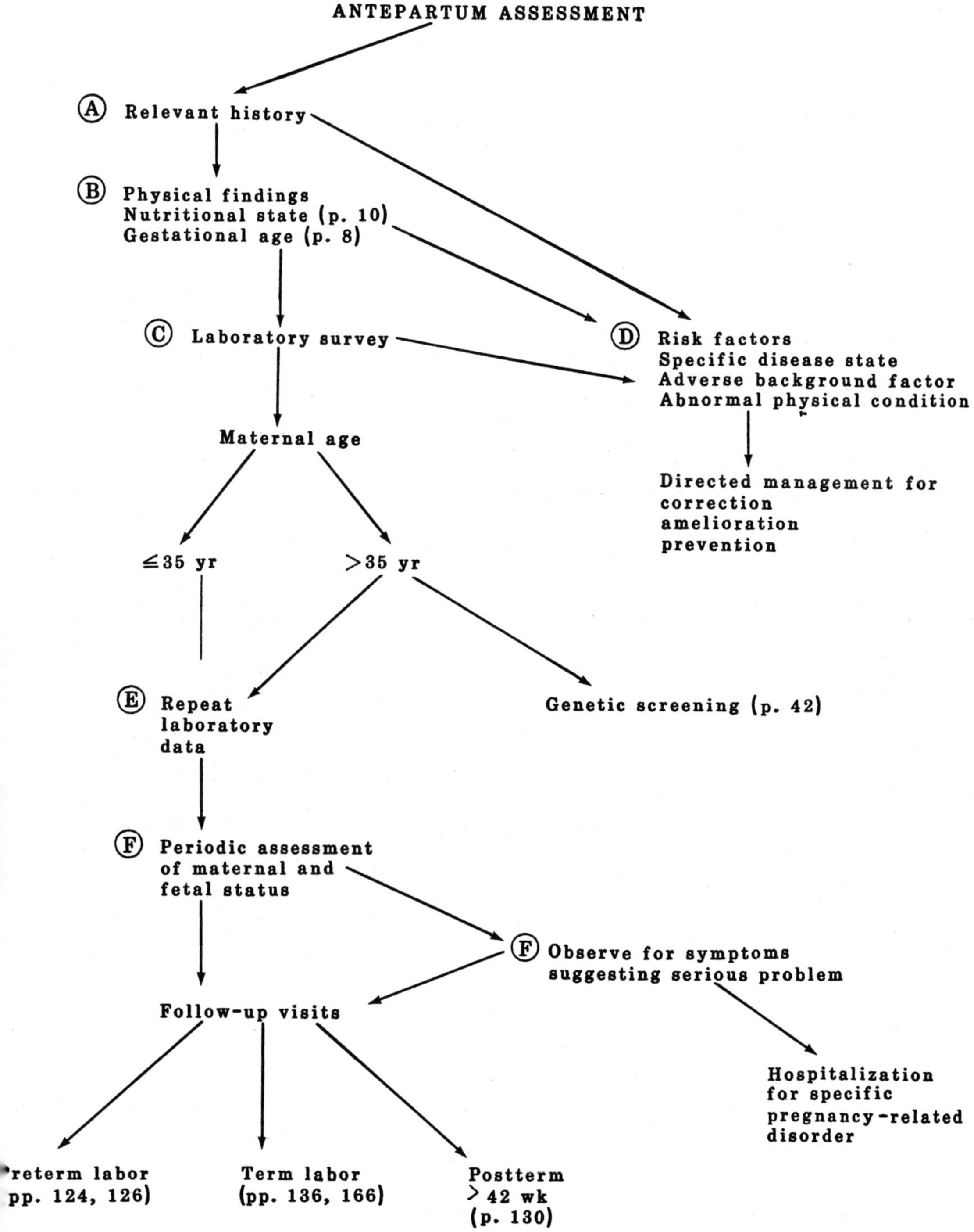
ANTEPARTUM ASSESSMENT
Ⓐ Relevant history
Ⓑ Physical findings
Nutritional state (p. 10)
Gestational age (p. 8)
Ⓒ Laboratory survey
Ⓓ Risk factors
Specific disease state
Adverse background factor
Abnormal physical condition
Directed management for
correction
amelioration
prevention
Maternal age
≤35 yr
>35 yr
Ⓔ Repeat
laboratory
data
Genetic screening (p. 42)
Ⓕ Periodic assessment
of maternal and
fetal status
Ⓕ Observe for symptoms
suggesting serious problem
Follow-up visits
Hospitalization
for specific
pregnancy-related
disorder
reterm labor
pp. 124, 126)
Term labor
(pp. 136, 166)
Postterm
> 42 wk
(p. 130)

NUTRITIONAL EVALUATION

Balmookoot Balgobin, M.D.

COMMENTS

A. Factors commonly associated with poor nutrition in pregnancy include adolescence (especially under age 16 years because of the gravida's own growth needs), prior poor obstetric outcome, rapid succession of deliveries, heavy smoking, chronic alcoholic intake, drug dependency, food faddism, indigency, debilitating disease, hyperemesis, multiple pregnancy, low prepregnancy weight (less than 85 percent of expected standard weight), inadequate weight gain in pregnancy (less than 0.5 lb per week or actual weight loss), and intrauterine growth retardation. Physical findings of overt malnutrition or specific nutritional deficiencies should be sought, including rare cutaneous and mucosal changes seen only in the severest cases.

B. There are few good laboratory indices of malnutrition, except anemia and hypoproteinemia. Sickle cell preparation is important in black women. Anemia (see p. 82) with blood indices showing microcytic, hypochromic erythrocytes warrants serum iron and total iron binding capacity; macrocytosis warrants serum and red cell folate levels. Other relevant investigations might include serum vitamin B_{12} concentrations, reticulocyte count, electrophoresis, and even bone marrow smear.

C. Protein malnutrition has a serious adverse impact on the fetus. It may be manifest in the gravida only by weight loss or inadequate weight gain. Severe hypoalbuminemia results in generalized edema. Inadequate protein stores are replenished by means of a high-protein diet containing at least 2 gm/kg daily. In rare cases of intense depletion, intravenous albumin and hyperalimentation may be indicated, but such measures are not without risk.

D. Therapy of anemia (see p. 82) should be specific if possible. Replacement and maintenance oral ferrous sulfate (or equivalent iron-containing product) for iron deficiency anemia plus special dietary correction are in order. Intravenous iron is seldom required. Similar programs are needed for the less common folate deficiencies. Whereas iron deficiency and folic acid deficiencies are usually separate entities, they may coexist with severe nutritional deficiencies.

E. Follow-up includes reassessment of and counselling in diet. Weight gain is an index of caloric intake, but it is not a reliable indicator of an adequate diet. Laboratory and clinical response to treatment is especially useful. Periodic laboratory studies ascertain whether anemia and/or hypoalbuminemia have been corrected. Intrauterine growth retardation should be searched for; at delivery, the baby's birth weight should be noted relative to length and gestational age. Postpartum re-evaluation of nutritional status is important as well, with advice on pregnancy spacing and contraception (see p. 214).

REFERENCES

American College of Obstetricians and Gynecologists, American Dietetic Association: Assessment of Maternal Nutrition. Technical Bulletin, 1978

Eastman N, Jackson E: Weight relationships in pregnancy. Obstet Gynecol Survey 23:1003, 1968

Mulvihill J, Yeager A: Fetal alcohol syndrome. Obstet Gynecol Survey 32:151, 1977

Rush D: Examination of the relationship between birthweight, cigarette smoking during pregnancy, and maternal weight gain. J Obstet Gynaecol Brit Cmwth 81:746, 1974

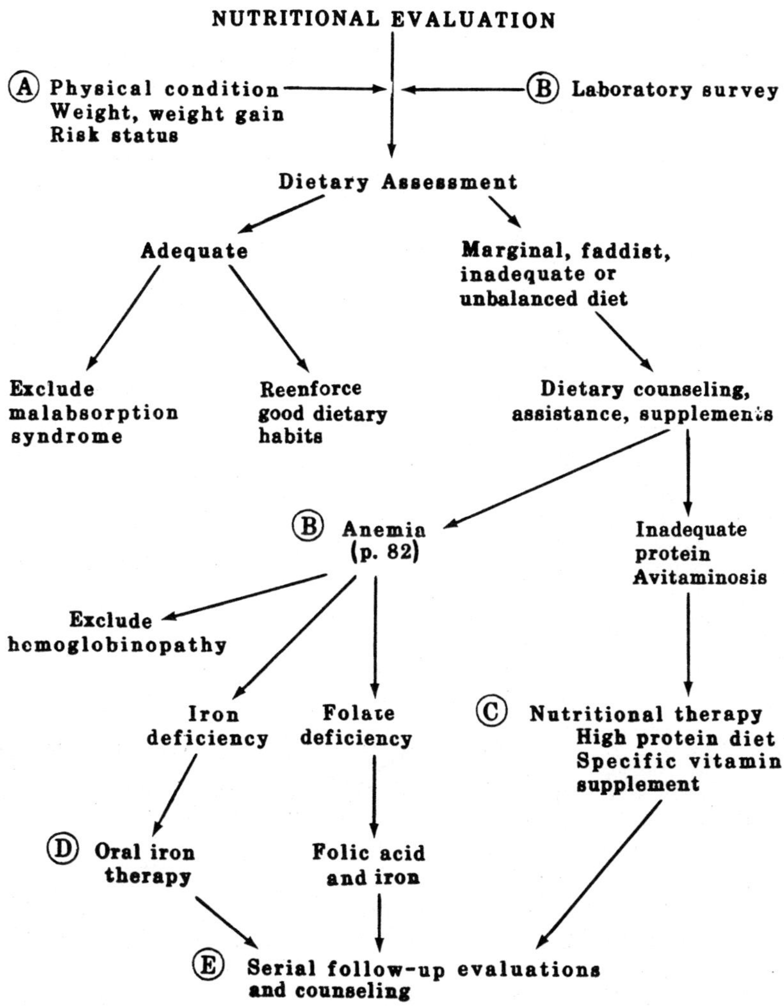
NUTRITIONAL EVALUATION
(A) Physical condition
Weight, weight gain
Risk status
(B) Laboratory survey
Dietary Assessment
Adequate
Marginal, faddist, inadequate or unbalanced diet
Exclude malabsorption syndrome
Reenforce good dietary habits
Dietary counseling, assistance, supplements
(B) Anemia (p. 82)
Inadequate protein Avitaminosis
Exclude hemoglobinopathy
Iron deficiency
Folate deficiency
(C) Nutritional therapy
High protein diet
Specific vitamin supplement
(D) Oral iron therapy
Folic acid and iron
(E) Serial follow-up evaluations and counseling

ADOLESCENT PREGNANCY

Johanna F. Perlmutter, M.D.

COMMENTS

A. Pregnancy in adolescents is a major societal problem today. More than 90 percent of teenagers are estimated to have been sexually active for about one year before seeking contraception, a fact which reflects their sense of denial ("it won't happen to me" syndrome). Unwanted pregnancy has an intense social and emotional impact on the young gravida. Physical effects relate to poor dietary habits, drug dependence, venereal disease, and concurrent medical conditions. The pregnant adolescent needs special attention as regards social service and psychologic, nutritional, medical, and obstetric factors.

B. Counseling is essential because recidivism is common. Even after an abortion, birth control measures may not be used, or not utilized effectively. To reduce the risk of repeat pregnancy, explore the reasons for the unintentional pregnancy before intervening. Induced abortion may not be the appropriate management for some of these patients.

C. It is often difficult to date the last menstrual period accurately. More objective means for dating the gestation (p. 6) may help to provide a good baseline in the event that intrauterine growth retardation, to which teenagers may be subject, develops later. Seek out underlying medical problems, particularly those known to affect young gravidas frequently: anemia based on poor nutrition and hypertension (both chronic and pregnancy-induced). Substandard eating habits are common. A nutritionist can work to make fad diets nutritionally acceptable, stressing protein intake.

D. Young gravidas need rigorous prenatal care. They should be seen often. Improved prenatal care and nutrition lead to fewer premature and low-birth-weight infants. One should be especially alert for early manifestations of pregnancy-induced hypertension (p. 58). Diastolic blood pressure levels of 80–85 mm Hg are in the hypertensive range in the young teenager. Hospitalize liberally to assess the status of mother and fetus and to manage these cases aggressively, because adolescents are not reliable enough to be followed on an ambulatory basis when such problems arise. Intrauterine growth retardation and premature labor are risks, making surveillance of fetal growth (p. 50) and well-being (p. 48) important.

E. Because the fetus is at risk from underlying maternal malnutrition or hypertension, intrapartum surveillance is prudent (p. 136). Prolonged labors have been reported in adolescents. One should be alert for the development of protraction disorders (p. 170).

REFERENCES

Edwards LE, Steinman ME, Arnold KA, Hakanson EY: Adolescent contraceptive use: Experience in 1,762 teenagers. Am J Obstet Gynecol 135:583, 1980

Ryan GM, Sweeney PJ: Attitudes of adolescents toward pregnancy and contraception. Am J Obstet Gynecol 137:358, 1980

Sherline DM, A-Davidson R: Adolescent pregnancy: The Jackson, Mississippi, experience. Am J Obstet Gynecol 132:245, 1978

Zelnick M, Kanter JF: Sexual activity, contraceptive use and pregnancy among metropolitan-area teenagers: 1971–1979. Fam Plan Perspect 12:230, 1980

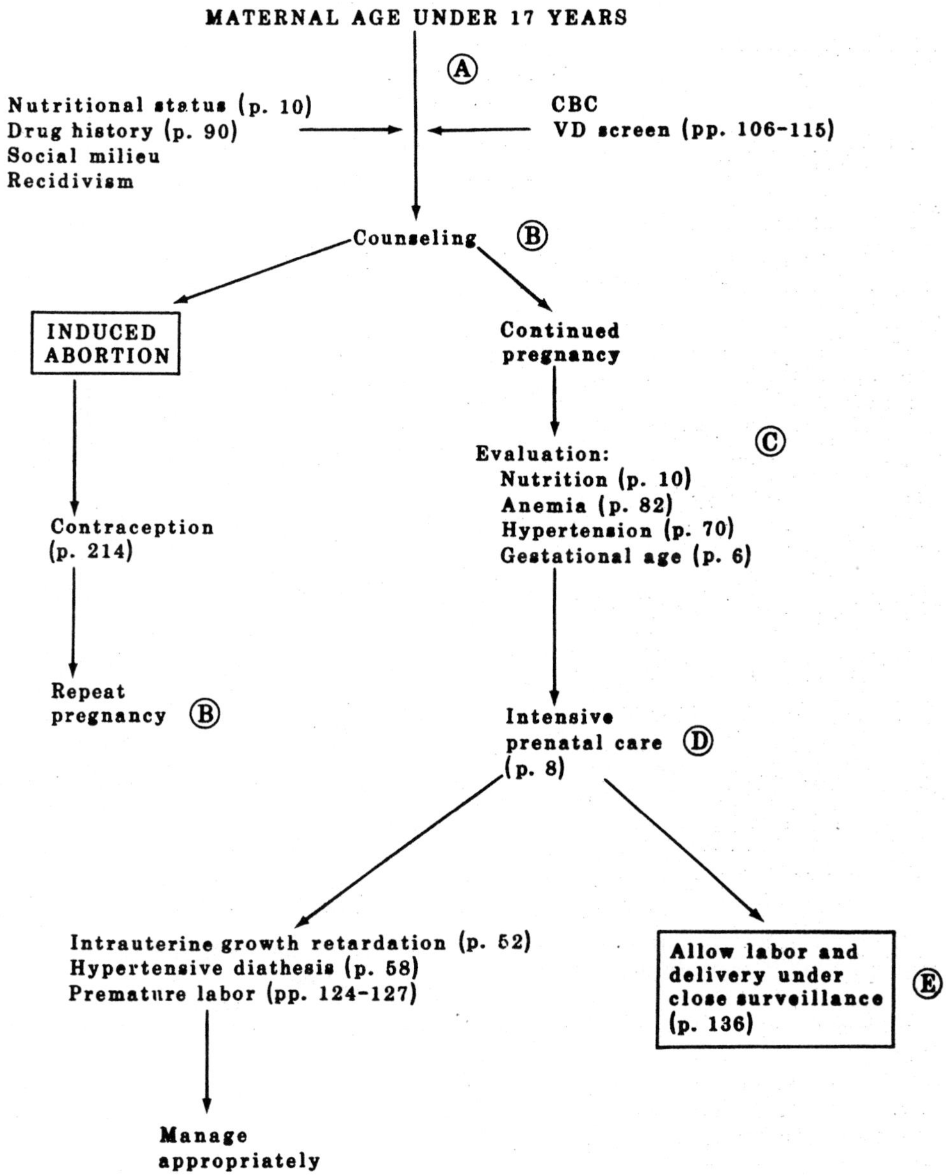
MATERNAL AGE UNDER 17 YEARS
Ⓐ
Nutritional status (p. 10)
Drug history (p. 90)
Social milieu
Recidivism
CBC
VD screen (pp. 106-115)
Counseling Ⓑ
INDUCED ABORTION
Continued pregnancy
Contraception (p. 214)
Repeat pregnancy Ⓑ
Evaluation:
Nutrition (p. 10)
Anemia (p. 82)
Hypertension (p. 70)
Gestational age (p. 6)
Ⓒ
Intensive prenatal care (p. 8) Ⓓ
Intrauterine growth retardation (p. 52)
Hypertensive diathesis (p. 58)
Premature labor (pp. 124-127)
Manage appropriately
Allow labor and delivery under close surveillance (p. 136)
Ⓔ

ELDERLY GRAVIDA

Selwyn P. Oskowitz, M.B.

COMMENTS

A. A gravida aged 35 years or more is considered elderly by most standards. Therefore, she is one who is at increased risk by virtue of age alone for maternal and fetal complications. This engenders anxiety in the patient and her family. In most cases the concerns are unwarranted. Various interventive measures undertaken strictly because of the risks of advanced maternal age cannot usually be justified, including induced abortion and cesarean section.

B. One should be alert to a history of infertility, especially if associated with prior extensive treatment programs, since this may enhance the risks of a pregnancy by yielding multiple pregnancy (especially after ovulation induction) or pregnancy loss (as with luteal phase deficiency). In addition, a poor reproductive background may reflect the existence of functional or anatomic defects. Habitual abortion (p. 36) places the patient at high risk as well.

C. Much misinformation prevails about the hazards of pregnancy in the elderly gravida. Therefore, such women need counseling and, in most cases, reassurance. They should be given realistic information concerning the genetic risks (p. 42). In the absence of underlying or intercurrent complicating conditions, there does not appear to be any other special hazard to pregnancy in these cases.

D. With advancing age, women increasingly develop various illnesses that may affect pregnancy or be adversely affected by pregnancy. Such disorders include hypertensive cardiovascular disease (p. 70), leiomyomata uteri, diabetes mellitus (p. 68), and malignancy, in descending order of frequency. Rh isoimmunization (p. 94) is related more to advancing parity than to age. Older gravidas do have an increased rate of hydatidiform mole (p. 54) and fetal genetic disorders (p. 42). Evaluations for these conditions are essential.

E. Intensive prenatal care has contributed substantially to improving maternal and fetal outcome in these cases. It may help uncover potentially serious conditions as they arise. Threatening premature labor may sometimes be effectively arrested (p. 124). Intrauterine growth retardation can be detected and managed appropriately (p. 52) so as to curtail its deleterious effects.

F. Because of the greater expectation of labor disorders, intrauterine growth retardation, and placental insufficiency (especially in hypertensive women), continuous electronic fetal heart rate monitoring is advisable (p. 136). It is prudent to have pediatric personnel available for care of the newborn infant. Puerperal sterilization (p. 216) may be considered, provided prenatal discussions and counseling have been done.

REFERENCES

Cohen WR, Newman L, Friedman EA: Risk of labor abnormalities with advancing age. Obstet Gynecol 55:414, 1980

Kajanoja D, Widholm O: Pregnancy and delivery in women aged 40 and over. Obstet Gynecol 51: 47, 1978

Kane SH: Advancing age and the primigravida. Obstet Gynecol 29:409, 1967

Kessler I, Lancet M: The problem of the older primipara. Obstet Gynecol 56:165, 1980

Morrison I: The elderly primigravida. Am J Obstet Gynecol 121:465, 1975

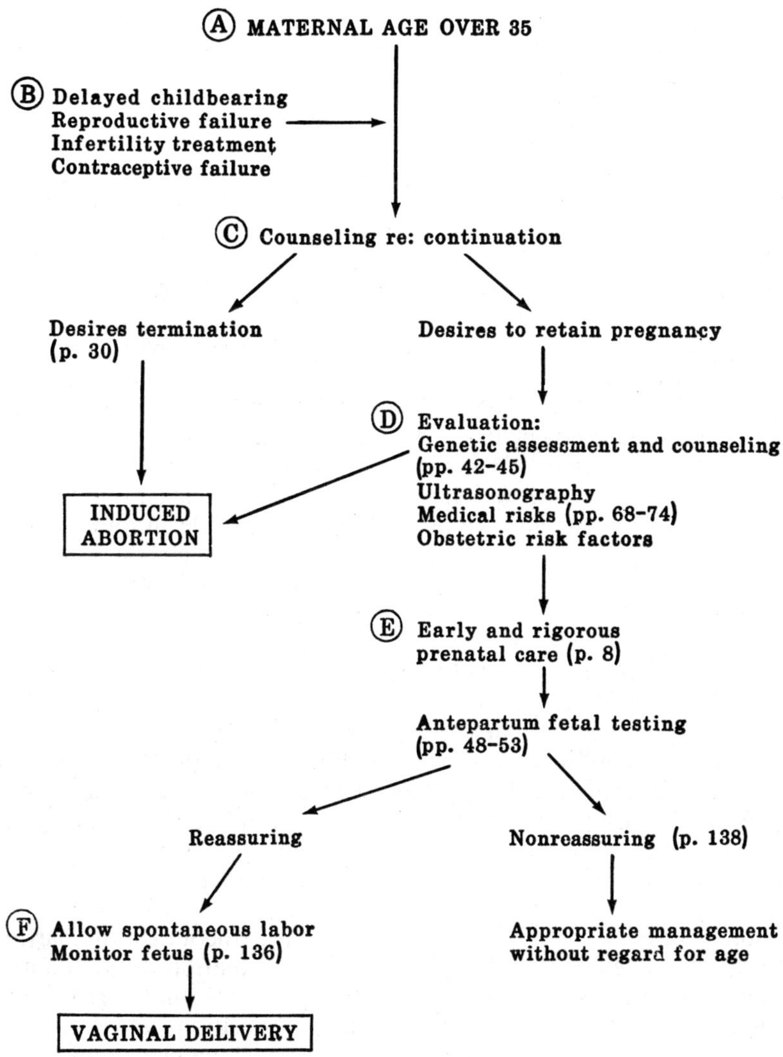
(A) MATERNAL AGE OVER 35
(B) Delayed childbearing
Reproductive failure
Infertility treatment
Contraceptive failure
(C) Counseling re: continuation
Desires termination (p. 30)
Desires to retain pregnancy
(D) Evaluation:
Genetic assessment and counseling (pp. 42-45)
Ultrasonography
Medical risks (pp. 68-74)
Obstetric risk factors
INDUCED ABORTION
(E) Early and rigorous prenatal care (p. 8)
Antepartum fetal testing (pp. 48-53)
Reassuring
Nonreassuring (p. 138)
(F) Allow spontaneous labor
Monitor fetus (p. 136)
Appropriate management without regard for age
VAGINAL DELIVERY

PSYCHOPROPHYLACTIC PREPARATION

Johanna F. Perlmutter, M.D. and
Catherine A. Keaney, R.N., B.S.N., M.S.

COMMENTS

A. Efforts should be made to develop a sense of trust before labor. Meeting new personnel mandates the establishment and reaffirmation of interpersonal relationships early in labor, if possible. Spend time discussing what to expect and explain the facilities and any procedure to be done. Try to understand the patient's preferences and needs. Encourage the couple to participate in decision-making. In early labor, allow them time for privacy within the constraints of safety. Keep a sense of humor and try to allay apprehensions. In early labor, it is important to foster ambulation and minimize attention to pain and discomfort. The patient should not be asked to time each contraction. Distractions should be encouraged. Breathing patterns should be reviewed in early labor because of the variety of techniques available. Patients should demonstrate those patterns and techniques with which they are familiar. Relaxation techniques can be rehearsed. Encourage slow deep breathing as long as possible. Avoid advancing too quickly to breathing techniques that ought to be reserved for later in labor. Exercises previously learned to prevent tension should be reviewed and discussed. Practicing during a contraction is useful.

B. In active labor, more support is needed. The patient should be told of her progress and verbally encouraged and complimented. As labor progresses, use active measures to relieve pain by trial and error, but there is no panacea. Try hot compresses to the back, cold compresses to the forehead, and ice chips by mouth. Stress relaxation between contractions. Maintain a calm, subdued environment with reduced noise and light. Limit the number of personnel in attendance. Combine breathing patterns as needed (e.g., slow chest breathing as the contraction begins, then rapid, shallow breathing at the peak, and slow chest breathing as the contraction subsides).

C. During transition, give concrete and specific instructions. Encourage the partner to be assertive and to participate actively. Focus the patient's attention during contractions. Act as a role model to increase eye contact, enhance touching, and perform breathing rituals with the patient. During the late active phase, transition, and second stage of labor, frequent position changes in bed or the use of a rocking chair may prove beneficial. Effective pushing can be done with the patient on her back, on her side, squatting, kneeling, or sitting on a commode, with traditional breath-holding and bearing down. A newer alternative method is "trumpet blowing," which involves slow exhalation while pushing.

COMMENTS

Lamaze F: *Painless Childbirth: Psychoprophylactic Method.* London: Burke Publishing Company, 1958

Sasmor JL: Stress adaptation: A theory for childbirth education. J Obstet Gynecol Nursing 2:48, 1973

Worthington EL, Martin GA: A laboratory analysis of response to pain after training in three Lamaze techniques. J Psychosom Res 24:106, 1980

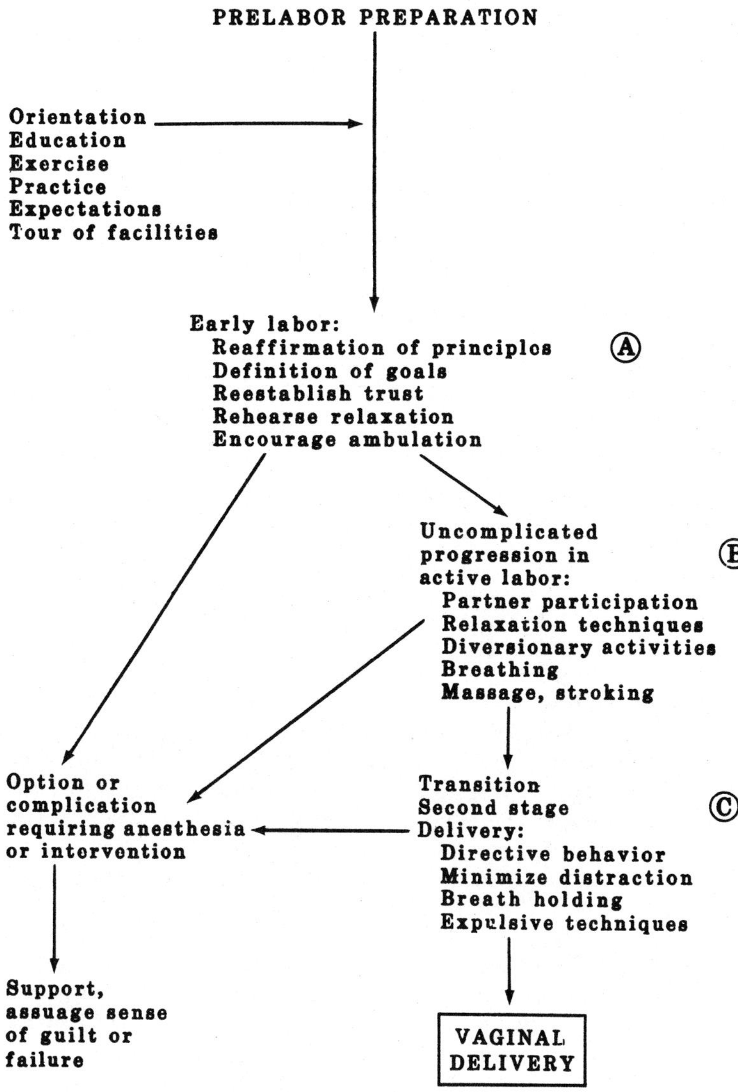
PRELABOR PREPARATION
Orientation
Education
Exercise
Practice
Expectations
Tour of facilities
Early labor:
Reaffirmation of principles
Definition of goals
Reestablish trust
Rehearse relaxation
Encourage ambulation
Ⓐ
Uncomplicated
progression in
active labor:
Partner participation
Relaxation techniques
Diversionary activities
Breathing
Massage, stroking
Ⓑ
Option or
complication
requiring anesthesia
or intervention
Transition
Second stage
Delivery:
Directive behavior
Minimize distraction
Breath holding
Expulsive techniques
Ⓒ
Support,
assuage sense
of guilt or
failure
VAGINAL
DELIVERY

CLINICAL CEPHALOPELVIMETRY

Lenard Simon, M.D.

COMMENTS

A. Assessing fetopelvic relationships is the keystone for many critical decisions related to the conduct of labor. Pelvic architecture and capacity are examined early in pregnancy. The features that flag the patient who may have an inadequate pelvis are: diagonal conjugate <12 cm, narrow subpubic arch, flat sacrum, bi-ischial diameter <8 cm, convergent sidewalls, prominent ischial spines, and sacrospinous ligament <2.5 cm. Screen all antepartum patients to identify those at risk. Re-evaluate late in pregnancy when the pelvic tissues soften.

B. Intrapartum examination reviews the pelvic architecture and relates the pelvic capacity to the presenting fetal head size. Any compensatory space should now be apparent. The labor pattern (p. 166) is important in identifying fetopelvic disproportion. One must be familiar with the way pelvic architecture affects the course of labor.

C. Abnormal labor patterns of protraction or arrest disorders (pp. 170, 172) signify serious risk regardless of the prior impression of the pelvis. Such patterns often signal a high degree of cephalopelvic disproportion. Clinical cephalopelvimetry demonstrating features of a small or unfavorably shaped pelvis in a patient who has a protraction or arrest disorder indicates a grave prognosis. These patients probably warrant delivery by cesarean section as opposed to vaginal operative procedures that are inherently more dangerous to both mother and fetus.

D. A useful clinical means for assessing cephalopelvic relationships is to determine the "thrust" of the fetal head in the birth canal. At the height of a uterine contraction augmented by the application of fundal pressure, vaginal palpation of the presenting part will demonstrate whether the head is tightly fixed in the pelvis or capable of further descent. Clear evidence of an obstruction tends to confirm the presence of disproportion, while advancement of the head in the pelvis rules out an obstruction at that pelvic station.

E. X-ray cephalopelvimetry should be reserved for objective documentation of an impediment detected by the dynamic test of pelvic capacity in cases with protraction or arrest disorders of labor. X-ray pelvimetry merely for the purpose of measuring pelvic dimensions (without simultaneously obtaining fetal head measurements) is not recommended. If techniques are not available for the simultaneous measurement of both fetal head and maternal pelvis and for comparing these measurements, it is preferable to bypass this step entirely.

REFERENCES

Friedman EA, Sachtleben MR: Station of the fetal presenting part: VI. Arrest of descent in multiparas. Obstet Gynecol 47:129, 1976

Friedman EA, Taylor MB: A modified nomographic aid for cephalopelvimetry. Am J Obstet Gynecol 105:1110, 1969; 106:884, 1970

Hillis DS: Diagnosis of contracted pelvis. Ill Med J 74:131, 1938

Klapholz H: A computerized aid to Ball pelvimetry. Am J Obstet Gynecol 121:1067, 1975

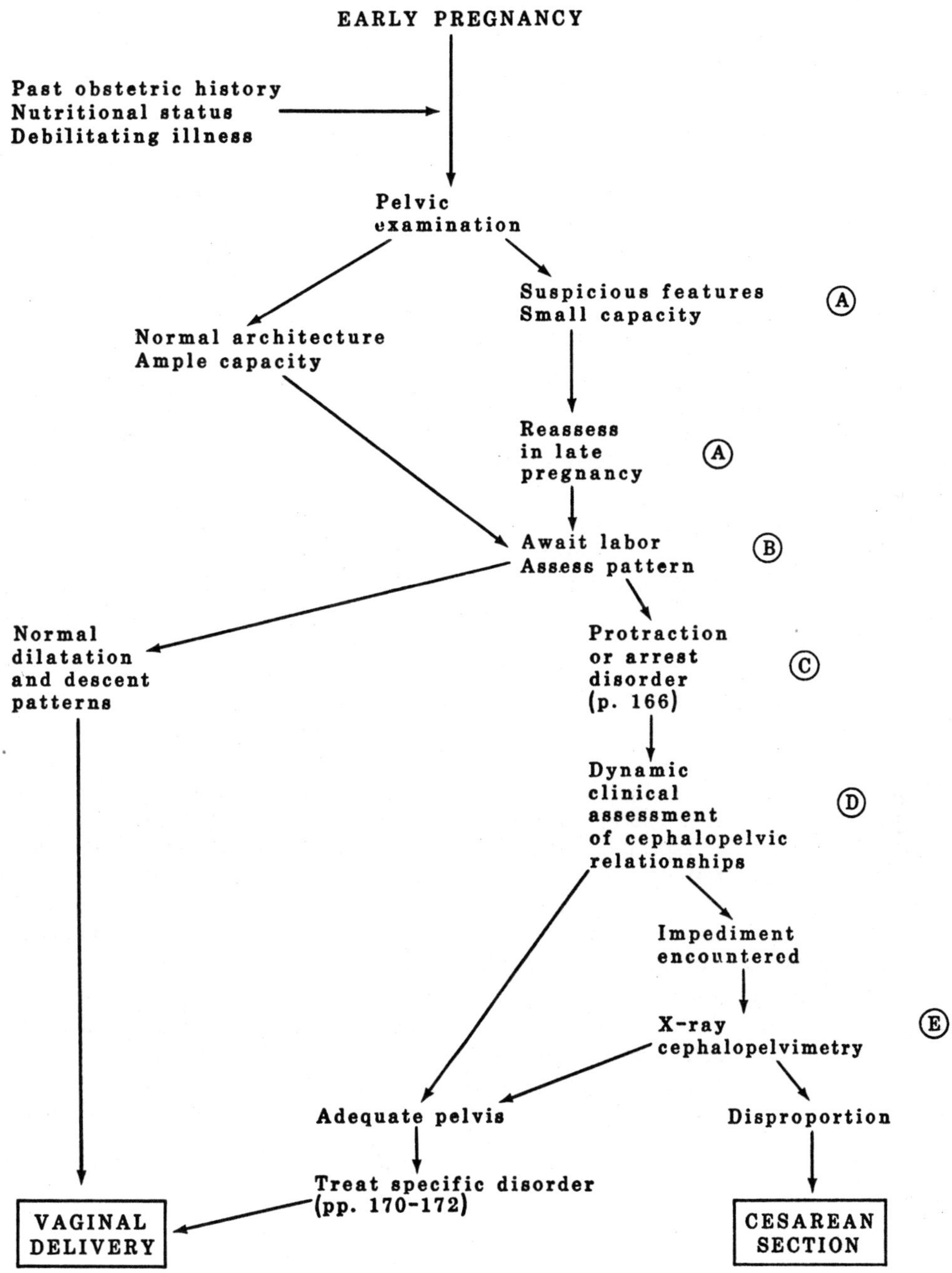
EARLY PREGNANCY
Past obstetric history
Nutritional status
Debilitating illness
Pelvic examination
Normal architecture
Ample capacity
Suspicious features
Small capacity
(A)
Reassess in late pregnancy
(A)
Await labor
Assess pattern
(B)
Normal dilatation and descent patterns
Protraction or arrest disorder (p. 166)
(C)
Dynamic clinical assessment of cephalopelvic relationships
(D)
Impediment encountered
X-ray cephalopelvimetry
(E)
Adequate pelvis
Disproportion
Treat specific disorder (pp. 170-172)
VAGINAL DELIVERY
CESAREAN SECTION

EXPOSURE TO RADIATION OR CHEMOTHERAPY

Lenard Simon, M.D.

COMMENTS

A. The adverse impact on the fetus of diagnostic levels of radiation is unproved. While no threshhold dose of radiation has been established, current objective data strongly suggest that exposures to less than 10 rads cause no apparent harm (and the "critical level" may be as much as 10 times higher). Few diagnostic x-ray studies today exceed one-tenth this level even when multiple exposures are made. This should not be interpreted to mean that unnecessary x-ray examinations are acceptable in pregnancy. The risk, however remote, must be weighed against possible benefit. Radioisotopic iodine (I^{131}) for thyroid function study is interdicted in pregnancy, especially after the fourteenth week, when the fetal thyroid gland is functioning sufficiently to concentrate this material.

B. The first trimester fetus is most sensitive to the teratogenic effects of both radiation and chemotherapy. Because of the theoretical extrapolation of risk to the immediate postconception period, it has been recommended that elective pelvic radiographic studies be limited to the first half of the menstrual cycle (since unrecognized pregnancy is possible in the second half). The basis for this practice is very dubious. Gravidas subjected to therapeutic radiation (not diagnostic levels) in the first trimester have a high frequency of fetal wastage, approaching 80 percent. Such women include patients with malignancies of breast, lymphoreticular system, gynecologic structures, bone, and those with skin melanoma.

C. Intense therapeutic exposure is likely to affect the pregnancy adversely. As with tumor cells, radiation and chemotherapy are quite active against the rapidly dividing cells of the fetus and placenta, especially during early organogenesis of the first trimester. In this regard, all chemotherapeutic agents and irradiation modalities are potentially mutagenic or teratogenic. The incidence of recessive mutations is entirely unknown; such mutations may not be manifest for several generations, although it is likely that significant adverse mutations will be lethal, and therefore unrecognized.

D. Continued pregnancy may affect the disease process for which the radiation or chemotherapy was given. For example, malignancies arising in tissues that are under endocrine control may be deleteriously affected by pregnancy. The anatomic or physiologic changes that occur during pregnancy may obscure subtle changes in malignancy, making clinical detection and periodic assessment difficult. Increased vascularity accompanying gestation may enhance early dissemination. In addition, the natural immunosuppression associated with pregnancy, especially when combined with the possibly immunosuppressive effects of chemotherapeutic agents or radiation therapy, may lead to widespread dissemination.

REFERENCES

Brent RL, Gorson RO: Radiation exposure in pregnancy. Curr Probl Radiol 2:1, 1972

Houston CS: Diagnostic irradiation of women during the reproductive period. Canad Med J Assoc 117:648, 1977

Lake FD: Radiation and women. Am Coll Radiol Bull 32:3, 1976

Oppenheimer BE, Griem ML, Meier P: The effects of diagnostic x-ray exposure on the human fetus: An examination of the evidence. Radiol 114:529, 1975

EXPOSURE TO RADIATION OR CHEMOTHERAPY

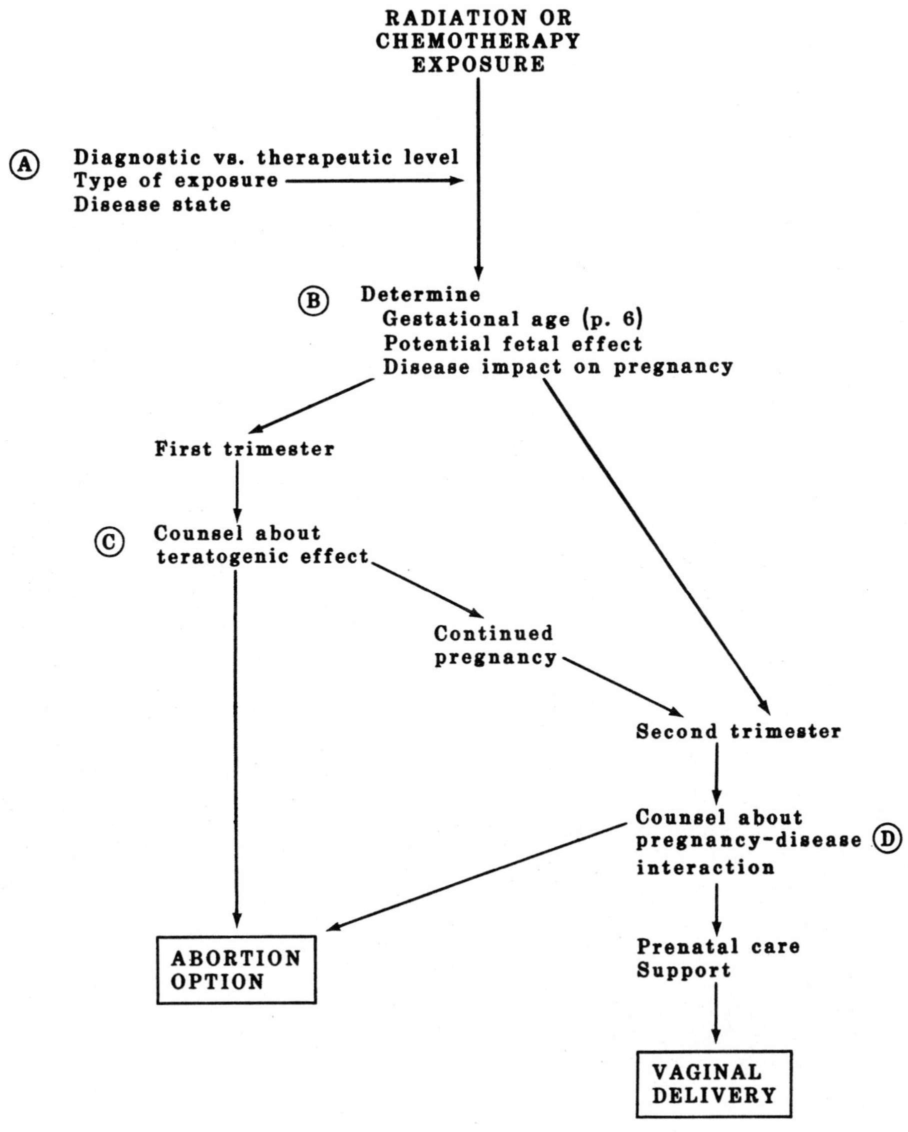

THREATENED ABORTION

Max Borten, M.D.

COMMENTS

A. Vaginal bleeding or staining, with or without uterine cramping, is the usual presenting manifestation of threatened abortion. About 20 percent of all pregnant women experience these symptoms, most often in the first trimester. Only half progress to spontaneous abortions.

B. If a gestational sac cannot be identified within the uterus, one must consider that an ectopic pregnancy may exist. Accordingly, hospitalization is in order for purposes of careful surveillance (p. 34).

C. Finding an intrauterine gestational sac by ultrasonography effectively rules out ectopic pregnancy. Rare exceptions are cases of heterotopic pregnancy with concomitant intrauterine pregnancies (1 in 10,000 ectopic pregnancies). In threatened abortion cases, one must try to ascertain whether the conceptus is "blighted" or the fetus is present and developing normally.

D. Prior to 8 weeks' gestational age (timing from the last menstrual period), B-scan or real-time ultrasonography is unreliable in this regard. Fetal motion is definitive evidence that the fetus is both present and alive (and, therefore, likely to be developing normally thus far). Absence of a fetus or failure to detect fetal motion before 8 weeks cannot be interpreted to mean that a fetus may not be present or that such a fetus may not be capable of continuing to develop. Therefore, one should consider re-examination after 8 weeks under these circumstances.

E. The very sensitive radioimmunoassay of beta-subunit of human chorionic gonadotropin (hCG) is useful in threatened abortion if serial tests are done. In early normal pregnancy, the quantitative levels rise rapidly; doubling time averages 2.2 days (standard deviation 1.0 day). Thus, two or more beta-subunit hCG assays will provide a reliable means for evaluating pregnancy prognosis, especially within the first 30 days of gestation (dating from conception).

F. As stated above, about half of these cases resolve, continuing to term with no further special problems. The other half progress to inevitable abortion (p. 24) and ultimately abort spontaneously. Use of progestational agents, once popular, has been shown to prolong the interval to spontaneous abortion even in cases of blighted ovum. However, it does not improve the outcome by way of salvage.

REFERENCES

Anderson SG: Management of threatened abortion with real time sonography. Obstet Gynecol 55: 259, 1980

Batzer FR, Schlaff S, Goldfarb AF, Corson SL: Serial β-subunit human chorionic gonadotropin doubling time as a prognosticator of pregnancy outcome in an infertile population. Fertil Steril 35:307, 1981

Jouppila P, Huhtaniemi I, Tapanainen J: Early pregnancy failure: Study by ultrasonic and hormonal methods. Obstet Gynecol 55:42, 1980

Smith C, Gregori CA, Breen JL: Ultrasonography in threatened abortion. Obstet Gynecol 51:173, 1978

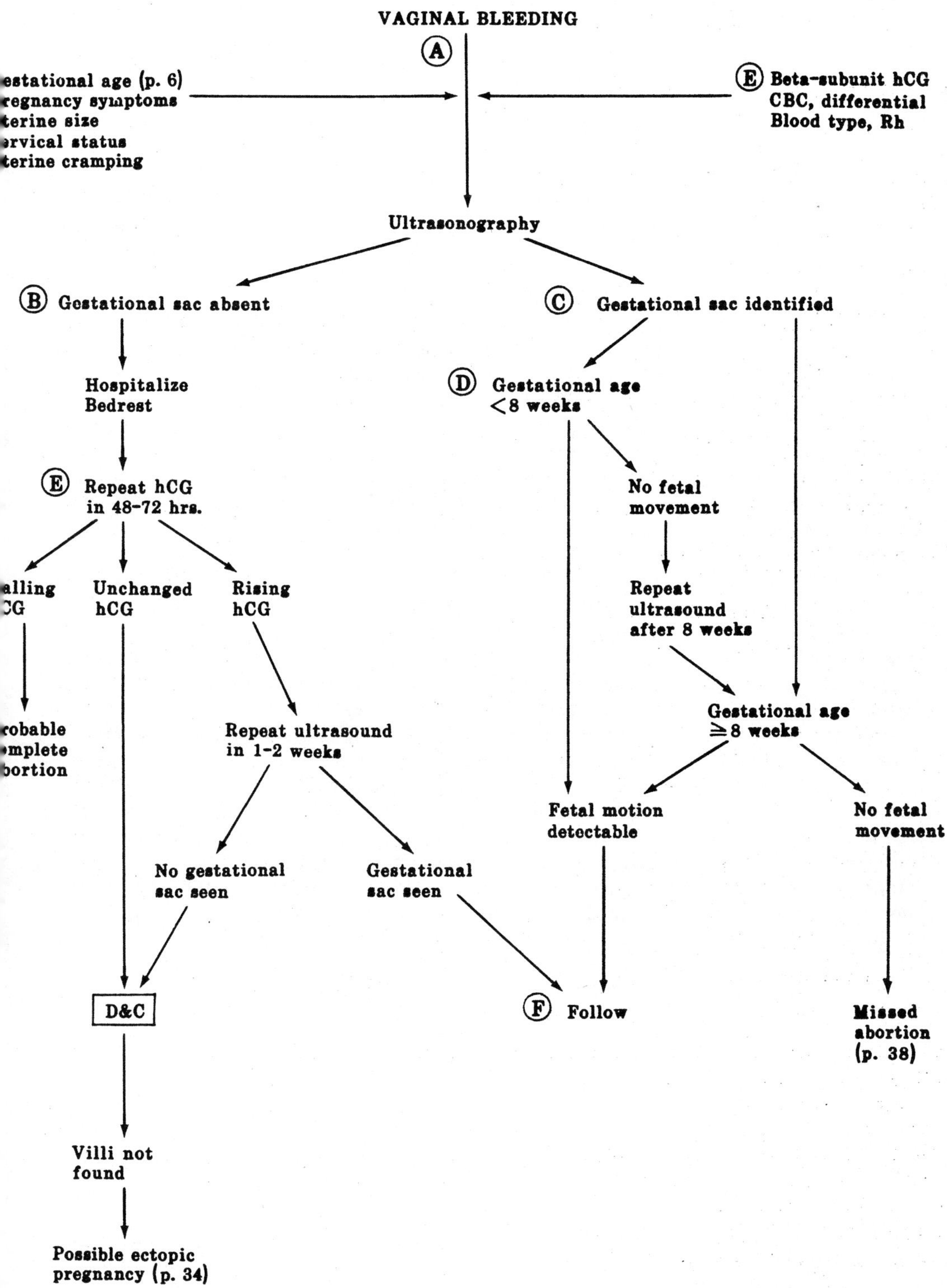
VAGINAL BLEEDING
A
estational age (p. 6)
regnancy symptoms
terine size
ervical status
terine cramping
E Beta-subunit hCG
CBC, differential
Blood type, Rh
Ultrasonography
B Gestational sac absent
C Gestational sac identified
Hospitalize
Bedrest
E Repeat hCG
in 48–72 hrs.
alling
CG
Unchanged
hCG
Rising
hCG
robable
mplete
bortion
Repeat ultrasound
in 1–2 weeks
No gestational
sac seen
Gestational
sac seen
D&C
Villi not
found
Possible ectopic
pregnancy (p. 34)
D Gestational age
<8 weeks
No fetal
movement
Repeat
ultrasound
after 8 weeks
Gestational age
≥8 weeks
Fetal motion
detectable
No fetal
movement
F Follow
Missed
abortion
(p. 38)

INCOMPLETE ABORTION

Max Borten, M.D.

COMMENTS

A. Merely because a pregnant woman has pelvic cramps and vaginal bleeding does not necessarily signify an incomplete abortion. Surgical intervention may not be indicated. This is of special concern for infertility patients who show signs of threatened abortion (p. 22) without passing tissue through the cervix. Some may have normal intrauterine pregnancy that will continue to term if left undisturbed.

B. Heavy bleeding, passage of tissue (especially if the fetus or the fetal sac is identified), cervical dilatation, and uterine size smaller than expected for gestational age make the diagnosis of incomplete abortion likely. Nonetheless, it is still important to try to confirm the diagnosis, especially if the patient's desire to retain the pregnancy and her current condition warrant it. Pathologic examination of the tissue is sometimes useful in this regard. If frozen-section study is contemplated, the tissue should be transported expediently in a fresh state or in normal saline. Formaldehyde fixation will preclude prompt histologic assessment. Verification of placental or fetal tissue warrants an evacuation procedure. Serial quantitative beta-subunit hCG assays will add information that may be helpful in determining whether or not the pregnancy is salvageable in doubtful cases.

C. Ultrasonography may also be useful. The fetal sac should be identifiable by B-scan by about 6 weeks from the last menstrual period. Similarly, the fetal heart should be detectable about the same time, especially by M-mode scanning. Absence of these signs supports a diagnosis of incomplete abortion or blighted ovum (p. 36). Ultrasonographic imaging can also be used to demonstrate anatomic changes in the lower uterine segment as well as dilatation of the internal cerivcal os.

D. Sharp curettage risks denuding the endometrial surface with subsequent synechiae formation. Suction curage is gentler, just as effective for evacuation of the uterus, somewhat safer in terms of risk of perforation, and it is therefore preferable.

E. Whereas women with complete abortion do not require further intervention, too often cases deemed to be complete are subsequently found to have retained placental tissue. Continued bleeding and infection signal this problem. If there is any doubt as to completeness of the spontaneous abortion process, therefore, evacuation should be done. Some even advocate instrumental evacuation for all such cases to ensure that none (or almost none) will be missed inadvertently. There is much to be said in support of this practice in terms of the substantive benefit relative to the negligible risk.

REFERENCES

Batzer FR, Schlaff S, Goldfarb AF, Corson SL: Serial β-subunit human chorionic gonadotropin doubling time as a prognosticator of pregnancy outcome in an infertile population. Fertil Steril 35:307, 1981

Corson SL, Batzer FR, Schlaff S: A comparison of serial quantitative serum and urine tests in early pregnancy. J Reprod Med 26:611, 1981

Donald J, Morley P, Barnett E: The diagnosis of blighted ovum by sonar. J Obstet Gynaecol Brit Comm 79:304, 1972

Hill DL: Management of incomplete abortion with vacuum curettage. Minn Med 54:225, 1971

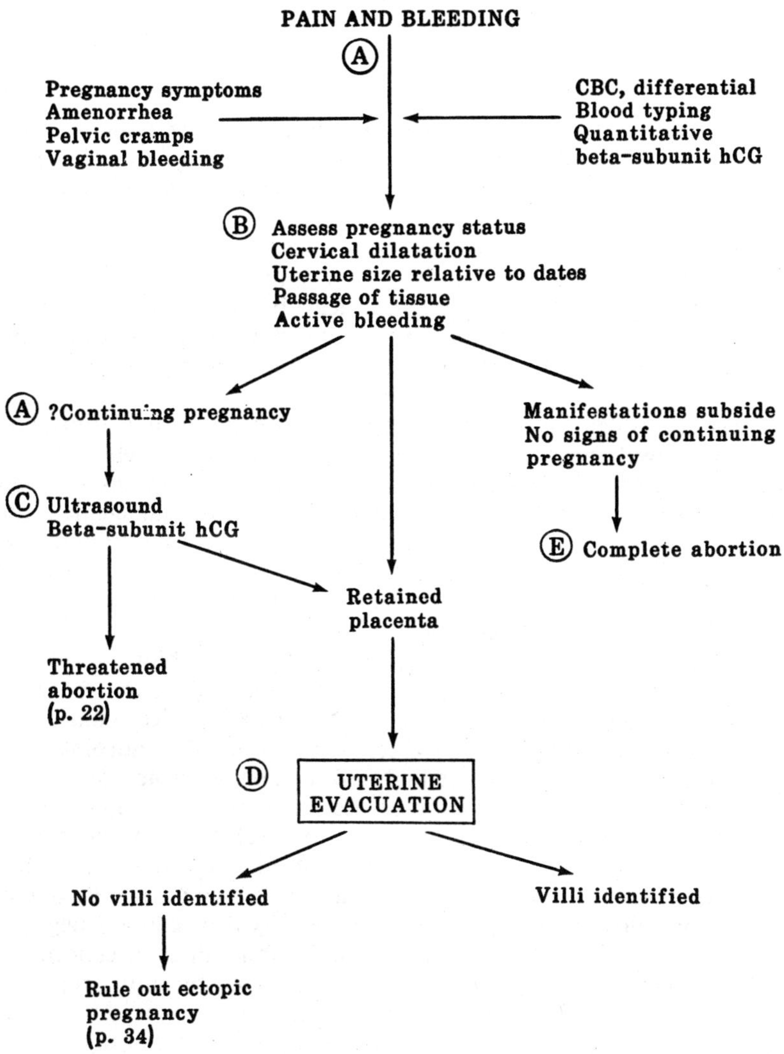
PAIN AND BLEEDING
A
Pregnancy symptoms
Amenorrhea
Pelvic cramps
Vaginal bleeding
CBC, differential
Blood typing
Quantitative
beta-subunit hCG
B
Assess pregnancy status
Cervical dilatation
Uterine size relative to dates
Passage of tissue
Active bleeding
A
?Continuing pregnancy
Manifestations subside
No signs of continuing
pregnancy
C
Ultrasound
Beta-subunit hCG
E
Complete abortion
Retained
placenta
Threatened
abortion
(p. 22)
D
UTERINE
EVACUATION
No villi identified
Villi identified
Rule out ectopic
pregnancy
(p. 34)

SEPTIC ABORTION

Max Borten, M.D.

COMMENTS

A. Suspect septic abortion in any woman who has fever, uterine cramps, and vaginal staining or bleeding. Recent instrumentation of uterine cavity may have occurred. Pregnancy with an IUD in situ is at serious risk of septic abortion, often with insidious onset and flu-like symptoms.

B. Initial Gram stain of a smear of cervical secretions will often give helpful information. It may serve to avoid surgical intervention, for example, if the intracellular Gram-negative dilplococci of gonorrhea are seen. Cervical, blood and urine cultures should be done before giving antibiotics. Both aerobic and anaerobic studies are important because anaerobes are common, especially in cases resistant to conservative medical management.

C. X-ray studies may reveal ileus or air under the diaphragm (in upright films) and should be done whenever bowel injury is suspected. Ultrasonography helps identify intrauterine gestational sac, retained placenta, adnexal mass and collections of blood or pus.

D. The patient's risk status will help choose between conservative management and intensive, expeditious intervention. The critical risk factors include a developing shock state (p. 198), peritonitis, intra-abdominal bleeding, or evidence of uterine perforation or bowel injury. Midtrimester septic abortion yields considerably greater risk than one in the first trimester, even with minimal clinical signs.

E. In the low-risk patient, await adequate circulating blood antibiotic levels and allow stabilization to take place. Under optimal anesthesia conditions, the uterus is evacuated. Suction is preferable to sharp curettage because there is less chance of uterine perforation or postoperative intrauterine synechiae (Asherman's syndrome).

F. Expeditious management is critical in the high-risk patient. Uterine evacuation is done if there are no peritoneal signs or suspicion of uterine or bowel injury. If the uterus is large, prostaglandin or oxytocin stimulation may be useful if time permits. Because urgency often prevails, however, operative intervention is usually required. Laparoscopic control helps ensure against uterine perforation. It may also guide one in evacuating a uterus that has already been perforated, especially if bleeding is negligible.

G. Laparotomy is done to ascertain the extent of intra-abdominal infection, injury, or bleeding. Bleeding from uterine perforation can be stemmed by suture repair or, if extensive or associated with myometrial necrosis or microabscesses, by hysterectomy. Damaged bowel must be repaired or resected (with diverting colostomy, if necessary). Drainage via abdominal stab incisions is essential.

REFERENCES

Cates WC, Ory HW, Rochat RW, Tyler CW: Intrauterine device and deaths from spontaneous abortion. New Engl J Med 295:1155, 1976

Cavanagh D, Rao PS, Comas MR: *Septic Shock in Obstetrics and Gynecology*. Philadelphia: WB Saunders Co, 1977

O'Neill RJ, Schwarz RH: Clostridial organisms in septic abortion. Obstet Gynecol 35:458, 1970

Studifford WE, Douglas GW: Placental bacteremia: A significant finding in septic abortion accompanied by vascular collapse. Am J Obstet Gynecol 71:842, 1956

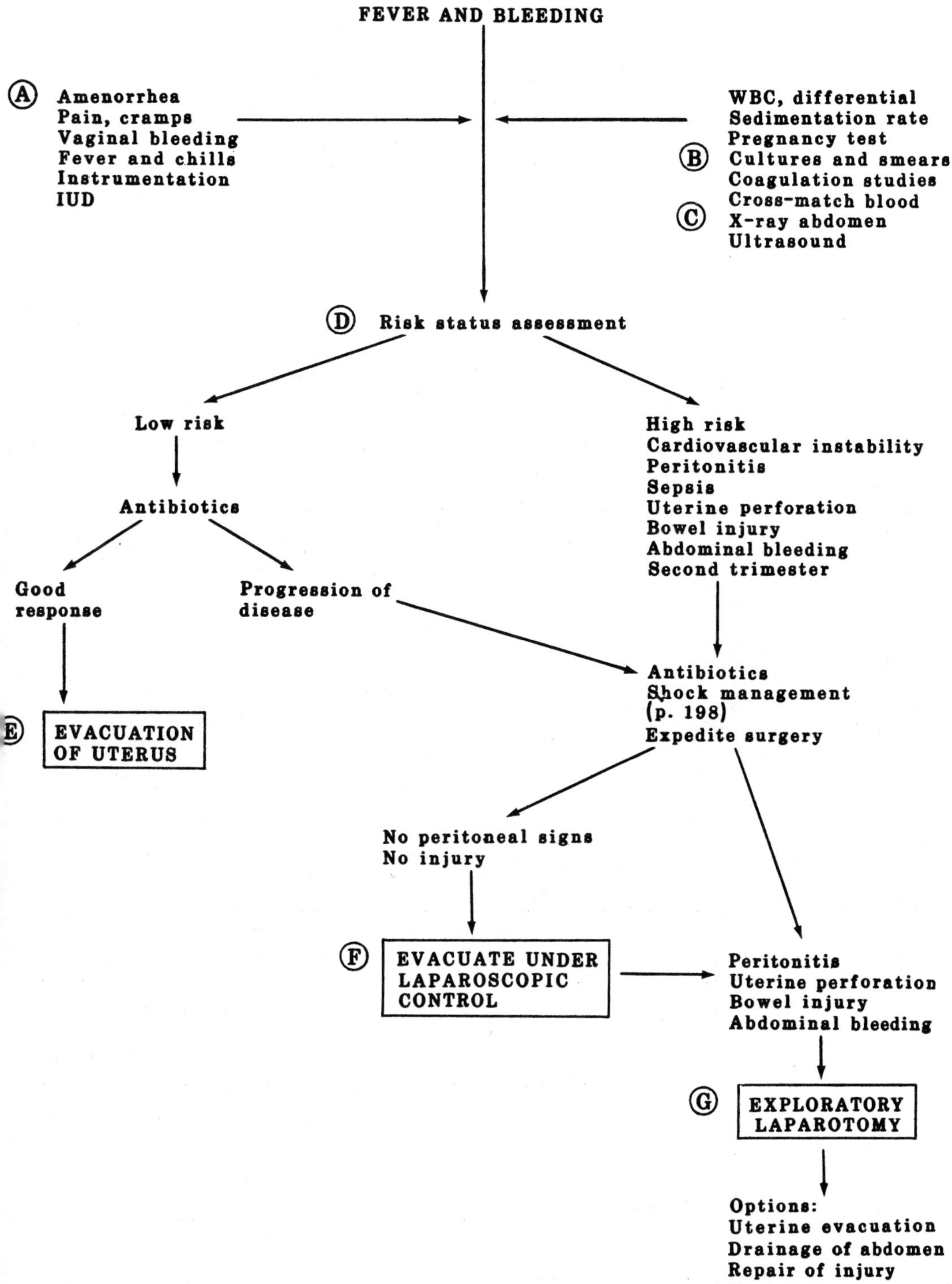
FEVER AND BLEEDING
Ⓐ Amenorrhea
Pain, cramps
Vaginal bleeding
Fever and chills
Instrumentation
IUD
WBC, differential
Sedimentation rate
Pregnancy test
Ⓑ Cultures and smears
Coagulation studies
Cross-match blood
Ⓒ X-ray abdomen
Ultrasound
Ⓓ Risk status assessment
Low risk
Antibiotics
Good response
Progression of disease
Ⓔ EVACUATION OF UTERUS
High risk
Cardiovascular instability
Peritonitis
Sepsis
Uterine perforation
Bowel injury
Abdominal bleeding
Second trimester
Antibiotics
Shock management (p. 198)
Expedite surgery
No peritoneal signs
No injury
Ⓕ EVACUATE UNDER LAPAROSCOPIC CONTROL
Peritonitis
Uterine perforation
Bowel injury
Abdominal bleeding
Ⓖ EXPLORATORY LAPAROTOMY
Options:
Uterine evacuation
Drainage of abdomen
Repair of injury
Hysterectomy

PREGNANCY WITH INTRAUTERINE DEVICE (IUD)

Johanna F. Perlmutter, M.D.

COMMENTS

A. B-scan ultrasonography may verify the pregnancy and locate the device. The device may have been expelled without the gravida being aware of it.

B. Although a string at the cervical os usually means the IUD is within the uterine cavity, it may have perforated into the broad ligament or even the abdominal cavity. Thus, there is a need for ultrasonography.

C. The greatest risks of an IUD in situ during pregnancy are sepsis and spontaneous abortion. More than half these patients will abort, and the majority of them will suffer from infection. The condition may be fatal, especially during the second trimester of the pregnancy. Therefore, induced abortion is recommended.

D. For the patient who does not want induced abortion, try to remove the device by traction on the exposed string. If successful, abortion will occur less than 30 percent of the time. Remaining pregnancies should carry to term with no further problems.

E. If the IUD is within the uterine cavity and the string is not found, it cannot be removed without disturbing the gestation. This leaves induced abortion and continuing the pregnancy as the only choices; abortion is preferable.

F. The patient who chooses to continue the pregnancy is at increased risk for spontaneous abortion, premature rupture of the membranes, bleeding complications, and stillbirth. She may develop potentially fatal sepsis. She must be followed very carefully for the development of subtle symptoms that may presage fulminating sepsis.

G. Copper-containing devices in the peritoneal cavity may cause an intense inflammatory reaction with adhesion formation. Progestasert is included among active devices because progesterone may affect the developing fetus.

H. An extrauterine IUD may be removed via laparoscopy, colpotomy, or laparotomy. The choice depends upon the site and device. For example, A Cu-7 fits through a laparoscope but embedment in omentum may make it inaccessible.

I. About 1 in 20 pregnancies with an IUD will be tubal in location, reflecting fewer intrauterine pregnancies rather than a real increase in ectopic pregnancies. For early diagnosis, one's index of suspicion should be high in these cases.

REFERENCES

Foreman H, Stadel BV, Schlesselman S: Intrauterine device usage and fetal loss. Obstet Gynecol 58:669, 1981

Gentile GP, Siegler A: The misplaced or missing IUD. Obstet Gynecol Survey 32:627, 1977

McArdle C: Ultrasonic localization of missing intrauterine contraceptive devices. Obstet Gynecol 51: 330, 1978

Perlmutter JF: Pregnancy and the IUD. J Reprod Med 20:133, 1978

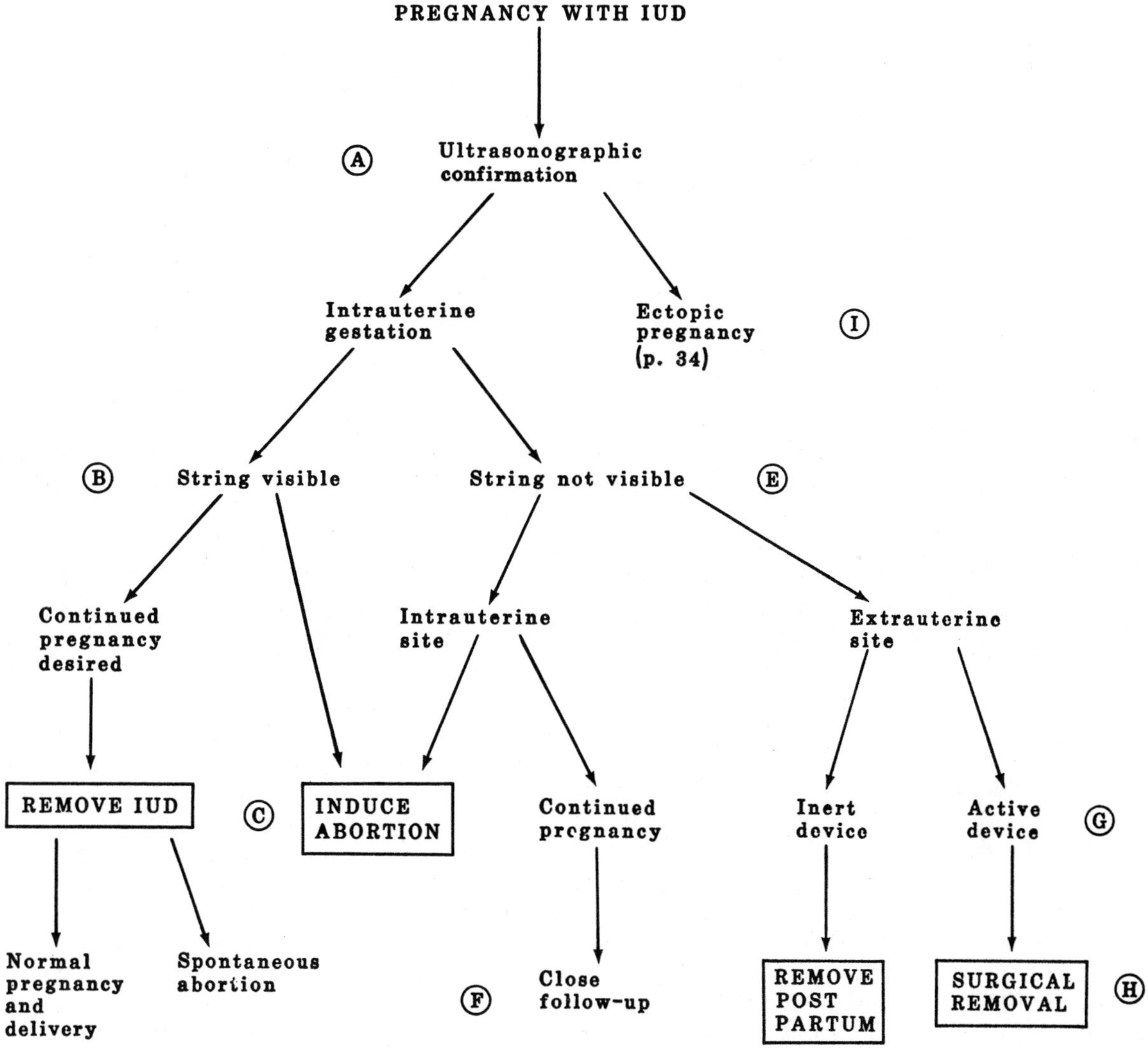
PREGNANCY WITH IUD
Ⓐ Ultrasonographic confirmation
Intrauterine gestation
Ectopic pregnancy (p. 34) Ⓘ
Ⓑ String visible
String not visible Ⓔ
Continued pregnancy desired
Intrauterine site
Extrauterine site
REMOVE IUD
Ⓒ INDUCE ABORTION
Continued pregnancy
Inert device
Active device Ⓖ
Normal pregnancy and delivery
Spontaneous abortion
Ⓕ Close follow-up
REMOVE POST PARTUM
SURGICAL REMOVAL Ⓗ

INDUCED ABORTION

Max Borten, M.D. and Selwyn P. Oskowitz, M.B.

COMMENTS

A. The gravida should be fully informed about alternative resources, safety and risks. Counseling is done at the first visit, as well as prior to the procedure itself and during the follow-up visit.

B. Screen candidates to uncover serious medical and psychiatric conditions. In addition to taking an in-depth social history, assess relationships with others, contraceptive history, attitudes about abortion, support systems, and life goals.

C. A wide range of advanced cardiac, metabolic, pulmonary, neurologic, and renal diseases put the gravida at high risk. Try to educate the patient so that she can make an informed decision. Patients at significant risk are best referred to regionalized centers for care. If the patient chooses to continue the pregnancy, intensive prenatal care is essential.

D. Preabortion counseling should be open and understanding. Deal with ambivalence, guilt, anger, shame, sadness, and sense of loss; emphasize contraception.

E. Menstrual extraction is useful for very early pregnancies (under 7 weeks). While low in risk and relatively inexpensive, it has a high failure rate. Moreover, many women may not be pregnant at all. Be alert for ectopic pregnancy.

F. Suction evacuation is commonly done. Paracervical anesthesia carries a very low risk. If general anesthesia must be used, avoid myometrial relaxing drugs (such as the halogenated agents), which may cause excessive blood loss. Most abortions can be performed in freestanding surgical units; it is prudent to hospitalize patients with risk factors. Suitable preparation and staff mobilization will anticipate complications.

G. Mid-trimester interruptions are done by inserting vaginal suppositories of prostaglandin E_2 (PGE_2) or transcervical evacuation. Common side effects with PGE_2 are nausea, vomiting, and diarrhea. The cervical dilatation needed for suction techniques may lead to cervical incompetence. Overall, early mid-trimester instrumentation may be safer (except for possible hemorrhage and perforation); patient acceptability is better and hospital stay shorter.

H. Intra-amniotic $PGF_{2\alpha}$ is also effective, but side effects are common. Live birth may be prevented by using PG with hypertonic saline (no more than 50 ml to avoid coagulopathy).

I. If the placenta is not expelled within two hours, suction curettage is done to reduce risks of blood loss and infection. It is also used if the placenta is expelled piecemeal or is not intact.

REFERENCES

Borten M: Use of combination prostaglandin $F_{2\alpha}$ and hypertonic saline for midtrimester abortion. Prostaglandins 12:625, 1976

Fielding WL, Lee SY, Friedman EA: Continued pregnancy after failed first trimester abortion. Obstet Gynecol 52:56, 1978

Grimes DA, Schulz KF, Cates W, Tyler CW: Local versus general anesthesia: Which is safer for performing suction curettage abortions? Am J Obstet Gynecol 135:1030, 1979

Hodari AA, Peralta J, Quiroga PJ, Gerbi EB: Dilatation and curettage for second-trimester abortions. Am J Obstet Gynecol 127:850, 1977

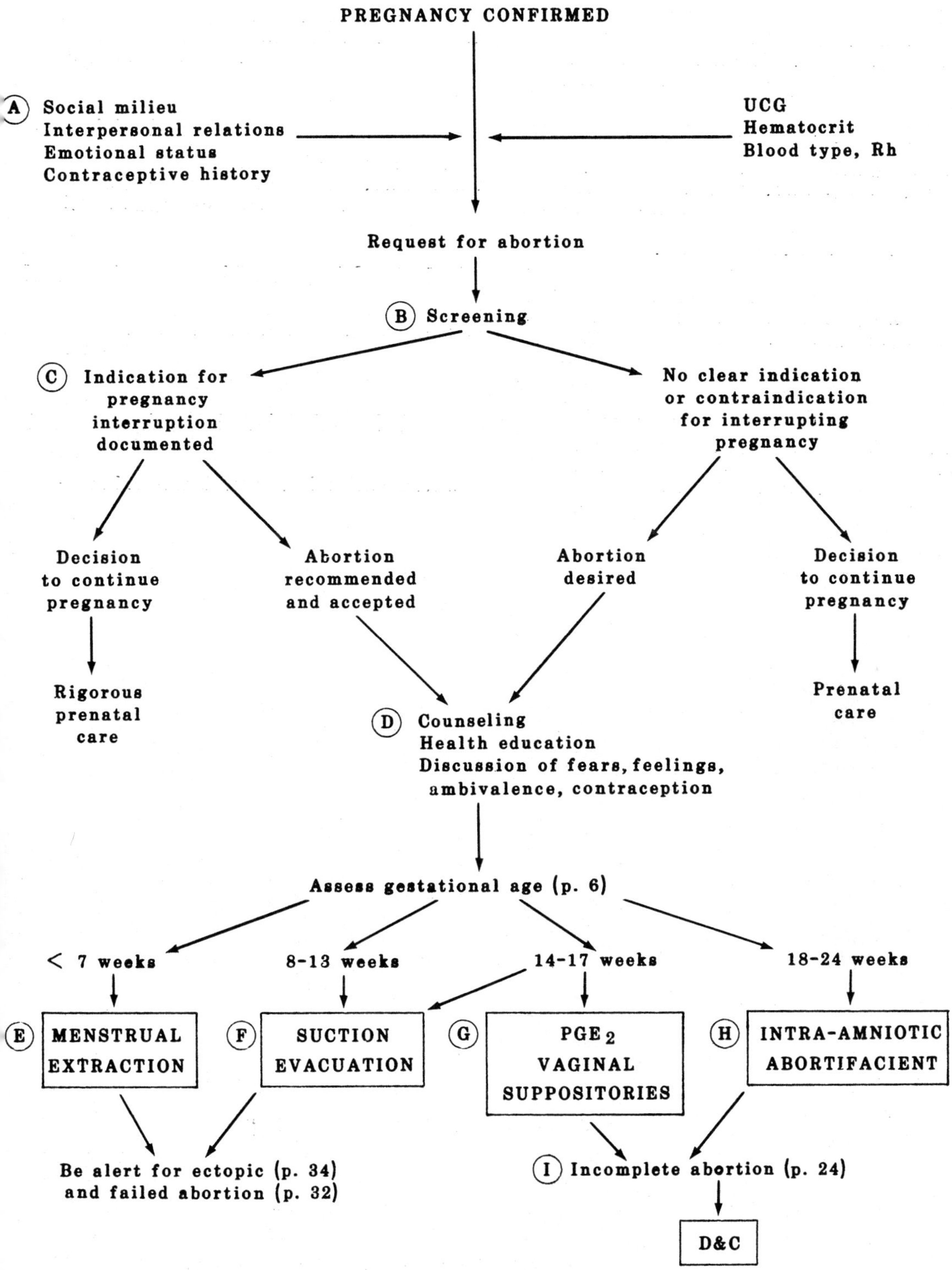
PREGNANCY CONFIRMED
(A) Social milieu
Interpersonal relations
Emotional status
Contraceptive history
UCG
Hematocrit
Blood type, Rh
Request for abortion
(B) Screening
(C) Indication for pregnancy interruption documented
No clear indication or contraindication for interrupting pregnancy
Decision to continue pregnancy
Abortion recommended and accepted
Abortion desired
Decision to continue pregnancy
Rigorous prenatal care
Prenatal care
(D) Counseling
Health education
Discussion of fears, feelings, ambivalence, contraception
Assess gestational age (p. 6)
< 7 weeks
8-13 weeks
14-17 weeks
18-24 weeks
(E) MENSTRUAL EXTRACTION
(F) SUCTION EVACUATION
(G) PGE 2 VAGINAL SUPPOSITORIES
(H) INTRA-AMNIOTIC ABORTIFACIENT
Be alert for ectopic (p. 34) and failed abortion (p. 32)
(I) Incomplete abortion (p. 24)
D&C

FAILED ABORTION

Selwyn P. Oskowitz, M.B.

COMMENTS

A. In less than 1 percent of well-conducted induced abortions, the procedure may fail and the pregnancy continue. One should be alert to this possibility during the course of an operation for instrumental evacuation. If the curettings are minimal, evacuation may not be complete. This applies particularly if the amount of tissue removed is less than one would expect for the gestational age. Efforts should be made to identify the gestational sac by floating the material in saline. Observing fetal parts is, of course, definitive. Pathologic examination of all specimens is especially valuable for confirming intrauterine pregnancy (that is, ruling out ectopic pregnancy, p. 34), but it cannot verify complete evacuation. If there is a discrepancy between the uterine size and gestational age, this may serve to signal a potential problem. Uterine malformations, especially with gestational implantation in one horn of a double uterus, place the patient at special risk for continued pregnancy.

B. Postoperatively, persistence of pregnancy-related signs and symptoms should raise one's index of suspicion. Continued bleeding, unrelieved morning nausea, and breast tenderness are important manifestations.

C. Re-examination should be done about two weeks after induced abortion so as to detect and manage any complications. Incomplete evacuation will usually result in continued bleeding, cramping, and in some instances fever and malaise. Continued pregnancy should be suspected if the uterus is still an appropriate size for the gestational age and soft in consistency. A positive urinary pregnancy test at this time will confirm the diagnosis.

D. Intensive counseling is important in these cases. Occasionally, a patient may have changed her mind with regard to interrupting the pregnancy. With the advancement of gestational age by two or more additional weeks, the procedure for interruption may now be more complicated and hazardous (or in some communities, no longer feasible as a consequence of legal constraints).

REFERENCES

Bozorgi N: Statistical analysis of first-trimester pregnancy termination in an ambulatory surgical center. Am J Obstet Gynecol 172:763, 1977

Fielding WL, Lee S, Friedman EA: Continued pregnancy after failed first trimester abortion. Obstet Gynecol 52:56, 1978

Hodgson JE, Portmann KC: Complications of 10,453 consecutive first-trimester abortions: A prospective study. Am J Obstet Gynecol 120:802, 1974

FAILED ABORTION

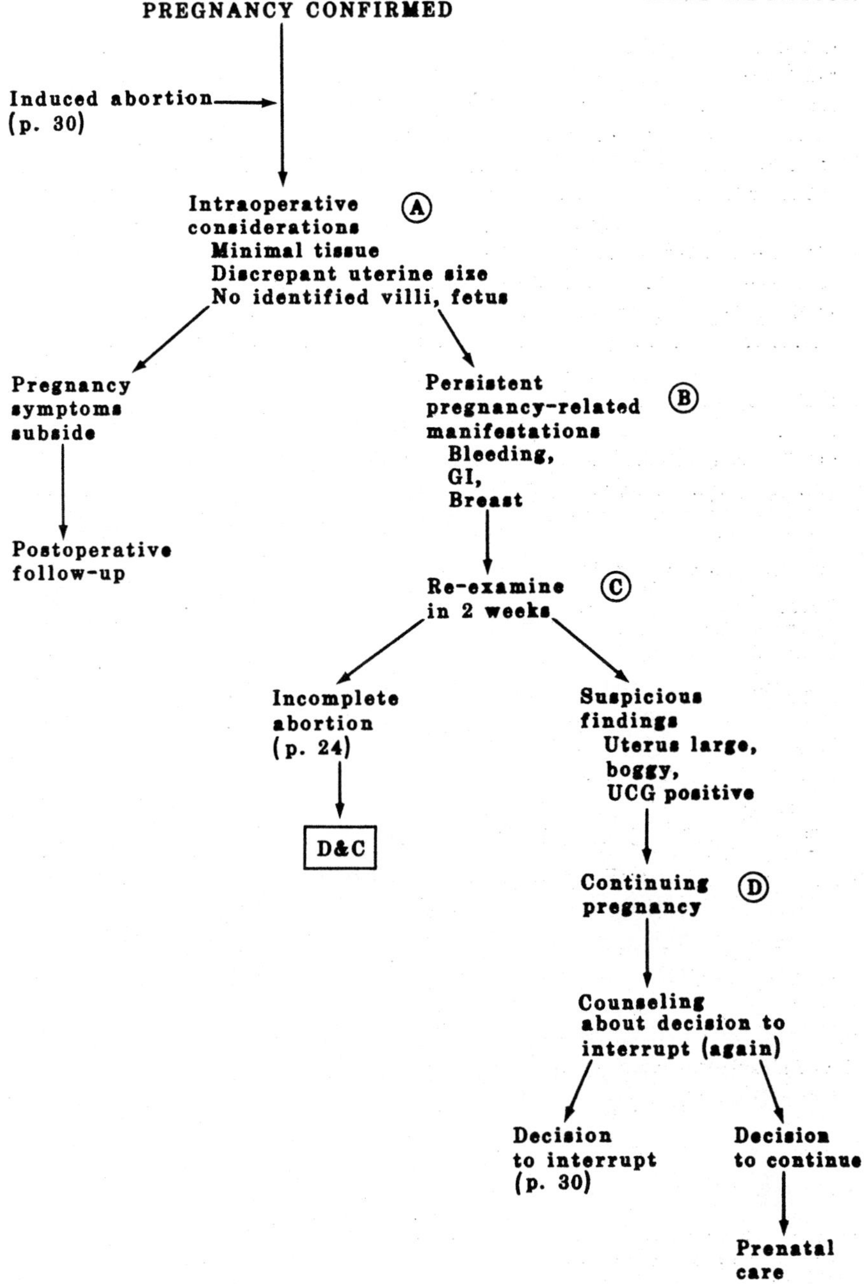

ECTOPIC PREGNANCY

Austin Wertheimer, M.D.

COMMENTS

A. A 50 percent incidence of falsely negative urine slide or tube pregnancy tests in association with ectopic pregnancy makes them unreliable for diagnosis. The much more sensitive β-subunit hCG is therefore preferable.

B. The incidence of heterotopic pregnancy, consisting of coexisting intrauterine and extrauterine pregnancy, is reportedly only 1 in 30,000.

C. Culdocentesis may be waived if there is poor patient or physician acceptability or if the uterus is sharply retroflexed so that the fundus is in the cul-de-sac. In such instances, one must assume the results to be negative and proceed to laparoscopy.

D. D & C may be substituted for ultrasound if pregnancy is not desired and induced abortion is acceptable. If chorionic villi are obtained as confirmed by gross inspection or microscopic study, intrauterine pregnancy is confirmed. Finding hypersecretory endometrium or decidua does *not* confirm the presence of intrauterine pregnancy.

E. The choice of salpingectomy versus salpingostomy depends on the condition of the opposite tube, the patient's desire for future childbearing, history of infertility, and operative feasibility.

REFERENCES

Schwartz RO, DiPietro DL: Beta-hCG as a diagnostic aid for suspected ectopic pregnancy. Obstet Gynecol 56:197, 1980

Mattingly RF: *TeLinde's Operative Gynecology*, 5th edition. Philadelphia: JB Lippincott, 1977, pp 367-383.

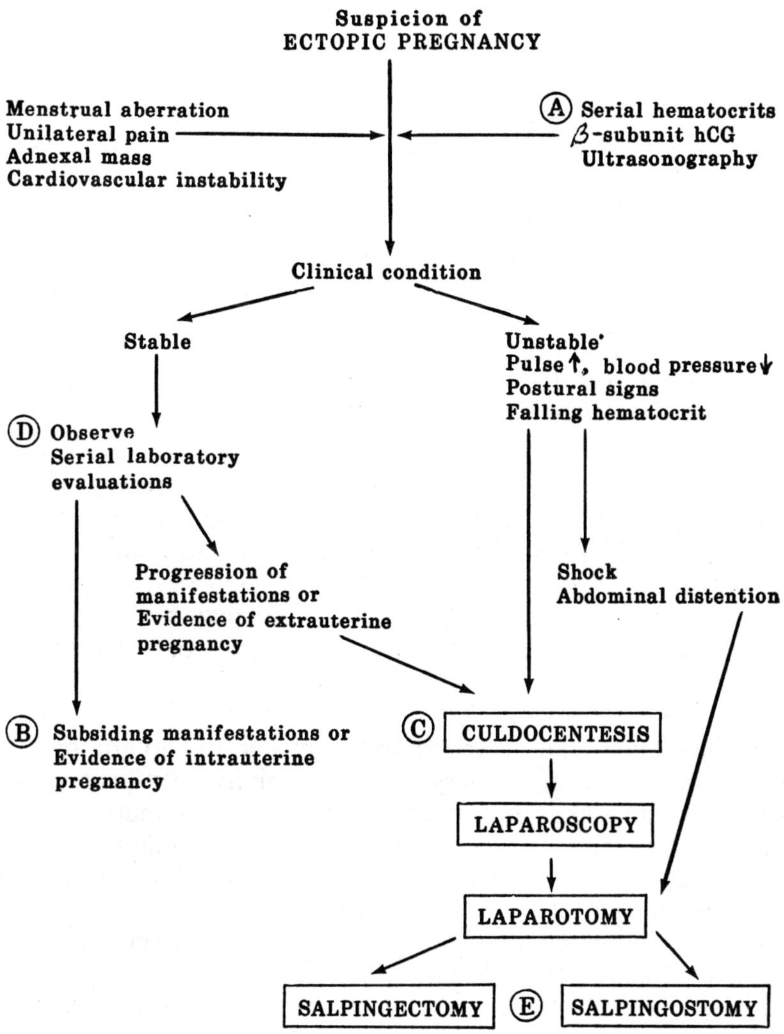
Suspicion of
ECTOPIC PREGNANCY
Menstrual aberration
Unilateral pain
Adnexal mass
Cardiovascular instability
(A) Serial hematocrits
β-subunit hCG
Ultrasonography
Clinical condition
Stable
Unstable
Pulse ↑, blood pressure ↓
Postural signs
Falling hematocrit
(D) Observe
Serial laboratory
evaluations
Progression of
manifestations or
Evidence of extrauterine
pregnancy
Shock
Abdominal distention
(B) Subsiding manifestations or
Evidence of intrauterine
pregnancy
(C) CULDOCENTESIS
LAPAROSCOPY
LAPAROTOMY
SALPINGECTOMY
(E)
SALPINGOSTOMY

HABITUAL ABORTION

Louis Burke, M.D.

COMMENTS

A. Habitual abortion (3 or more first trimester abortions) comprises 5 percent of all spontaneous abortions and 0.2–0.4 percent of pregnancies. Careful evaluation reveals reproductive system or fetal pathology in only 15 percent of cases.

B. Fetal wastage confined to the first trimester may be related to problems of conception and embryogenesis, and second trimester losses to uterine anomalies and cervical incompetence. Prior curettage, particularly if done in pregnancy, suggests cervical trauma. In utero exposure to DES may cause uterine defects leading to premature delivery and fetal loss.

C. Blighted ova are common among abortions. Couples with repeated early loss have up to a 60 percent chance of having identifiable chromosomal disorders. Chromosomal studies should be done on both fetus and placenta, and parents should be checked for balanced translocation. Genetic screening and counselling are useful (p. 42). Some habitual abortions may be due to immunologic rejection (absence of serum lymphocytic blocking factors specific for paternal antigen).

D. Cervical incompetence, characterized by silent cervical dilatation, may result from the cervical trauma of delivery, abortion, or forceful instrumental dilatation. Intrauterine DES exposure increases the risk of prematurity from associated congenital uterine and cervical defects. Uterine anomalies increase the risk of cervical incompetence. In most cases the cause is unknown. Try to uncover and treat subtle factors such as poor nutritional state, thyroid disorder, luteal phase deficiency, increased capillary fragility (perhaps related to vitamin C deficiency), hypofibrinogenemia, and Rh isoimmunization. Consider possible psychogenic influences; supportive psychotherapy and counseling help allay anxiety (the 80 percent reported rate of success is comparable to that of placebo trials).

REFERENCES

Glass RH, Golbus MS: Habitual abortion. Fertil Steril 29:257, 1978

Herbst AL, Hubby MM, Blough RR, Azizi F: A comparison of pregnancy experience in DES-exposed and DES-unexposed daughters. J Reprod Med 24:62, 1980

Horta JLH: Direct evidence of luteal insufficiency in women with habitual abortion. Obstet Gynecol 49:705, 1977

Rochlin RE, Kitzmiller JL, Carpenter CB, Garvoy MR, David JR: Absence of an immunologic factor from the sera of women with chronic abortion. New Engl J Med 295: 1209, 1976

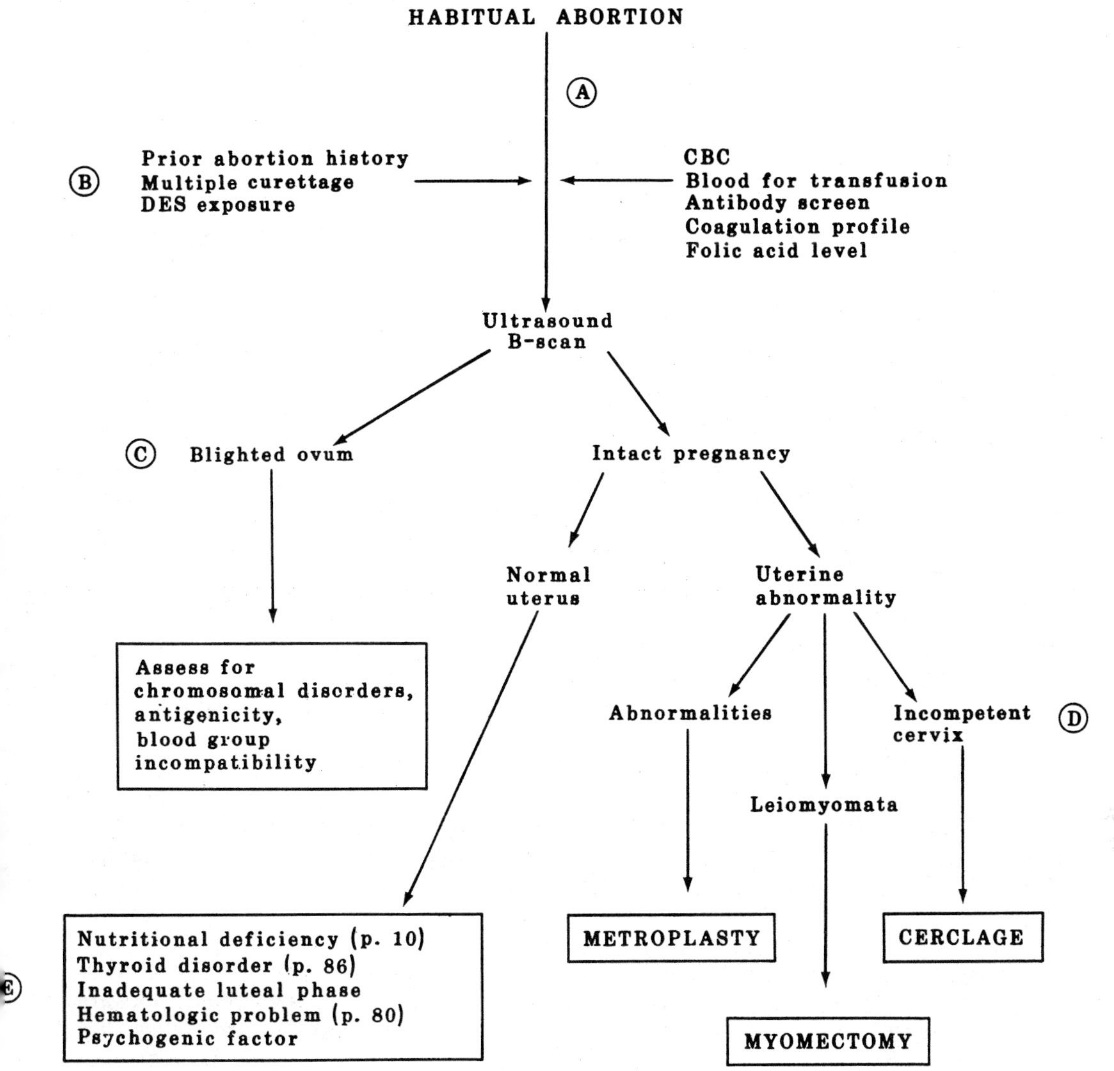
HABITUAL ABORTION
A
B
Prior abortion history
Multiple curettage
DES exposure
CBC
Blood for transfusion
Antibody screen
Coagulation profile
Folic acid level
Ultrasound
B-scan
C
Blighted ovum
Intact pregnancy
Normal
uterus
Uterine
abnormality
Assess for
chromosomal disorders,
antigenicity,
blood group
incompatibility
Abnormalities
Incompetent
cervix
D
Leiomyomata
Nutritional deficiency (p. 10)
Thyroid disorder (p. 86)
Inadequate luteal phase
Hematologic problem (p. 80)
Psychogenic factor
E
METROPLASTY
CERCLAGE
MYOMECTOMY

MISSED ABORTION

Max Borten, M.D.

COMMENTS

A. Although missed abortion is still formally defined as retention of a dead abortus for more than 8 weeks, the term is now commonly applied to intrauterine retention of a dead conceptus when the diagnosis is verified by ultrasonography. It is often associated with stable or falling beta-subunit hCG levels (recognizing that levels are expected to fall normally toward the end of the first trimester) and cessation of uterine growth. Sometimes uterine size actually diminishes. The reliability of uterine growth for diagnosis, however, is marginal.

B. Baseline coagulation studies (p. 84) should be obtained whenever missed abortion is entertained as part of the differential diagnosis. Although overt manifestations of disseminated intravascular coagulation (DIC) are seldom seen until 4–6 weeks after fetal death, difficulty in assessing the exact time of demise makes it important to begin coagulation studies early and to repeat them periodically. DIC is the most feared complication of a retained dead fetus.

C. B-scan, real-time, and M-mode ultrasonographic techniques have made it possible to diagnose fetal death with a high degree of reliability. Delay in regard to intervention in the past was based on our appropriate unwillingness to interrupt a pregnancy in which a diagnosis of fetal death may have been made incorrectly. Further, the techniques for interrupting such pregnancies were more hazardous and less reliable than those available to us today.

D. When ultrasound is not readily available, it is best to wait at least 4–6 weeks before taking action (unless some complication arises to force one's hand, of course), because lack of uterine growth cannot be considered a reliable indicator of fetal death. Even in normal pregnancies, the uterus need not appear to be growing at a constant rate. During this observation period, periodic bimanual abdominopelvic examinations should be done to evaluate uterine size. Urinary chorionic gonadotropin determinations may provide information on the presence of active trophoblastic tissue.

E. The techniques outlined for induced abortion (p. 30) are generally applicable here as well. In second trimester missed abortion, use of prostaglandin E_2 vaginal suppositories has proved to be an effective noninvasive method. Nonetheless, the frequency of side effects is high, especially those related to gastrointestinal symptoms. If instrumentation proves to be necessary, suction curage is preferable to sharp curettage. Decidual necrosis often accompanies missed abortion, and the basalis layer of endometrium may thus be readily injured by the sharp curette. Suction evacuation might avert the postcurettage synechiae characteristic of Asherman's syndrome.

REFERENCES

Gustavii B: Missed abortion and uterine contractility. Am J Obstet Gynecol 130:18, 1978

Hunter C, Picker RH: Ultrasound in management of threatened abortion. Austr NZ J Obstet Gynaecol 17:192, 1977

Lauersen NH, Wilson KH: Induction of labor in patients with missed abortion and fetal death in utero with prostaglandin E_2 suppositories. Am J Obstet Gynecol 127:609, 1977

Phelan JP, Meguiar RV, Matey D, Newman C: Dramatic pyresic and cardiovascular response to intravaginal prostaglandin E_2 (PGE_2). Am J Obstet Gynecol 132:28, 1978

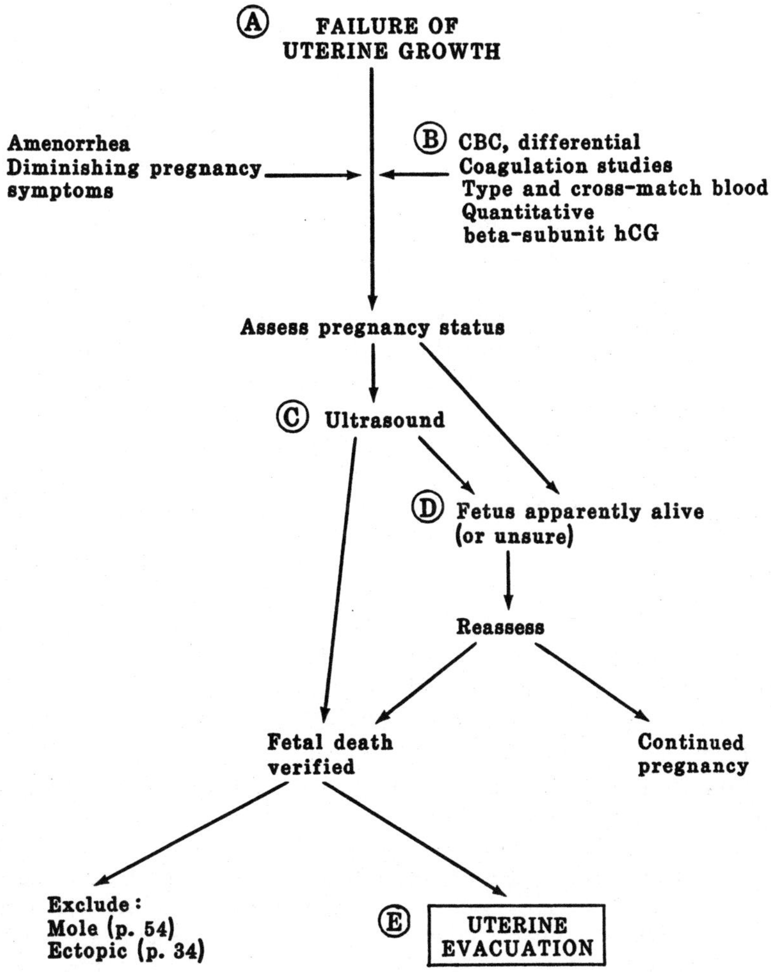
(A) FAILURE OF UTERINE GROWTH
Amenorrhea
Diminishing pregnancy symptoms
(B) CBC, differential
Coagulation studies
Type and cross-match blood
Quantitative beta-subunit hCG
Assess pregnancy status
(C) Ultrasound
(D) Fetus apparently alive (or unsure)
Reassess
Fetal death verified
Continued pregnancy
Exclude:
Mole (p. 54)
Ectopic (p. 34)
(E) UTERINE EVACUATION

CERVICAL INCOMPETENCE

Selwyn P. Oskowitz, M.B.

COMMENTS

A. Suspect cervical incompetence on the basis of prior mid-trimester spontaneous abortion; rapid previable labor with little uterine contractility; or cervical trauma or surgical procedures that left scarring, shortening, distortion, or absence. Evaluate by thorough history and physical examination; assess thyroid function, infection past or present, glucose tolerance, hysterosalpingography, and sound the internal os for patulousness (to the passage of a #8 size Hegar dilator) prior to the next pregnancy.

B. Ultrasonography is useful for determining whether or not the fetus is normal. Ensure that the membranes are intact, because there is a serious risk of infection.

C. Cerclage will fail in the presence of perceptible uterine contractions unless the contractions stop spontaneously or can be stopped by tocolytic agents.

D. The prognosis is best if the cervix has not yet effaced or dilated. This applies especially if the intact membranes balloon out in hourglass fashion.

E. Conservative measures are sometimes effective when the surgical approach is unfeasible. Prolonged bedrest may work by neutralizing gravity and perhaps reversing the dynamics of the condition, especially in the head-down Trendelenburg position (which is poorly tolerated). A vaginal pessary (Hodge-Smith) may also allow the cervix to reform so that it becomes more amenable to cerclage.

F. Cerclage is used once the cervix begins its characteristic dilatation and effacement, in the absence of contractions and other causes of premature labor. The success rate is about 40 percent. Higher success rates are obtained if cerclage is utilized before the cervix has begun to dilate or efface (or prior to conception), because some of these cases may not require it at all. Among the techniques available, McDonald and Shirodkar procedures are equally effective. McDonald cerclage places a nonabsorbable purse-string suture around the cervix as close to the internal os as possible without reflecting the bladder, while Shirodkar cerclage advances the bladder first. An abdominal approach may be considered if the cervix is destroyed.

G. Cesarean section may be done at or near term if the cerclage suture has been effective and is still in situ. If labor begins earlier, cut the suture to allow the cervix to dilate and the fetus to deliver vaginally.

REFERENCES

Harger JH: Comparison of success and morbidity in cervical cerclage procedures. Obstet Gynecol 56: 543, 1980

McDonald IA: Cervical cerclage. Clin Obstet Gynaecol 7:461, 1980

Shirodkar VN: A new method of operative treatment for habitual abortion in the second trimester of pregnancy. Antisept 52:229, 1955

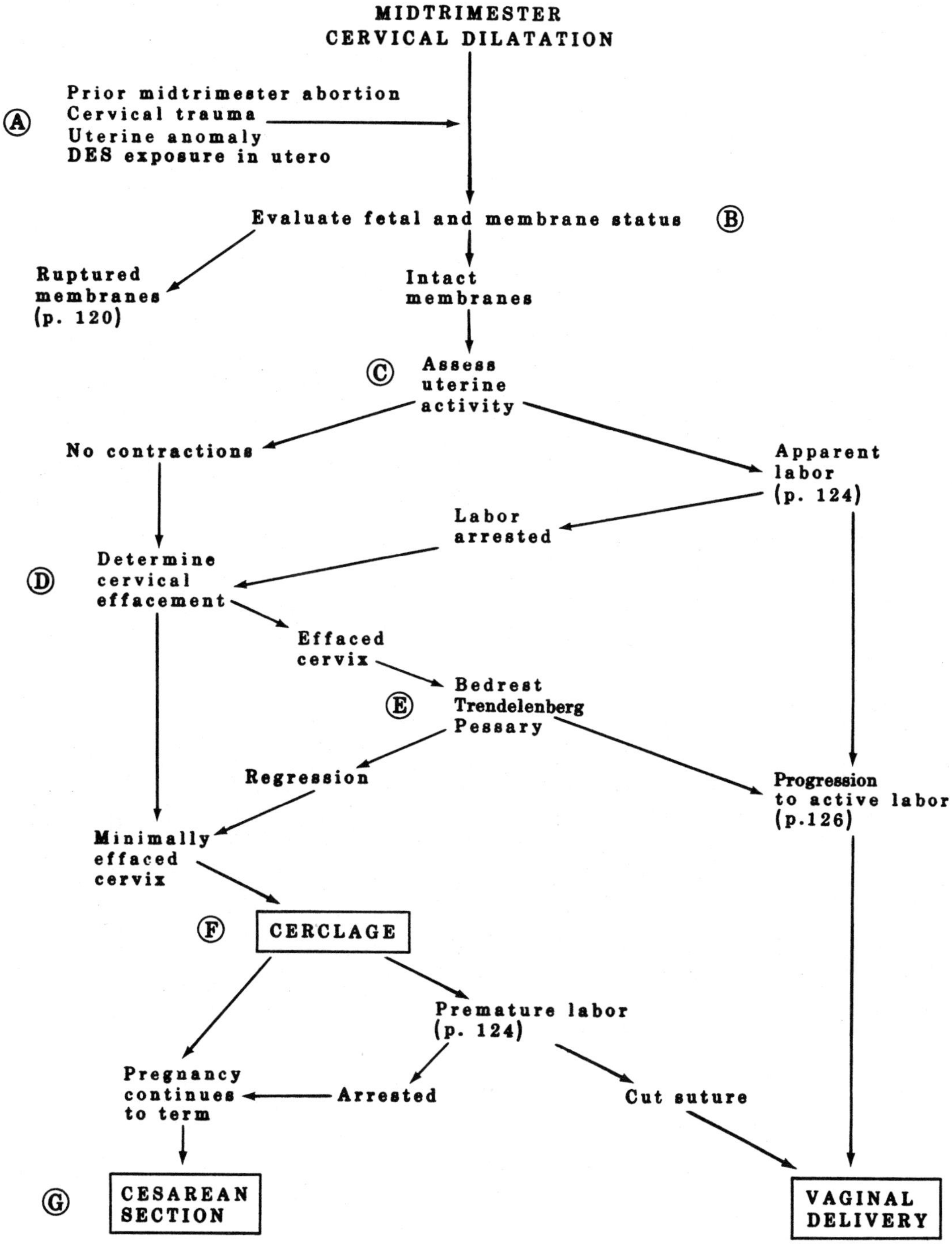
MIDTRIMESTER
CERVICAL DILATATION
Ⓐ
Prior midtrimester abortion
Cervical trauma
Uterine anomaly
DES exposure in utero
Evaluate fetal and membrane status
Ⓑ
Ruptured membranes (p. 120)
Intact membranes
Ⓒ
Assess uterine activity
No contractions
Apparent labor (p. 124)
Labor arrested
Ⓓ
Determine cervical effacement
Effaced cervix
Ⓔ
Bedrest
Trendelenberg
Pessary
Regression
Progression to active labor (p.126)
Minimally effaced cervix
Ⓕ
CERCLAGE
Premature labor (p. 124)
Pregnancy continues to term
Arrested
Cut suture
Ⓖ
CESAREAN SECTION
VAGINAL DELIVERY

PRENATAL GENETIC SCREENING

Wayne Miller, M.D.

COMMENTS

A. The factors that place the fetus at substantive risk include: (1) maternal age over 35; (2) a previous child with a chromosome abnormality; (3) either parent a carrier of a balanced chromosome translocation; (4) a family history of an inborn error of metabolism that is diagnosable prenatally; (5) a previous child with a neural tube defect; and (6) mother a carrier of an X-linked disorder.

B. The more remote risk factors include: (1) obstetric history of repeated fetal or infant loss; (2) previous birth of a child with malformations; (3) a family history of a recurrent disorder; and (4) exposure to teratogens during pregnancy.

C. Ultrasonography should be used in conjunction with amniocentesis to estimate gestational age correctly; this determines timing of amniocentesis and allows proper interpretation of alpha-fetoprotein. In addition it will help identify multiple gestation, locate the placenta, and localize the site for amniocentesis needle insertion. It can also be used alone for visualization of certain fetal malformations.

D. Fetal visualization is often difficult and incomplete. Fetoscopy is more useful for fetal blood sampling, which can be used for diagnosis of thalassemia, sickle cell anemia, and hemophilia. Fetal skin biopsy is possible in some types of serious dermatologic disorders.

REFERENCES

Elias S, Masur M, Simpson JL: Prenatal diagnosis of ichthyosis congenita. Am J Hum Genet 31:70A, 1979

Hobbins JC, Winsberg F, Blanchett M, Bennett M, Boisvert J, Hunter A, Melancon S, Miskin M, Whethan J: Fetal imaging. Prenatal Diagn 1:35, 1980

Kan YW, Golbus MS, Trecartin RF, Filly RA, Valenti C, Furbetta M, Cao A: Prenatal diagnosis of B-thalassaemia and sickle-cell anaemia. Lancet 1:269, 1977

Mibashan RS, Rodeck CH, Thumpston JK, Edwards RJ, Singer JD, White JM, Campbell S: Plasma assay of fetal factors VIIIC and IX for prenatal diagnosis of haemophilia. Lancet 1:1309, 1979

Miller WA, Erbe RW: Genetic counseling for the obstetrician-gynecologist. Current Probl Obstet Gynecol 2(3):1, 1979

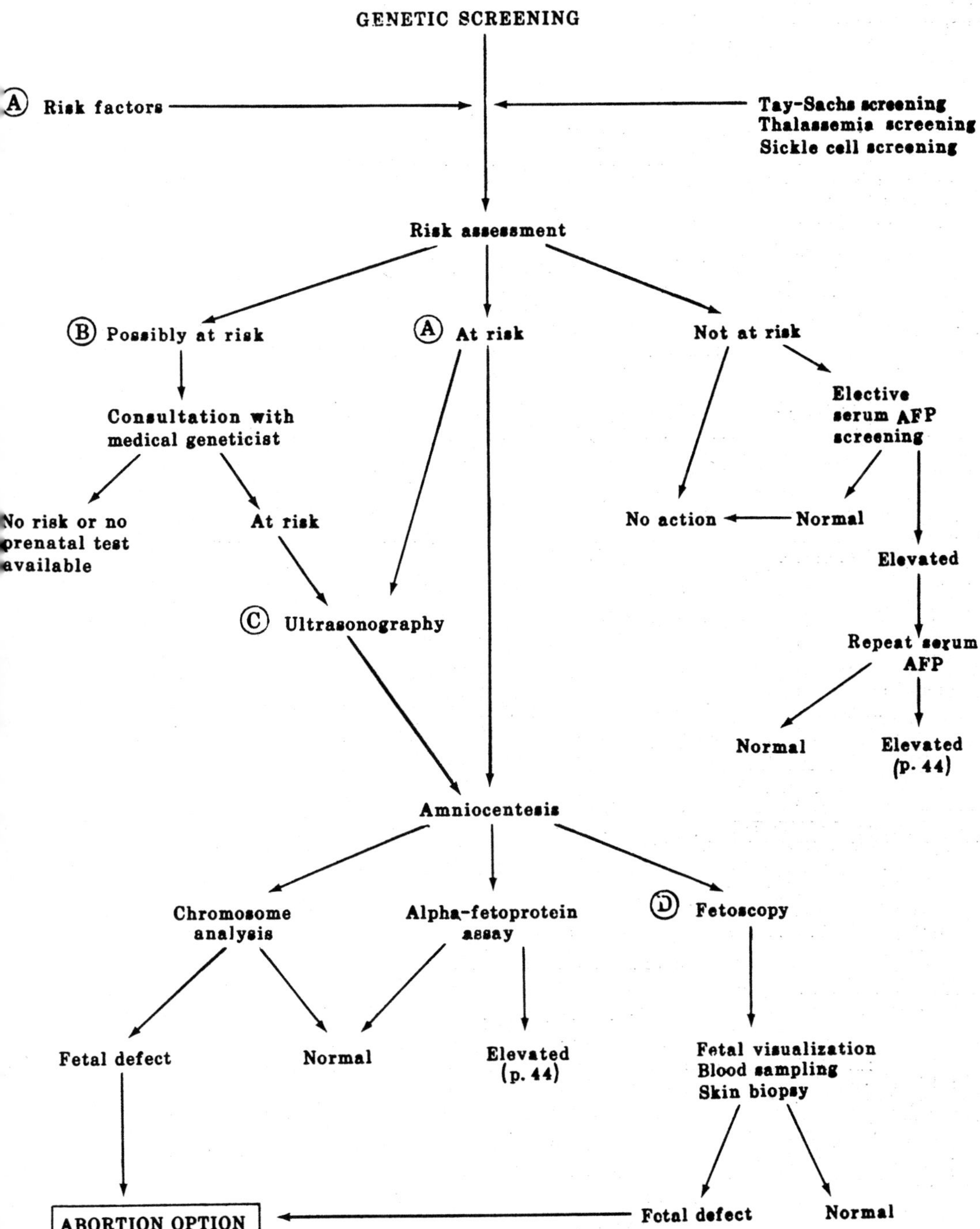
GENETIC SCREENING
(A) Risk factors
Tay-Sachs screening
Thalassemia screening
Sickle cell screening
Risk assessment
(B) Possibly at risk
(A) At risk
Not at risk
Consultation with medical geneticist
Elective serum AFP screening
No risk or no prenatal test available
At risk
No action
Normal
Elevated
(C) Ultrasonography
Repeat serum AFP
Normal
Elevated (p. 44)
Amniocentesis
Chromosome analysis
Alpha-fetoprotein assay
(D) Fetoscopy
Fetal defect
Normal
Elevated (p. 44)
Fetal visualization
Blood sampling
Skin biopsy
ABORTION OPTION
Fetal defect
Normal

ALPHA-FETOPROTEIN ASSESSMENT

Wayne Miller, M.D.

COMMENTS

A. Hemoglobin F and/or Kleihauer acid elution analysis should be performed on all amniotic fluid samples with elevated AFP. Contamination of the sample with fetal blood is the most common cause of false positive elevations of amniotic fluid AFP.

B. In this situation, the most likely lesion is a small spina bifida. Recognition of such subtle lesions requires sophisticated equipment and an experienced observer.

C. Lesions here are unlikely to be open neural tube defects but rather omphalocele, gastroschisis, anal atresia, duodenal atresia, sacrococcygeal teratoma, and so on.

D. Consideration at this point must be given to situations such as congenital nephrosis, impending fetal demise, placental abnormalities, and occult tumor (maternal or fetal).

E. The measured values of AFP should be reinterpreted given the new information. Many laboratories have constructed normal ranges for twin gestations. Since serum AFP increases with advancing gestation, incorrect estimation of gestational age can lead to misinterpretation of the measured value of AFP.

F. Women with elevated serum AFP and normal amniotic fluid AFP, though not at increased risk for a child with an open neural tube defect, do have an increased risk of obstetric complications. This risk is directly proportional to the degree of AFP elevation.

REFERENCES

Brock DJH, Barron L, Duncan P, Scrimgeour JB, Watt M: Significance of elevated midtrimester maternal plasma alpha-fetoprotein values. Lancet 1:1281, 1979

Haddow JE, Morin ME, Holman MS, Miller WA: Acetylcholinesterase and fetal malformations: A qualitative technique for diagnosis of neural tube defects. J Biochem 27: 61, 1980

Miller WA, Erbe RW: Genetic counseling for the obstetrician-gynecologist. Current Probl Obstet Gynecol 2(3):1, 1979

Report of United Kingdom collaborative study on alpha-fetoprotein in relation to neural tube defects: Maternal serum alpha-fetoprotein measurement in antenatal screening for anencephaly and spina bifida in early pregnancy. Lancet 1:1323, 1977

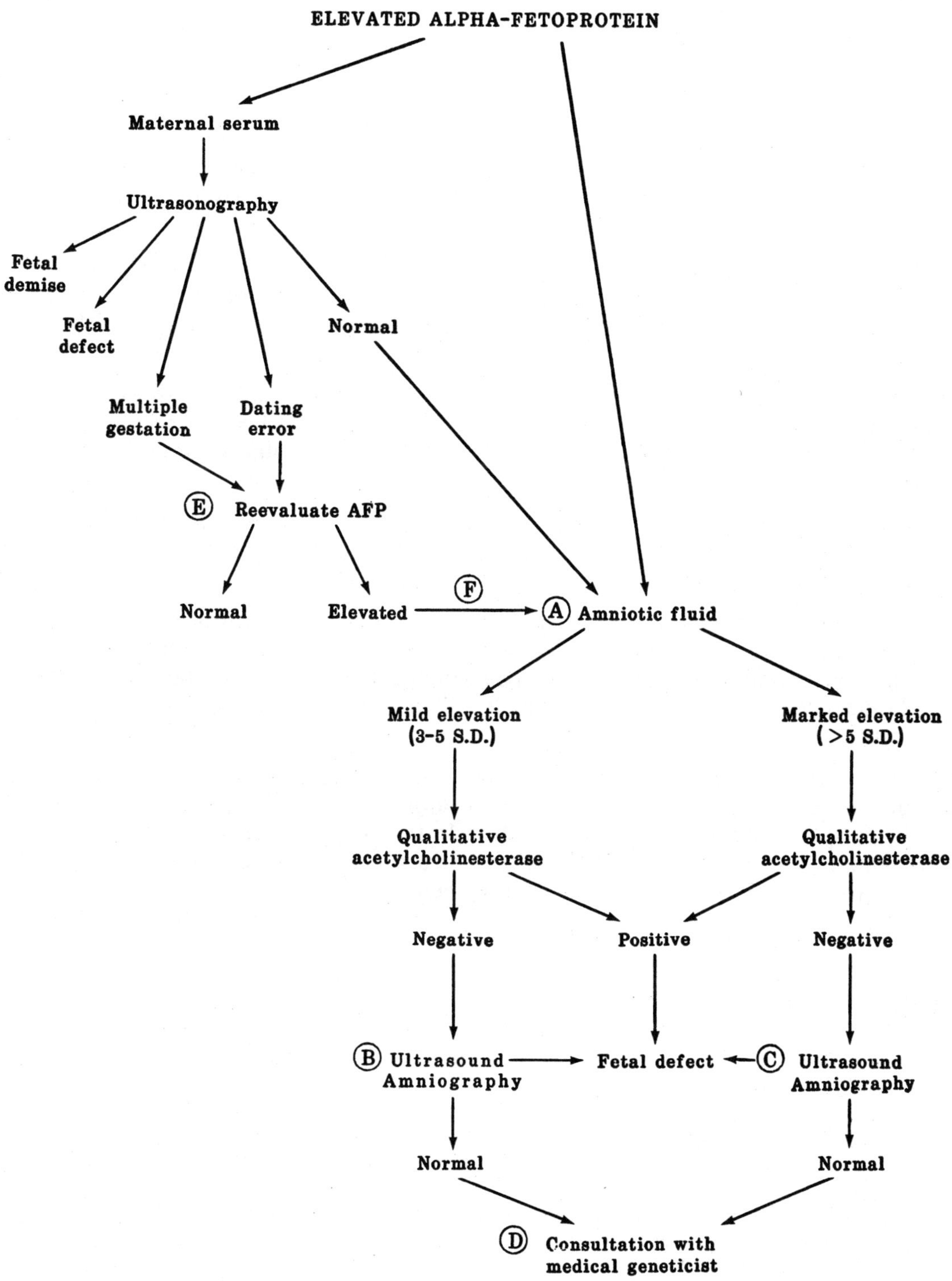
ELEVATED ALPHA-FETOPROTEIN
Maternal serum
Ultrasonography
Fetal demise
Fetal defect
Multiple gestation
Dating error
Normal
E Reevaluate AFP
Normal
Elevated
F
A Amniotic fluid
Mild elevation (3-5 S.D.)
Marked elevation (>5 S.D.)
Qualitative acetylcholinesterase
Qualitative acetylcholinesterase
Negative
Positive
Negative
B Ultrasound Amniography
Fetal defect
C Ultrasound Amniography
Normal
Normal
D Consultation with medical geneticist

HORMONE EXPOSURE

Johanna F. Perlmutter, M.D.

COMMENTS

A. In the past, progesterone (for pregnancy maintenance) and progestins (as a pregnancy test by invoking withdrawal) have been given early in the first trimester during the critical period of fetal organogenesis. Available limited data do not appear to implicate progesterone as causing any fetal anomalies.

B. Progestins, synthetic progesterone congeners included in birth control pills, may be taken inadvertently in early pregnancy. Abnormalities have been reported.

C. The fetal risks of progestins are unclear. Retrospective analyses show a wide variety of defects, but only genital changes (and perhaps heart defects) can be confirmed. Based on our current knowledge, one can equally support the patient's decision to continue the pregnancy or not to continue.

D. Estrogens (mostly DES) were once widely used for pregnancy maintenance and they were given throughout pregnancy for this purpose. They are no longer used because of fetal sequelae and ineffectiveness.

E. Although no longer recommended for clinical practice, high doses of estrogen given within 72 hours of unprotected coitus have been used effectively to prevent conception. Risks to the fetus from such exposure are not known, but one should try to ensure that the woman will accept abortion should pregnancy occur.

F. Only reproductive tract anomalies have been reported thus far in both male and female offspring. In males, benign nodulation of the epididymis and reduced sperm count may cause infertility. In females, clear cell carcinoma of the vagina is a very infrequent but serious occurrence; more common are vaginal adenosis and deformed lower uterine segment.

REFERENCES

Chez RA: Proceedings of the symposium "Progesterone, progestins, and fetal development." Fertil Steril 30:16, 1978

Driscoll SG, Taylor SH: Effects of prenatal maternal estrogens on the male urogenital system. Obstet Gynecol 56:537, 1980

Herbst AL: Diethylstilbestrol and other sex hormones during pregnancy. Obstet Gynecol 58:35s, 1981

Schardein JL: Congenital abnormalities and hormones during pregnancy: A clinical review. Teratol 22:251, 1980

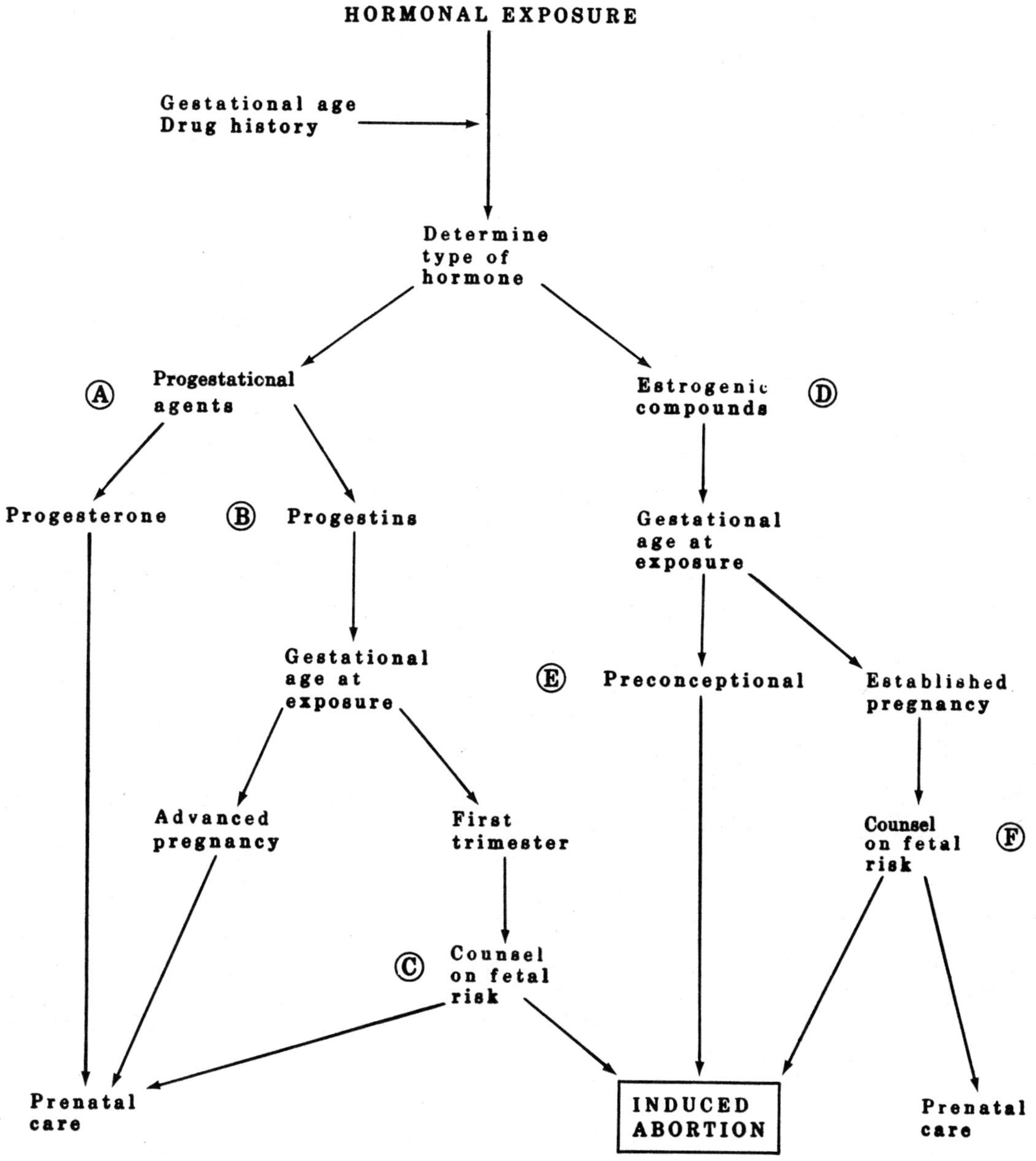
HORMONAL EXPOSURE
Gestational age
Drug history
Determine type of hormone
Progestational agents
A
Estrogenic compounds
D
Progesterone
B
Progestins
Gestational age at exposure
Gestational age at exposure
E
Preconceptional
Established pregnancy
Advanced pregnancy
First trimester
Counsel on fetal risk
F
C
Counsel on fetal risk
Prenatal care
INDUCED ABORTION
Prenatal care

ASSESSING FETAL WELL-BEING

Henry Klapholz, M.D.

COMMENTS

A. All fetuses at risk (p. 8) warrant routine testing. If the risk status reverts to normal (that is, if the mother's condition is corrected), further testing may no longer be indicated.

B. B-mode ultrasonographic scanning reliably measures the fetal biparietal diameter (within 1-2 mm). Expected growth up to about 34 weeks is 2-3 mm per week; later in pregnancy, growth slows. Abnormally slow growth is an alert (p. 52).

C. Fetal activity assessment is subjective. The gravida should count and record the movements she feels in a half-hour period 2-3 times daily. The fetus tends to be most active during the first half hour after a meal.

D. Serum or urinary estriol assays help. Drugs may interfere with the urinary tests (e.g., ampicillin, aspirin, and steroids). Inadequate collection of a full 24-hour specimen can be corrected by using the estriol-to-creatinine ratio. Single estriol levels are not useful unless very low; trends are valuable. Elevations occur with twins, diabetes, and Rh disease. Low values are seen with anencephaly, adrenal hypoplasia, and placental sulfatase deficiency.

E. Nonstress test consists of external electronic FHR monitoring to detect FHR acceleration with fetal movements. A reactive test is one with accelerations to at least two fetal movements.

F. Reassessment frequency depends on the nature of the risk factor. In general, ultrasound studies are done at 2-week intervals; fetal activity every 6 hours. Nonstress tests are repeated weekly, but 2- to 3-day intervals may be more appropriate in sick patients; estriol determinations every 1-2 days.

G. Oxytocin challenge test monitors the FHR response to oxytocin-induced uterine contractions. Give oxytocin by controlled intravenous drip or preferably pump. Late FHR decelerations are ominous, although false-positive results are common.

H. Fetal lung maturity is tested in amniotic fluid samples by L/S or DSPC. Low levels (less than L/S 2.0 and DSPC 800) indicate the likelihood of severe respiratory distress.

I. Use of corticosteroids to accelerate fetal lung maturity seems helpful at 27-32 weeks. We use dexamethasone 24 mg, orally or parenterally, divided over a 48-hour period (4 mg every 8 hours).

J. For the fetus in jeopardy, delivery is indicated. Induction is often successful (p. 128), although careful monitoring is essential. Thus, cesarean section may not be required.

REFERENCES

Goebelsmann U: Protein and steroid hormones in pregnancy. J Reprod Med 23:166, 1979

Hobbins JC, Berkowitz RL: Ultrasonography in the diagnosis of intrauterine growth retardation. Clin Obstet Gynecol 20:957, 1977

Phelan JP: The nonstress test: A review of 3,000 tests. Am J Obstet Gynecol 139:7, 1981

Timor-Tritsch IE, Dierker LJ Jr, Hertz RH, Rosen MG: Fetal movement: A brief review. Clin Obstet Gynecol 22:583, 1979

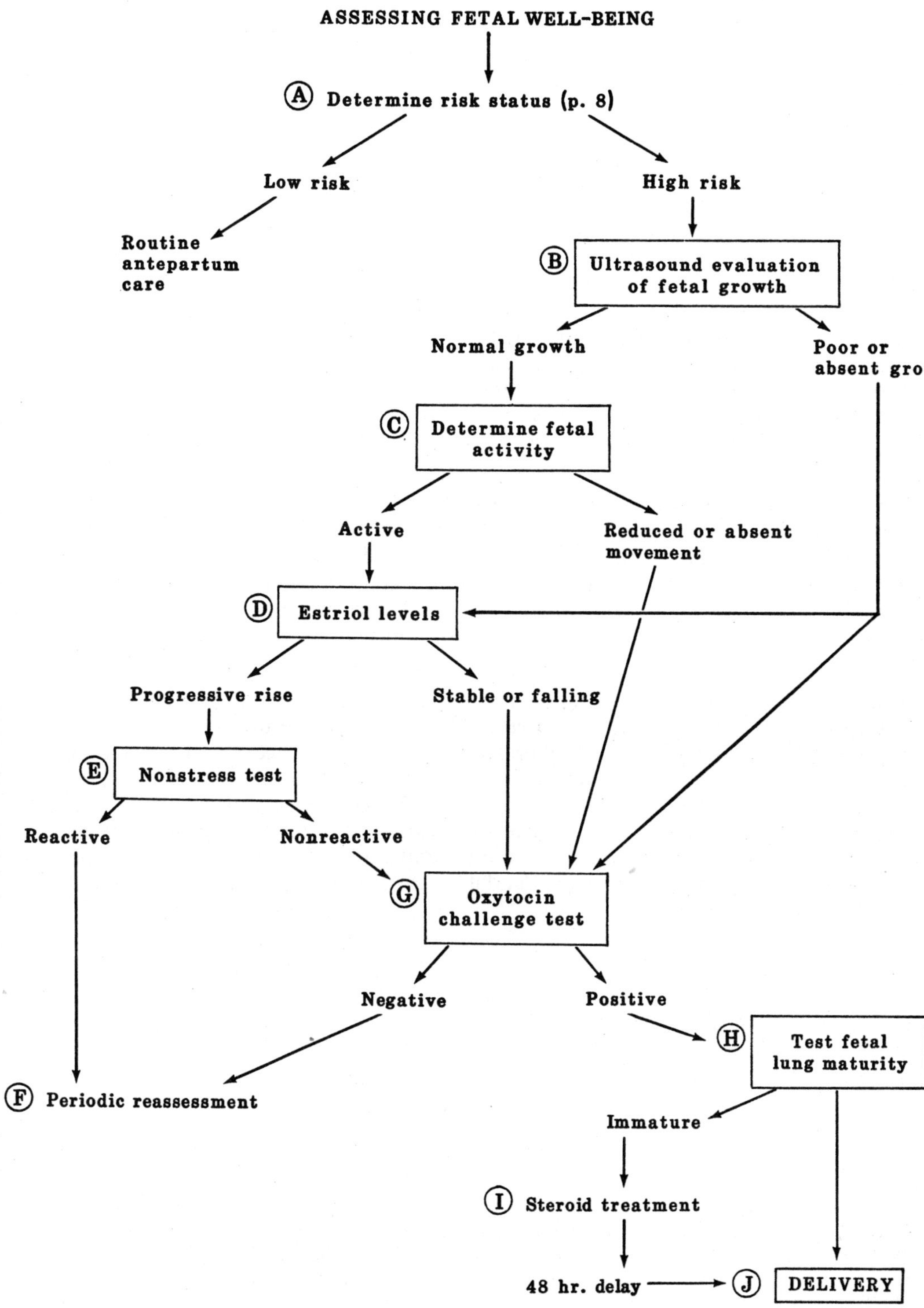
ASSESSING FETAL WELL-BEING
(A) Determine risk status (p. 8)
Low risk
High risk
Routine antepartum care
(B) Ultrasound evaluation of fetal growth
Normal growth
Poor or absent growth
(C) Determine fetal activity
Active
Reduced or absent movement
(D) Estriol levels
Progressive rise
Stable or falling
(E) Nonstress test
Reactive
Nonreactive
(G) Oxytocin challenge test
Negative
Positive
(H) Test fetal lung maturity
(F) Periodic reassessment
Immature
(I) Steroid treatment
48 hr. delay
(J) DELIVERY

ASSESSING FETAL GROWTH

Henry Klapholz, M.D.

COMMENTS

A. High-risk background factors mandating close surveillance include prior delivery of a premature or growth-retarded infant, perinatal loss, and recurrent late abortion. Assess nutritional factors even though only extreme malnutrition affects fetal growth significantly. Calorie supplementation may increase birth weight, but starvation causes little intellectual impairment. Weight gain of at least 15 pounds is optimal (p. 10). Social status may be an index of nutritional deprivation. Watch for relevant illnesses: hemoglobinopathies, cyanotic heart disease, hepatitis, hypertension, antepartum hemorrhage, vascular disease, Rh isoimmunization, and diabetes mellitus. About 35 percent of all growth-retarded infants are associated with placental vascular insufficiency attributable to hypertension or related disorders of placental perfusion.

B. Chromosomal variants account for fewer than 10 percent of affected fetuses. Maternal smoking reduces average fetal weight, as do high altitude and chronic exposure to carbon monoxide. Toxoplasmosis, cytomegalovirus, and rubella infection may reduce fetal growth and brain development. Even without fetal infection, placental infection may retard growth. Potentially teratogenic alcohol, Coumadin, hydantoin, heroin, methadone, nicotine, and antimetabolites can also impede fetal development.

C. Measurement of uterine size is of limited value, but sequential observations at each prenatal visit help assess growth objectively. Measure from the upper margin of the symphysis pubis to the fundus; a calibrated caliper is more accurate than a tape. Relating the fundal height to a landmark, such as the umbilicus or xiphoid, is a poor practice. During 20–36 weeks, uterine size increases 3.5 cm per month, reaching about 35 cm. Obesity, distended bowel, full bladder, hydramnios, multiple gestation, transverse lie, and pendulous abdomen obscure the significance of fundal height measurement as a signal of poor fetal growth. Fundal height may recede near term with fetal engagement.

D. Accurate and reliable measures of fetal growth are serial ultrasonographic determinations of biparietal diameter. Accuracy of 2 mm is possible for gestational age estimates within 2 weeks. Failure of growth can thus be ascertained reliably. Because the fetal head is larger than the abdomen until about 36 weeks, the head-to-abdomen ratio may help distinguish symmetric from asymmetric (head-sparing) growth retardation (p. 52).

REFERENCES

Brown JE, Jacobson HN, Askue LH, Peieck MG: Influence of pregnancy weight gain on the size of infants born to underweight women. Obstet Gynecol 57:13, 1981

Jones OW: Genetic factors in the determination of fetal size. J Reprod Med 21:305, 1978

Knox GE: Influence of infection on fetal growth and development. J Reprod Med 21:352, 1978

Redmond GP: Effect of drugs on intrauterine growth. Clin Perinat 6:15, 1979

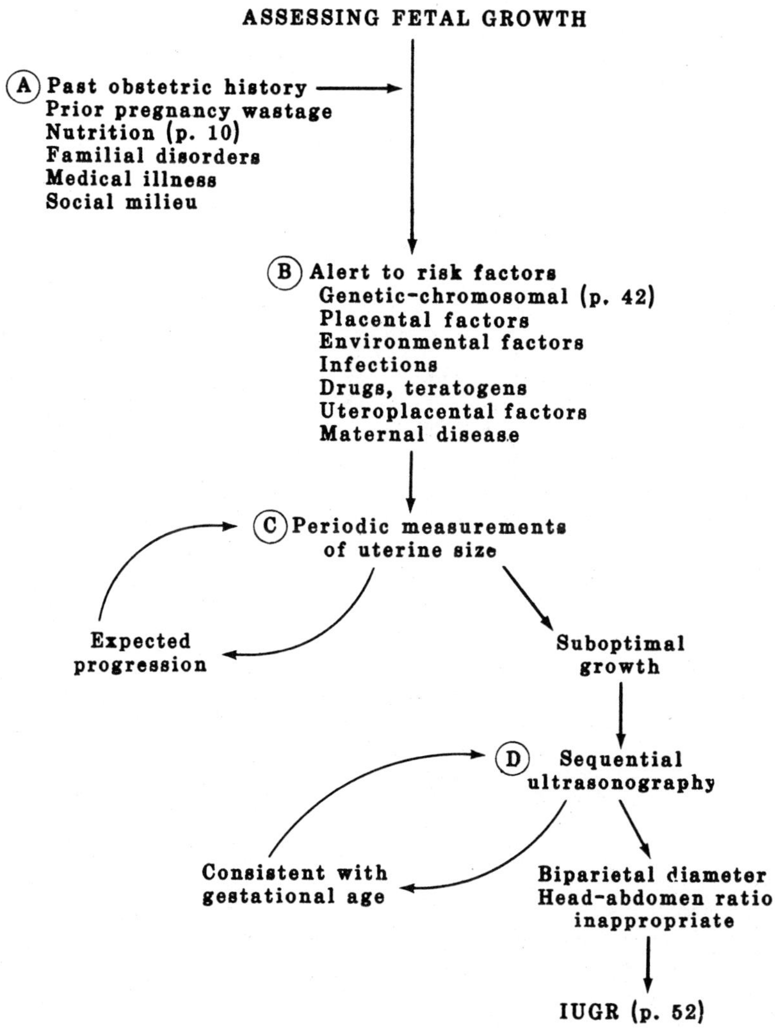
ASSESSING FETAL GROWTH
(A) Past obstetric history
Prior pregnancy wastage
Nutrition (p. 10)
Familial disorders
Medical illness
Social milieu
(B) Alert to risk factors
Genetic-chromosomal (p. 42)
Placental factors
Environmental factors
Infections
Drugs, teratogens
Uteroplacental factors
Maternal disease
(C) Periodic measurements of uterine size
Expected progression
Suboptimal growth
(D) Sequential ultrasonography
Consistent with gestational age
Biparietal diameter
Head-abdomen ratio
inappropriate
IUGR (p. 52)

INTRAUTERINE GROWTH RETARDATION (IUGR)

Henry Klapholz, M.D.

COMMENTS

A. Risk factors for IUGR as determined at the initial prenatal visit include prior fetal growth retardation, twins, maternal disease, malnutrition, smoking, and inadequate weight gain.

B. Quantitative fetal growth evaluation is usually done every 2–3 weeks during the last trimester. Failure of the uterine fundus to grow (p. 50) requires confirmation by ultrasonography. Fetal biparietal diameter (BPD) measurements are easily made. BPD growth slows from 3–3.5 mm per week at 28 weeks to 2.5 mm per week at 28–32 weeks, and 1.7 mm per week to term. Since the ultrasound error is about 2 mm, we need 3-week intervals to differentiate true growth retardation. Brain sparing in early pregnancy (asymmetric IUGR) shows normal head growth in a fetus smaller than expected. Serial measurements of thorax or abdomen diameters provide head-to-abdomen or head-to-thorax ratios. Most IUGR cases show head-to-thorax ratios above the 95th percentile for the gestational age. Symmetric IUGR is often seen earlier in pregnancy, resulting from chronic infection, chromosomal anomalies, and cigarette smoking. These infants tend to have poorer long-term prognosis. Total intrauterine volume obtained by ultrasound may help assess overall uterine growth and in detecting oligohydramnios or polyhydramnios associated with poor fetal development. Total fetal weight assessment requires complex calculations based on multiple ultrasound images of the fetal thorax and abdomen. Correlations within 10 percent of actual fetal weight can be achieved by measuring abdominal circumference and BPD.

C. Complete cessation of growth over a 2- to 3-week interval is serious. Consider delivery at once if the fetus is physiologically mature as determined by amniotic fluid L/S ratio, disaturated phosphatidylcholine, or the ratio of phosphatidylinositol to phosphatidylglycerol.

D. Reduced fetal growth is detectable by periodic antepartum testing. Evidence of placental insufficiency should prompt delivery. In the face of rising estriol levels and persistently reactive nonstress or negative contraction stress tests, allow the pregnancy to continue until spontaneous labor begins. Use fetal monitoring throughout the labor to detect fetal hypoxia based on placental insufficiency.

E. Induction of labor and subsequent vaginal delivery are preferable to cesarean section; however, associated placental insufficiency may make it impossible to effect strong uterine contractions without producing fetal hypoxia (p. 136) and necessitate abdominal delivery for fetal salvage.

REFERENCES

Bowes WA: Delivery of the low birth weight infant. Clin Perinat 8:183, 1980

Cook LN: Intrauterine and extrauterine recognition and management of deviant fetal growth. Pediatr Clin North Am 24:431, 1977

Frigoletto FD, Rothchild SB: Altered fetal growth: An overview. Clin Obstet Gynecol 20:915, 1977

Koops BL: Neurologic sequelae in infants with intrauterine growth retardation. J Reprod Med 21: 343, 1978

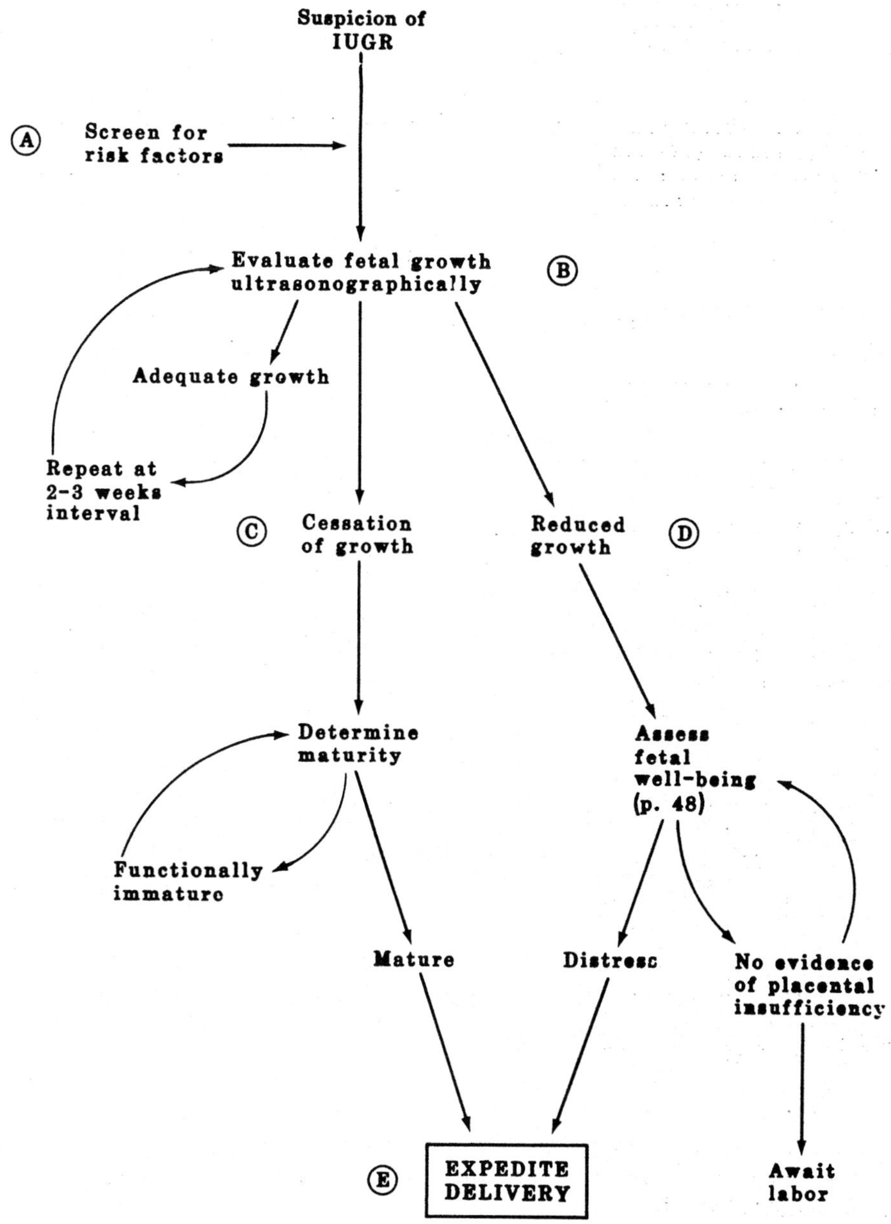
Suspicion of IUGR
A
Screen for risk factors
Evaluate fetal growth ultrasonographically
B
Adequate growth
Repeat at 2-3 weeks interval
C
Cessation of growth
Reduced growth
D
Determine maturity
Assess fetal well-being (p. 48)
Functionally immature
Mature
Distress
No evidence of placental insufficiency
E
EXPEDITE DELIVERY
Await labor

MOLAR PREGNANCY

Lenard Simon, M.D.

COMMENTS

A. Suspect a mole if uterine growth is excessively rapid and if no fetal heart can be heard with ultrasound (Doptone) after 10 weeks. The possibility of a mole is suggested by prolonged and heavy vaginal bleeding, anemia, excessive uterine enlargement, hyperemesis gravidarum, hypertension in the first or second trimester, hyperthyroidism, hemoptysis, cough, dyspnea, or chest pain.

B. Prior history of gestational trophoblastic neoplasms (GTN) should alert the physician. B-scan ultrasonography is usually reliable in showing absence of a gestational sac and scattered uterine echoes. Quantitative beta-subunit hCG may be helpful if markedly elevated; however, it need not always be elevated, especially with rapidly proliferating neoplastic tissue undergoing necrosis.

C. Assess risk status by pretreatment evaluation of hCG level, liver function, thyroid status, coagulation profile, chest x-ray, stool guaiac, and, where indicated, studies of lung, brain, and liver for metastasis by tomography, arteriography, or CT scan. Comorbid conditions include hyperthyroidism, pregnancy-induced hypertension, trophoblastic embolization, and disseminated intravascular coagulation.

D. Treatment of metastatic GTN is preferably done at regionalized centers. A combination of methotrexate with citrovorum factor rescue is the regimen of choice. Actinomycin D is used in place of the potentially hepatotoxic methotrexate in women with liver dysfunction. Actinomycin D may also be used prophylactically in high-risk cases to avert metastatic sequelae; the benefits seem to outweigh the risks in them. Prophylactic use should begin 3 days before evacuation, if possible.

E. Weekly beta-subunit hCG is done for 3 consecutive weeks and then monthly until normal for 6 months. Obtain chest x-rays before treatment and after 4 weeks. The patient should avoid subsequent pregnancy during the follow-up interval so as not to interfere with interpretation of follow-up hCG levels. Contraception should be used until the hCG levels have been normal for at least 6 months.

F. Give a subsequent course of therapy if the hCG levels remain stable for more than 2 weeks, if the levels rise, or if metastases appear. The regimen for repeat treatment is actinomycin D. Cases failing to respond should be considered for multiple agent chemotherapy.

REFERENCES

Bagshawe KD: Treatment of trophoblastic tumors. Ann Acad Med 5:273, 1976

Goldstein DP: Prevention of gestational trophoblastic disease by use of actinomycin D in molar pregnancies. Obstet Gynecol 43:475, 1974

Goldstein DP, Berkowitz RS: *Gestational Trophoblastic Neoplasms.* Philadelphia: WB Saunders Co, 1982

Hammond CB, Borchert LG, Tyrey L, Creasman WT, Parker RT: Treatment of metastatic trophoblastic disease: Good and bad prognosis. Am J Obstet Gynecol 115:451, 1973

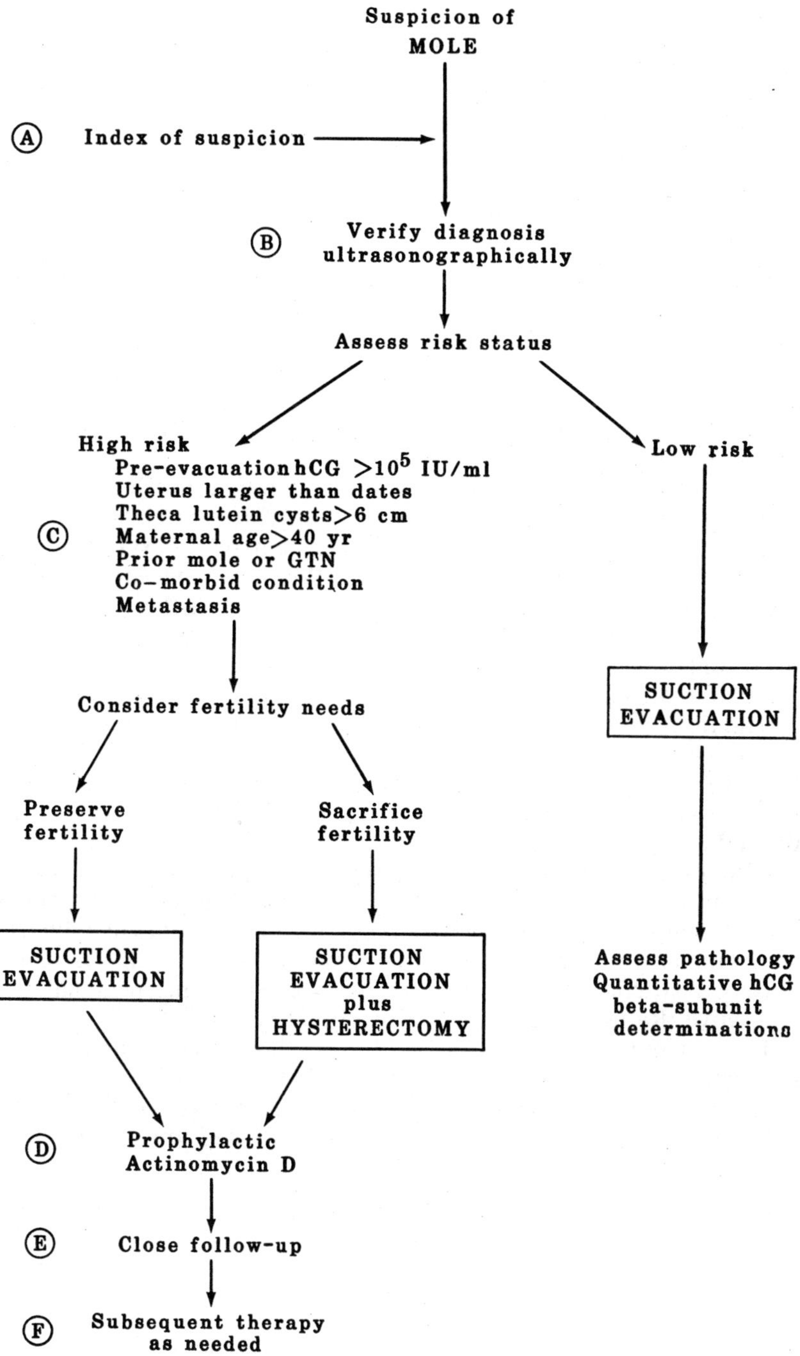
Suspicion of
MOLE
Ⓐ Index of suspicion
Ⓑ Verify diagnosis ultrasonographically
Assess risk status
High risk
Pre-evacuation hCG >10^5 IU/ml
Uterus larger than dates
Theca lutein cysts>6 cm
Ⓒ Maternal age>40 yr
Prior mole or GTN
Co-morbid condition
Metastasis
Low risk
Consider fertility needs
Preserve fertility
Sacrifice fertility
SUCTION EVACUATION
SUCTION EVACUATION plus HYSTERECTOMY
SUCTION EVACUATION
Assess pathology
Quantitative hCG beta-subunit determinations
Ⓓ Prophylactic Actinomycin D
Ⓔ Close follow-up
Ⓕ Subsequent therapy as needed

HYPEREMESIS GRAVIDARUM

Selwyn P. Oskowitz, M.B.

COMMENTS

A. Nausea and vomiting of pregnancy are usually self-limiting, rarely continuing beyond 18 weeks. Fluid and electrolyte disturbances may occur. Serious complications include rupture of esophageal vessels or of the esophagus itself and aspiration pneumonitis.

B. Hyperemesis gravidarum is increasingly seen among patients with ambivalence toward pregnancy, with previous stress-related gastrointestinal disturbances or with immature and dependent personalities. It is not apparently related to parity, illegitimate pregnancy, or overt desire for abortion.

C. Hospitalization is warranted for patients who are dehydrated and have ketoacidosis and electrolyte disturbances. They may show evidence of chronic weight loss and other features of inanition. Other severe manifestations include hyperpyrexia, dental erosion (from chronic oral acidity), peripheral neuropathy, Wernicke's encephalopathy, liver cell necrosis or fatty infiltration, retinal hemorrhages, and even hepatorenal failure, coma, and death.

D. Most patients do well with minor dietary modifications, such as small frequent feedings. They usually tolerate bland, dry foods best.

E. A number of conditions may invoke nausea and vomiting. They encompass a host of intercurrent disease states, including urinary and respiratory tract infections, gastroenteritis, appendicitis, peptic ulcer, intestinal obstruction, hepatitis, cholelithiasis, pancreatitis, yellow atrophy of the liver, diabetic ketoacidosis, uremia, twisted adnexa, ovarian tumor, and even cerebral tumor.

F. Hospital care includes intravenous fluids, glucose, electrolytes and vitamins based on appropriate monitoring of the patient's hydration, ketones, electrolytes, and blood gases. Oral intake is initially restricted. Nasogastric suction and antiemetic agents are given. Gradual increments in oral intake follow. Counseling or psychiatric care may be required. Visitor restriction may have to be imposed where interpersonal relations appear to be causative. Rarely is a therapeutic abortion indicated.

G. Risks of any drugs in pregnancy must be carefully weighed. Doxylamine succinate, meclizine, or prochlorperazine may be considered. Many studies have shown no adverse effects from these drugs in pregnancy, although isolated reports suggest potential fetal danger. Use of these agents should, therefore, be restricted to cases in which they are clearly indicated.

REFERENCES

Fairweather DVI: Nausea and vomiting in pregnancy. Am J Obstet Gynecol 102:135, 1968

Sheehan HL: The pathology of hyperemesis and vomiting of late pregnancy. J Obstet Gynaecol Brit Emp 46:685, 1939

Yerushalmy J, Milkovich L: Evaluation of the teratogenetic effect of meclizine in man. Am J Obstet Gynecol 93:553, 1965

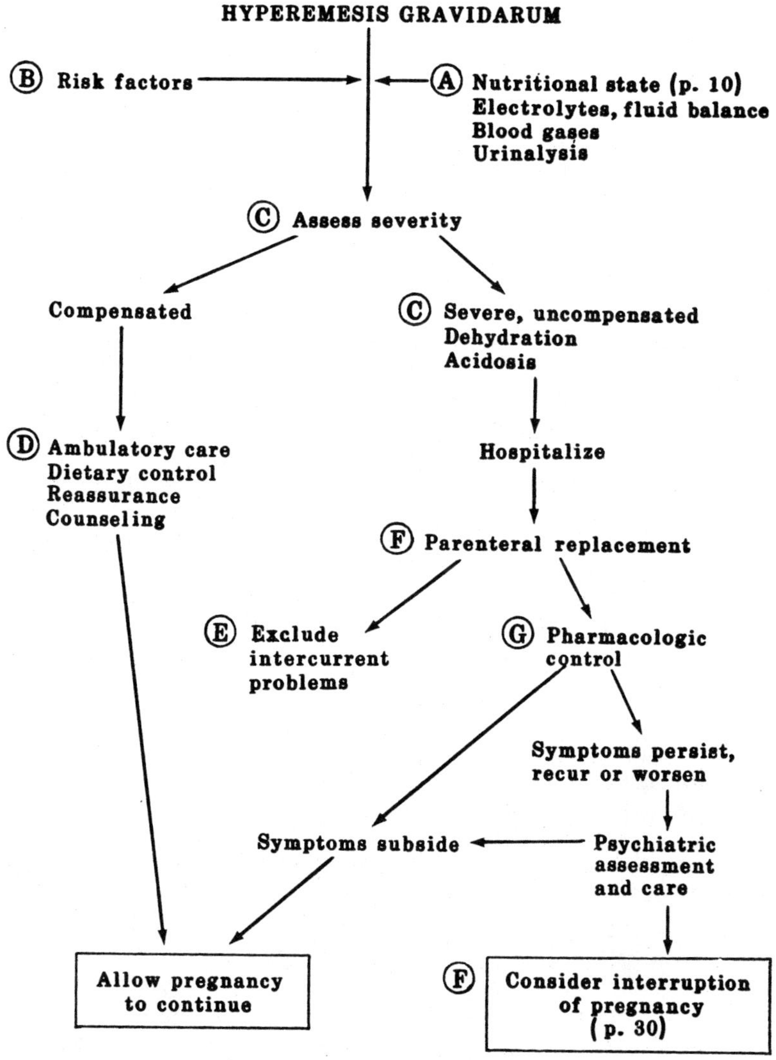
HYPEREMESIS GRAVIDARUM
(B) Risk factors
(A) Nutritional state (p. 10)
Electrolytes, fluid balance
Blood gases
Urinalysis
(C) Assess severity
Compensated
(C) Severe, uncompensated
Dehydration
Acidosis
(D) Ambulatory care
Dietary control
Reassurance
Counseling
Hospitalize
(F) Parenteral replacement
(E) Exclude intercurrent problems
(G) Pharmacologic control
Symptoms persist, recur or worsen
Symptoms subside
Psychiatric assessment and care
Allow pregnancy to continue
(F) Consider interruption of pregnancy (p. 30)

PREGNANCY-INDUCED HYPERTENSION

Emanuel A. Friedman, M.D.

COMMENTS

A. Risk factors include diabetes mellitus, renal disease, and pyelonephritis, as well as a family background of hypertension.

B. Mid-trimester levels of mean arterial blood pressure (MAP = diastolic + 1/3 difference between diastolic and systolic) of 90 mm Hg or more presage PIH. In the third trimester, blood pressure levels exceeding 135/85 should be considered abnormal. The "classic" limit of 140/90 for normal is too high. Increases of 15 mm Hg diastolic or 30 mm Hg systolic serve as comparable signals. Similarly, any proteinuria more than trace warrants attention. Neither salt restriction nor administration of diuretics is of any value in preventing PIH. The same applies to weight control measures.

C. Because PIH can be fulminating with rapid progression over a period of hours to convulsion, coma, and death, hospitalization is essential. Until the patient is stabilized, frequent observations of blood pressure, urinary output, reflexes, retina for vasospasm, condition of sensorium, etc. are required.

D. Cases with severe manifestations include those with systolic blood pressure >160 mm Hg or diastolic >100 mm Hg. Oliguria <30 ml/hr is ominous. Symptoms of an advanced PIH state include hyperreflexia, visual disturbances, epigastric pain, cyanosis, dyspnea, and obtunded sensorium.

E. Progressive hyperreflexia with clonus generally precedes the seizure. Aggressive intervention is mandatory, aimed at stopping the convulsions, maintaining adequate oxygenation, avoiding tracheobronchial aspiration, preventing or treating heart failure, and emptying the uterus as soon as it is safe to do so in the interests of both mother and baby.

F. Magnesium sulfate is the primary treatment of PIH. An initial loading dose of 20 ml 20 percent solution is given very slowly by intravenous push over at least a 3-minute period, testing the knee jerk and watching the respirations. Stop the administration when the deep tendon reflexes diminish. Have calcium gluconate available to counteract the magnesium effect if respirations should stop (a sign of overdose). Supplemental $MgSO_4$ can be given by intravenous drip or by periodic intramuscular injections, titrated according to the return of hyperreflexia. If the intramuscular route is chosen, 10 ml 50% $MgSO_4$ is given deeply into each buttock and followed at 4-hourly intervals with 10 ml 50% $MgSO_4$ in alternating buttocks.

G. The underlying PIH process continues until the pregnancy ends. Because the patient remains at high risk, careful, frequent follow-up is essential, with rehospitalization at the earliest sign.

H. Once the patient's condition is stabilized, one should try to maintain control with $MgSO_4$ and proceed in 12–24 hours to conclude the pregnancy. Even under suboptimal conditions (e.g., unripe cervix), labor induction with carefully titrated oxytocin infusion (see p. 128) may prove unexpectedly successful. Continuous electronic fetal heart rate monitoring is essential. If induction fails, cesarean section can be done for patients with severe PIH. Postpartum observations must continue to detect and manage exacerbations expediently.

REFERENCES

Chesley LC: *Hypertensive Disorders in Pregnancy.* New York: Appleton-Century-Crofts, 1978

Friedman EA, Neff RK: *Pregnancy Hypertension.* Littleton, Mass.: PSG Publishing Co, 1977

Pritchard JA: The use of magnesium sulfate in preeclampsia-eclampsia. J Reprod Med 23:107, 1979

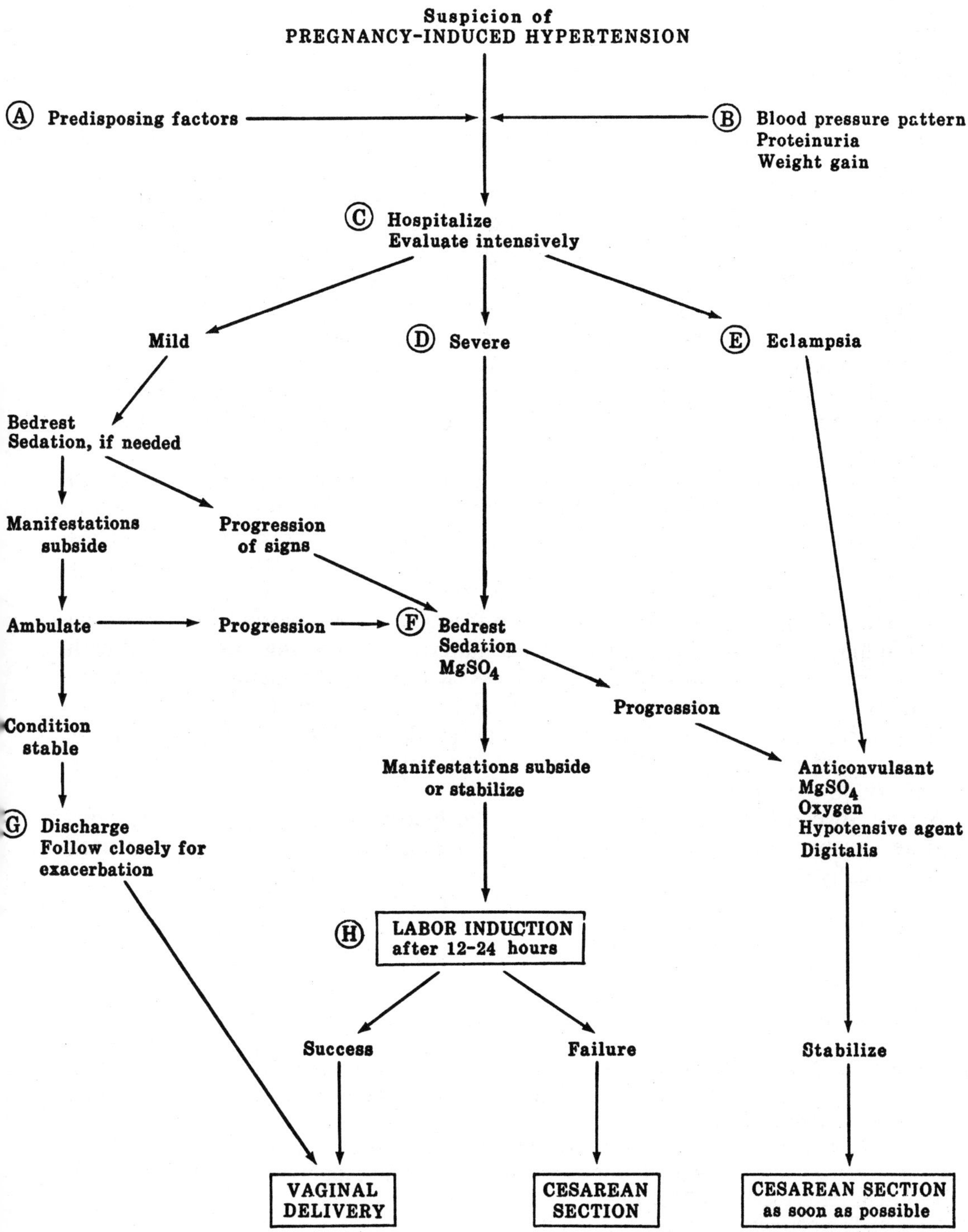
Suspicion of
PREGNANCY-INDUCED HYPERTENSION
(A) Predisposing factors
(B) Blood pressure pattern
Proteinuria
Weight gain
(C) Hospitalize
Evaluate intensively
Mild
(D) Severe
(E) Eclampsia
Bedrest
Sedation, if needed
Manifestations subside
Progression of signs
Ambulate
Progression
(F) Bedrest
Sedation
MgSO4
Progression
Condition stable
Manifestations subside or stabilize
Anticonvulsant
MgSO4
Oxygen
Hypotensive agent
Digitalis
(G) Discharge
Follow closely for exacerbation
(H) LABOR INDUCTION
after 12-24 hours
Success
Failure
Stabilize
VAGINAL DELIVERY
CESAREAN SECTION
CESAREAN SECTION
as soon as possible

PLACENTA PREVIA

Harold Rubin, M.D.

COMMENTS

A. The first episode of bleeding is rarely profuse. However, this does not eliminate the potential catastrophic nature of the problem.
B. Speculum examination is done to rule out local sources of bleeding, such as cervical polyp, cancer, vaginal varix, and so on. It should be done gently and with great care to avoid traumatizing the placental site. No other form of intravaginal examination or manipulation is permissible. Digital vaginal or rectal examinations can cause torrential hemorrhage.
C. Ultrasonography is very useful for confirming the presence of a placenta previa. It is also helpful in assessing fetal size and status.
D. Profuse bleeding is life-threatening to the mother. It may jeopardize the fetus as well, because 10 percent of blood lost is fetal in origin. Therefore, all deliberate speed is imperative.
E. All invasive procedures (except gentle speculum examination) must be done in the operating room with patient fully informed and everything in readiness for immediate surgery. Preparation includes: (1) intravenous lines open, (2) blood immediately available, (3) instruments and scrub nurse ready, (4) assistants scrubbed and gowned, and (5) anesthesia prepared for immediate action.
F. Induction of labor should be undertaken if the cervix is favorable and bleeding is minimal or absent. Constant fetal and maternal monitoring are essential with the operating room and blood in readiness. Rupturing the membranes may aid in tamponading the fetal head against the edge of the placenta.
G. If possible, expectant management is desirable until fetal maturity can be documented by L/S ratio. Amniocentesis for this purpose is always done with ultrasound guidance.
H. As the lower uterine segment develops, the placental site may appear to "migrate" away from the internal os. Therefore, ultrasound should be repeated periodically if bleeding begins early.

REFERENCES

Crenshaw C Jr, Jones DED, Parker RT: Placenta previa: A survey of twenty years experience with improved survival by expectant therapy and cesarean delivery. Obstet Gynecol Survey 28:461, 1973
King DL: Placental migration demonstrated by ultrasonography. Radiol 109:167, 1973
Wexler P, Gottesfeld KR: Second-trimester placenta previa: Apparently normal placentation. Obstet Gynecol 50:706, 1977
Young GB: The peripatetic placenta. Radiol 128:183, 1978

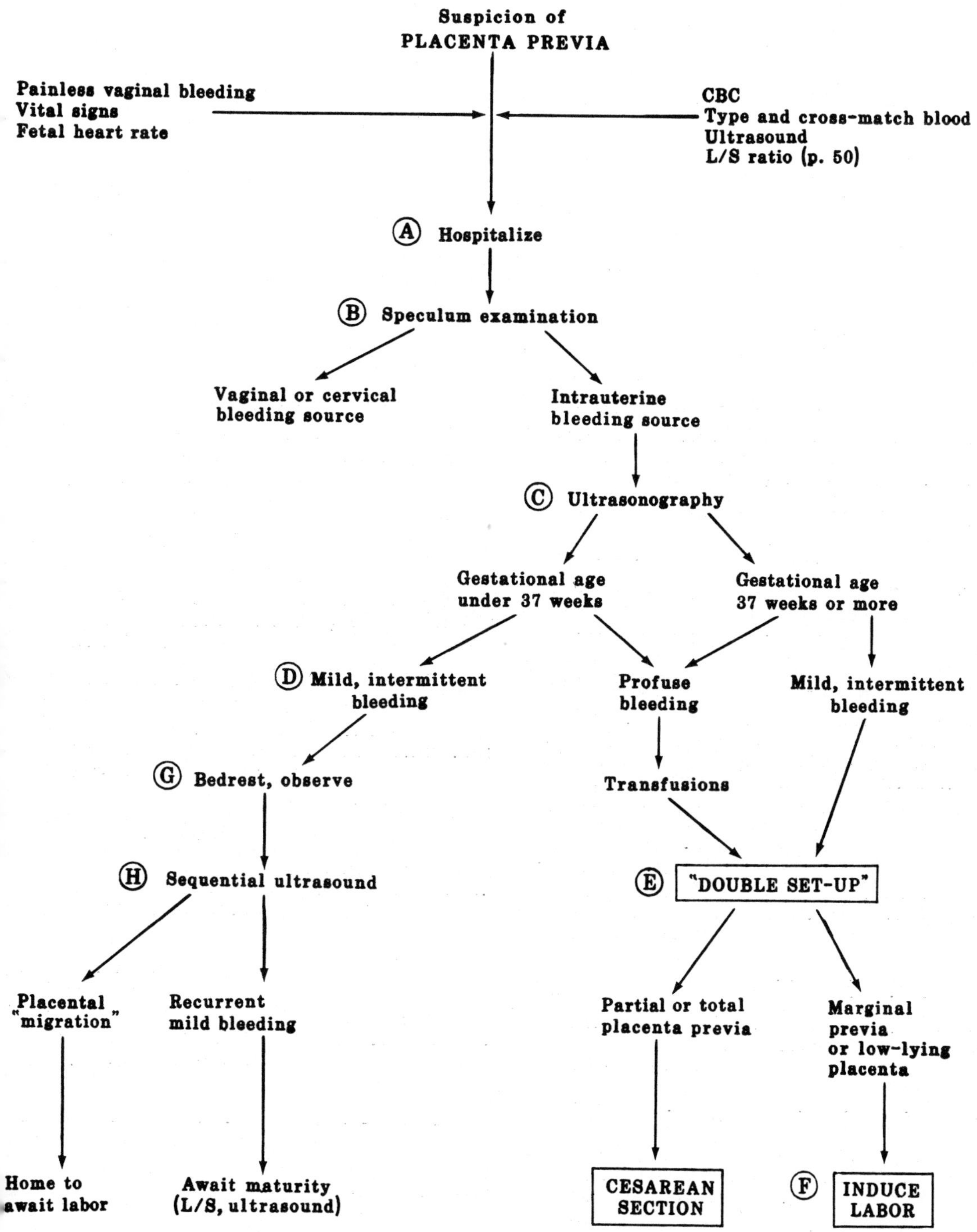
Suspicion of
PLACENTA PREVIA
Painless vaginal bleeding
Vital signs
Fetal heart rate
CBC
Type and cross-match blood
Ultrasound
L/S ratio (p. 50)
(A) Hospitalize
(B) Speculum examination
Vaginal or cervical bleeding source
Intrauterine bleeding source
(C) Ultrasonography
Gestational age under 37 weeks
Gestational age 37 weeks or more
(D) Mild, intermittent bleeding
Profuse bleeding
Mild, intermittent bleeding
(G) Bedrest, observe
Transfusions
(H) Sequential ultrasound
(E) "DOUBLE SET-UP"
Placental "migration"
Recurrent mild bleeding
Partial or total placenta previa
Marginal previa or low-lying placenta
Home to await labor
Await maturity (L/S, ultrasound)
CESAREAN SECTION
(F) INDUCE LABOR

PLACENTA ACCRETA

Harold Rubin, M.D.

COMMENTS

A. This condition represents abnormal adherence of all or part of placenta to the abdominal wall. Definitive diagnosis is made on microscopic examination that reveals complete or partial absence of the decidua basalis. There are three types of placenta accreta: (1) placenta accreta, in which the placenta is adherent to the myometrium; (2) placenta increta, in which the uterine wall is invaded; (3) placenta percreta, in which the uterine wall is invaded to the serosa.

B. Past history of placenta previa, prior cesarean section, uterine malformation, myomectomy, manual removal of the placenta, uterine infection, retained placenta, hemorrhage, and postpartum or postabortal curettage should alert one to the possibility of a placenta accreta.

C. To establish the diagnosis of placenta accreta clinically, manual removal is attempted. In the case of total accreta, no cleavage plane is found; in partial accreta, the cleavage plane is found but removal cannot be completed. The exploration of the uterus is performed in the operating room with anesthetist in attendance, anesthesia being given as needed, blood ready or actually infusing, assistants scrubbed and gowned, and nurses with instruments for abdominal surgery in readiness.

D. Complete (total) placenta accreta is generally asymptomatic. Since there is no separation unless a false plane is artificially made, there is no bleeding.

E. Partial placenta accreta usually presents as a partially separated placenta with acute hemorrhage.

F. Emergency measures are often necessary to maintain cardiovascular integrity, including rapid administration of volume expanders and blood replacement coupled with bilateral internal iliac artery ligation, for example.

G. It has been well established that, once the clinical diagnosis of placenta accreta is made, the best results are obtained when a hysterectomy is performed (about 6.1 percent mortality rate); by contrast, the mortality rate for patients treated conservatively is 4 times as great (25.6 percent).

REFERENCES

Breen JL, Neubecker R, Gregori CA, Franklin JE Jr: Placenta accreta, increta and percreta: Survey of 40 cases. Obstet Gynecol 49:43, 1977

Fox H: Placenta accreta, 1945–1969. Obstet Gynecol Survey 27:475, 1972

Hammond H: Death from obstetrical hemorrhage. Calif Med 117:16, 1972

Weeks LR, Greig LB: Placenta accreta: A twenty year review. Am J Obset Gynecol 113: 76, 1972

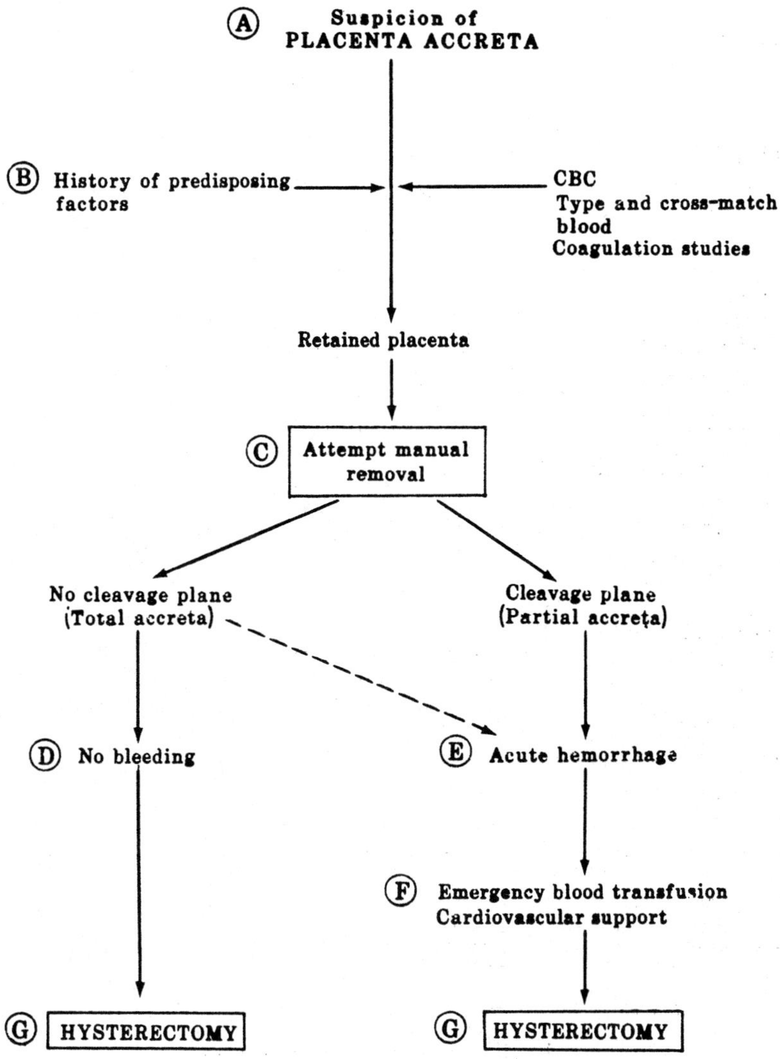
Ⓐ Suspicion of PLACENTA ACCRETA
Ⓑ History of predisposing factors
CBC
Type and cross-match blood
Coagulation studies
Retained placenta
Ⓒ Attempt manual removal
No cleavage plane (Total accreta)
Cleavage plane (Partial accreta)
Ⓓ No bleeding
Ⓔ Acute hemorrhage
Ⓕ Emergency blood transfusion
Cardiovascular support
Ⓖ HYSTERECTOMY
Ⓖ HYSTERECTOMY

ABRUPTIO PLACENTAE

Louis Burke, M.D.

COMMENTS

A. Although the etiologic factors in premature separation of the placenta are unclear, it is associated with high parity, chronic hypertension, pregnancy-induced hypertension, inferior vena caval compression, uterine trauma, short umbilical cord, sudden uterine decompression, uterine anomaly, and (perhaps) folic acid deficiency. Women with previous abruptio placentae may be at increased risk for recurrence. The condition should be considered in a gravida who develops sudden, intense, usually focalized uterine pain with or without vaginal bleeding. Characteristically, the uterus is quite tender, with increased tone, often of a boardlike nature. Occult retroplacental bleeding may produce a shock state out of proportion to the vaginal bleeding. Disseminated intravascular coagulation may develop, especially in the more severe cases. Although the clinical picture is usually clear-cut, ultrasound B-scan study may be able to demonstrate the site of retroplacental hematoma formation.

B. It is useful to divide cases according to clinical severity. In the mild form, placental separation is minimal, involving less than one-sixth of the surface. Bleeding is generally less than 500 ml. The maternal condition remains good, and the fetus demonstrates no evidence of any adverse effect. In general, no intervention is necessary for mild cases, although hospitalization can be foreshortened if definitive care is rendered to those at term (by means of labor induction). Severe abruptio placentae involves separation of more than two-thirds of the placenta accompanied by severe pain, tetanic uterine contractions, and fetal distress or intrauterine death. The maternal condition may be unstable, with hypotension, tachycardia, coagulopathy, and even renal failure. In such cases, intervention is mandatory in the interests of the mother and, if the fetus is alive and sufficiently mature, of the fetus as well. Moderately severe cases show blood loss of 500–1000 ml, uterine irritability, and incipient cardiovascular instability, although fetal distress is not usually present.

C. After placenta previa has been ruled out by "double-setup" examination (p. 60), amniotomy should be done and oxytocin infusion begun. Titrated oxytocin stimulation of labor (p. 30), even under suboptimal cervical conditions, is usually effective in promoting vaginal delivery. The process may be interrupted at any time in favor of cesarean section should there be evidence of deterioration of maternal or fetal condition. In some severe cases, cesarean section may be indicated as the primary approach because of maternal jeopardy, regardless of fetal status.

REFERENCES

Knab DR: Abruptio placentae: An assessment of the time and method of delivery. Obstet Gynecol 52:625, 1978

Notelovitz M, Bottoms SF, Dase DF, Leichter PJ: Painless abruptio placentae. Obstet Gynecol 53: 270, 1979

Sher G: Pathogenesis and management of uterine inertia complicating abruptio placentae with consumption coagulopathy. Am J Obstet Gynecol 129:164, 1977

Sher G: A rational basis for the management of abruptio placentae. J Reprod Med 21:123, 1978

Spirt RA, Kagan EH, Rozanski RM: Abruptio placentae: Sonographic and pathologic correlation. Am J Roentgenol 133:877, 1979

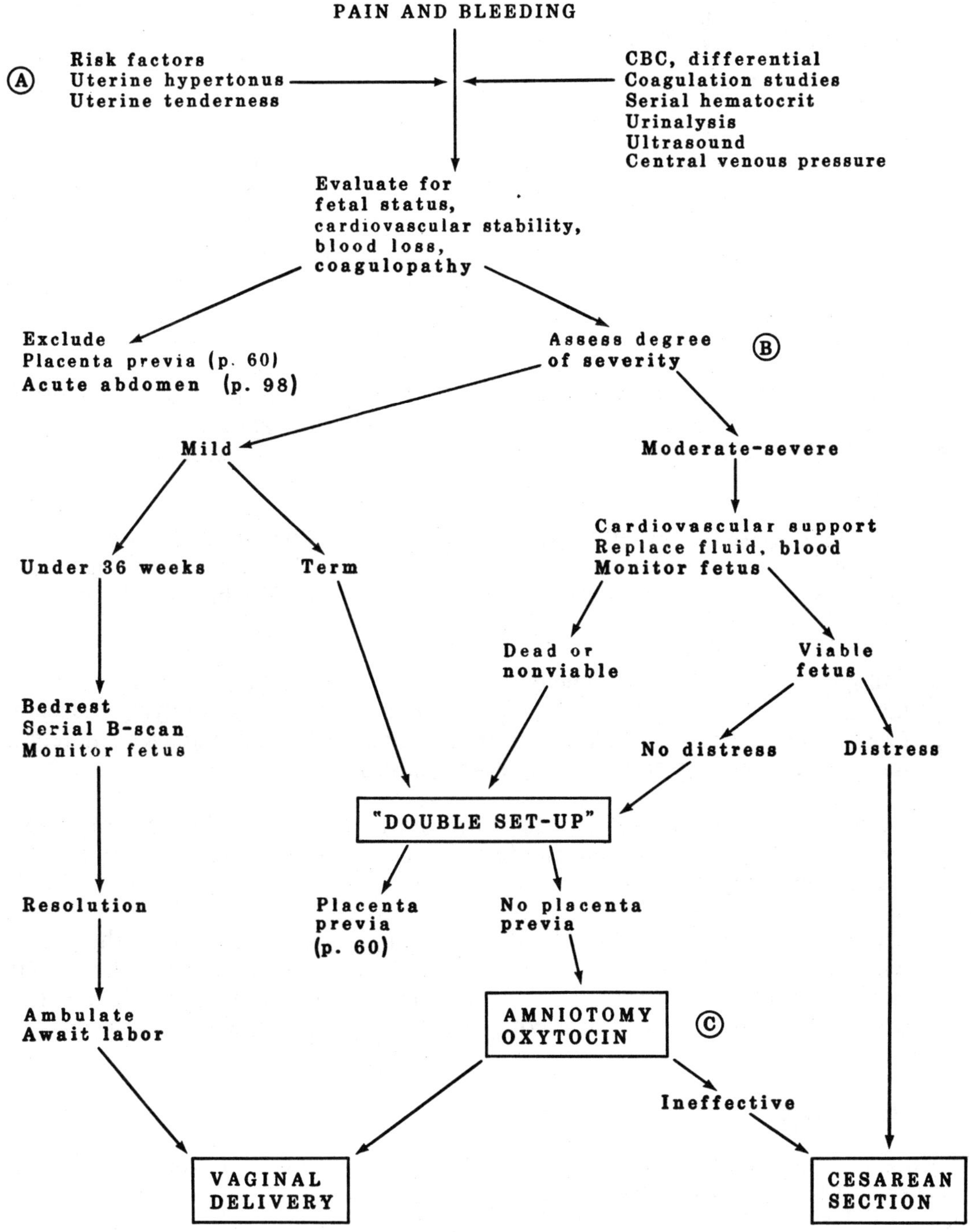
PAIN AND BLEEDING
(A)
Risk factors
Uterine hypertonus
Uterine tenderness
CBC, differential
Coagulation studies
Serial hematocrit
Urinalysis
Ultrasound
Central venous pressure
Evaluate for
fetal status,
cardiovascular stability,
blood loss,
coagulopathy
Exclude
Placenta previa (p. 60)
Acute abdomen (p. 98)
Assess degree
of severity
(B)
Mild
Moderate-severe
Under 36 weeks
Term
Cardiovascular support
Replace fluid, blood
Monitor fetus
Dead or
nonviable
Viable
fetus
Bedrest
Serial B-scan
Monitor fetus
No distress
Distress
"DOUBLE SET-UP"
Resolution
Placenta
previa
(p. 60)
No placenta
previa
Ambulate
Await labor
AMNIOTOMY
OXYTOCIN
(C)
Ineffective
VAGINAL
DELIVERY
CESAREAN
SECTION

VASA PREVIA

Harold Rubin, M.D.

COMMENTS

A. Vasa previa derives from velamentous fetal umbilical vessels that course in front of the presenting part. It is usually associated with a velamentous cord, bilobate placenta, succenturiate lobe, or twins. It occurs once in 2,500–3,000 deliveries.

B. Vaginal bleeding is accompanied by profound changes in fetal heart rate after rupture of membranes. Signs of placenta previa and abruptio placentae are absent. This constellation should create a high index of suspicion for vasa previa.

C. The blood that is lost is 100 percent fetal in origin. The Apt test, based on the resistance of fetal hemoglobin to alkali, distinguishes fetal from maternal hemoglobin. Finding nucleated red blood cells in a Wright-stained smear is helpful.

D. Uterine tenderness, hypertonicity and hypercontractility, plus cardiovascular instability (see Abruptio Placentae) or evidence suggesting forelying placenta (see Placenta Previa) warrant appropriate evaluation and management (e.g., ultrasonography and double set-up examination).

E. Gestational age, fetal size, and fetal life can be determined by ultrasound examination if it is unclear that the fetus is alive and sufficiently mature to survive if delivered.

F. The demonstration that the blood is fetal in origin indicates that the fetus, which cannot withstand an appreciable loss of blood, is in great danger (60 percent fetal mortality rate). Immediate delivery by cesarean section is essential unless vaginal delivery can be accomplished atraumatically almost at once.

REFERENCES

Naftolin F, Mishell DR: Vasa previa: Report of 3 cases. Obstet Gynecol 26:561, 1965

Pallewela CS: Antepartum diagnosis of vasa previa: Report of a case causing sudden foetal death. Postgrad Med J 50:723, 1974

Smith JJ, Benjamin F: Post-hemorrhagic anemia and shock in the newborn at birth: A review and etiologic classification. Obstet Gynecol Survey 23:511, 1968

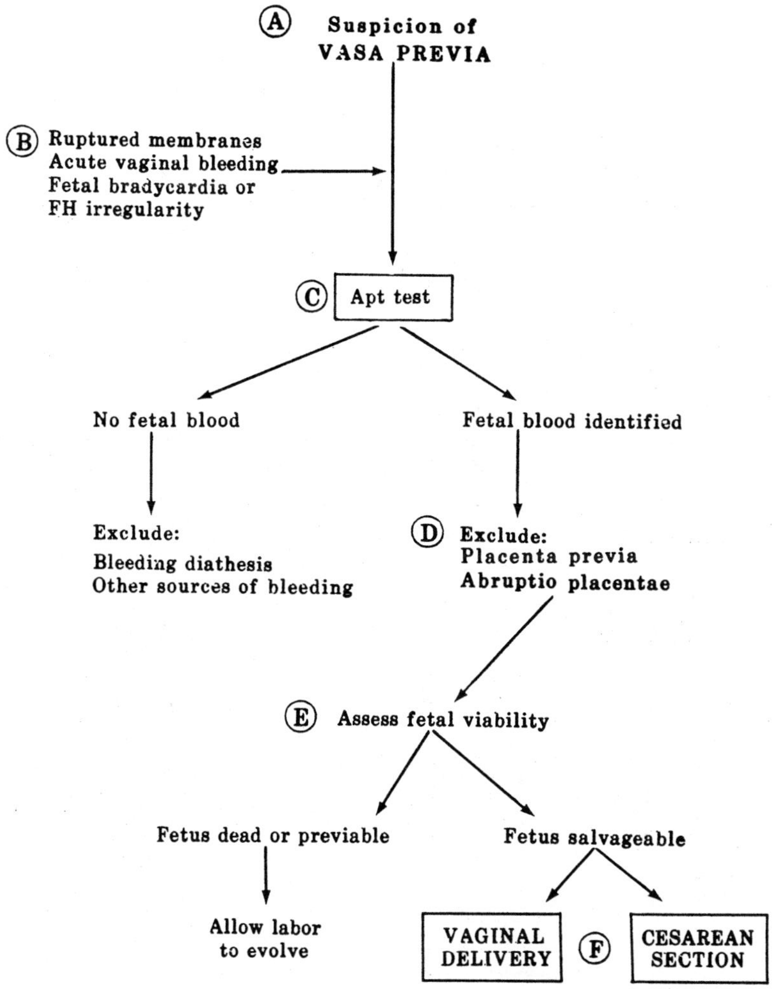
A Suspicion of VASA PREVIA
B Ruptured membranes
Acute vaginal bleeding
Fetal bradycardia or
FH irregularity
C Apt test
No fetal blood
Fetal blood identified
Exclude:
Bleeding diathesis
Other sources of bleeding
D Exclude:
Placenta previa
Abruptio placentae
E Assess fetal viability
Fetus dead or previable
Fetus salvageable
Allow labor
to evolve
VAGINAL DELIVERY
F
CESAREAN SECTION

DIABETES MELLITUS

Henry Klapholz, M.D.

COMMENTS

A. Be alert to history of prior stillbirth, traumatic delivery, infant with congenital anomaly or one weighing over 9 pounds, as well as elevated blood sugar, glycosuria, or recurrent moniliasis.

B. At each visit, evaluate for glycosuria, fetal growth, and hydramnios.

C. Blood sugar level 2 hours after the oral administration of 100 g of glucose is a useful screen. Levels greater than 120 mg percent require glucose tolerance test (GTT).

D. Maximum glucose levels after 100 g glucose intake are:

	Fasting	*1 hour*	*2 hours*	*3 hours*
Whole blood	90	165	145	125
Plasma	110	200	150	130

Any two abnormal values constitute an abnormal GTT. Diagnose class A diabetes if fasting level (FBS) is normal, and at least class B if FBS is abnormal.

E. Class A diabetes needs close observation and dietary control (2000–2200 calorie ADA diet). Patients are seen every 2 weeks. Outcome is usually good. Delivery is undertaken at 40 weeks to avoid post-term pregnancy and macrosomia. Eschew premature induction in these cases.

F. At special risk are those with elevated FBS (class B or worse) or those who develop pregnancy-induced hypertension or hydramnios.

G. Brief hospitalization is needed to evaluate daily blood sugar patterns and provide baseline renal function studies, retinal examination, urinalysis, and urine cultures.

H. Frequent antepartum testing must be done because the fetus may deteriorate very rapidly: urinary estriols 3 times weekly, nonstress and oxytocin challenge tests twice weekly, ultrasound for fetal growth every 3 weeks, and renal function studies monthly.

I. Hospitalize the diabetic patient at 34 weeks. Provide insulin as needed in divided doses to regulate blood sugars to normal levels (FBS 100 mg percent or less), aiming at daylong stability.

J. Amniocentesis at 36 weeks checks lung maturity. For diabetics, L/S ratios of 4.0 or greater should be achieved; better yet, DSPC of at least 800 and preferably 1200 mg percent ensures against neonatal respiratory distress.

K. Deliver as soon as the fetus is fully mature. If the fetus is deteriorating, interrupt earlier. Induction is preferred, but cesarean section may be needed.

L. Regulate blood sugar around 100 mg percent with intravenous insulin (4-hour intervals or continuous infusion at 2–8 U/hr), while giving 5 percent glucose (150 ml/hr). Monitor blood sugars every 4 hours and titrate insulin accordingly.

REFERENCES

Barden TP, Knowles HC: Diagnosis of diabetes in pregnancy. Clin Obstet Gynecol 24:3, 1981

Cohen AW, Gabbe SG: Intrapartum management of the diabetic patient. Clin Perinat 8:165, 1980

Lowensohn RI, Gabbe SG: The value of lecithin/sphingomyelin ratios in diabetes: A critical review. Am J Obstet Gynecol 134:702, 1979

West TE, Lowy C: Control of blood glucose during labour in diabetic women with combined glucose and low-dose insulin infusion. Brit Med J 1:1252, 1977

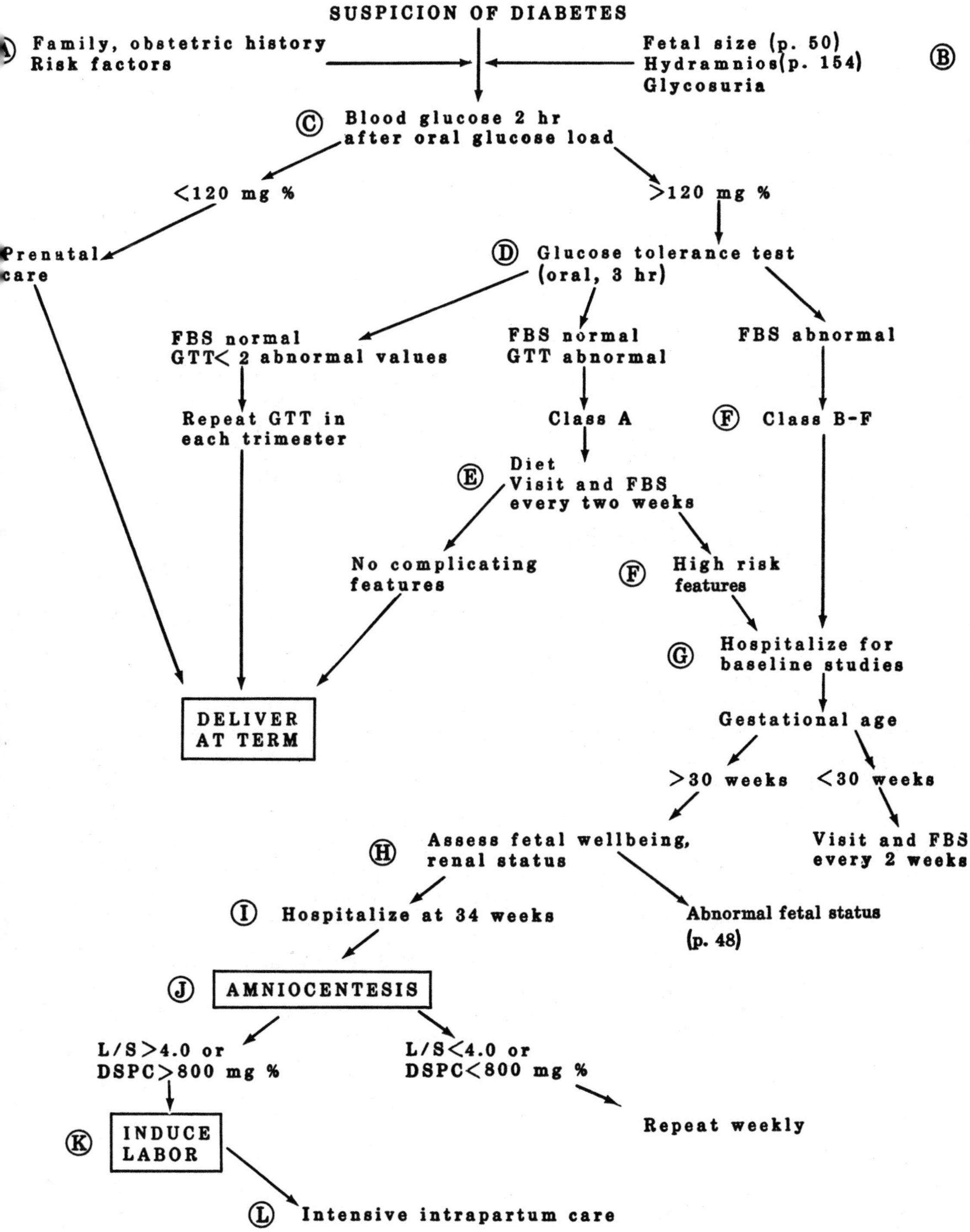
SUSPICION OF DIABETES
Ⓐ Family, obstetric history
Risk factors
Fetal size (p. 50)
Hydramnios(p. 154)
Glycosuria
Ⓑ
Ⓒ Blood glucose 2 hr
after oral glucose load
<120 mg %
>120 mg %
Prenatal
care
Ⓓ Glucose tolerance test
(oral, 3 hr)
FBS normal
GTT< 2 abnormal values
FBS normal
GTT abnormal
FBS abnormal
Repeat GTT in
each trimester
Class A
Ⓕ Class B-F
Diet
Ⓔ Visit and FBS
every two weeks
No complicating
features
Ⓕ High risk
features
Ⓖ Hospitalize for
baseline studies
DELIVER
AT TERM
Gestational age
>30 weeks
<30 weeks
Ⓗ Assess fetal wellbeing,
renal status
Visit and FBS
every 2 weeks
Ⓘ Hospitalize at 34 weeks
Abnormal fetal status
(p. 48)
Ⓙ AMNIOCENTESIS
L/S>4.0 or
DSPC>800 mg %
L/S<4.0 or
DSPC<800 mg %
Repeat weekly
Ⓚ INDUCE
LABOR
Ⓛ Intensive intrapartum care

CHRONIC HYPERTENSIVE DISEASE

Henry Klapholz, M.D.

COMMENTS

A. Be alert to family history of hypertension, labile hypertension early in childhood, renal disease, hematuria, frequent urinary tract infections, and childhood nephritis. Characteristic symptoms include recurrent headaches and nosebleeds. It is essential that women at risk be identified as early in pregnancy as possible.

B. Thorough baseline evaluation should be done when the patient is first seen. Complete renal evaluation (except for x-ray studies) includes microscopic urinalysis and examination of 24-hour urine collection for protein, catecholamine, and VMA, plus blood urea nitrogen, uric acid, electrolytes, and creatinine clearance. Renal ultrasound may also help. Examine the abdomen to detect renal artery bruits associated with arterial stenosis. Bear in mind that the normal values in pregnancy are influenced by increased glomerular filtration rate. Examine the retina to assess for hemorrhages, exudates, and vascular changes.

C. Treatment of patients with blood pressures less than 170/110 does not improve fetal outcome. Higher blood pressures, however, yield poor fetal results and may cause a cerebrovascular event, particularly if there is an area of vascular compromise, such as arteriovenous malformation or aneurysm. The risk of sudden placental abruption mandates treatment of such patients.

D. Avoid the use of thiazides in pregnancy, because severe fetal and maternal electrolyte imbalance may result. Hemorrhagic pancreatitis is a further risk. Propranolol has been shown to be an effective hypotensive agent with little apparent risk. Alpha-methyldopa and hydralazine are acceptable alternatives. None of these agents will prevent superimposed pregnancy-induced hypertension (PIH).

E. Since these patients are at fivefold risk of developing superimposed PIH, they have to be followed closely. They should be seen at least at 2-week intervals until 36 weeks and then weekly or more often until term. Be alert for failing cardiac and renal reserve. Repeat renal function studies at intervals of no more than two months, including creatinine clearance, blood urea nitrogen, and full urinalysis.

F. Begin testing fetal status at 30 weeks. Deterioration (2 or more abnormal test results) calls for delivery. A single suspicious test of fetal status warrants amniocentesis and evaluation of fetal maturity. Deliver a fetus documented to be mature. If the dates are well documented, hypertensive women should not be permitted to go beyond term. If in doubt, amniocentesis is done to evaluate fetal pulmonary maturity.

REFERENCES

Bear RA: Pregnancy in patients with renal disease: A study of 44 cases. Obstet Gynecol 48:13, 1976

De Alvarez RR: Preeclampsia-eclampsia and renal disease in pregnancy. Clin Obstet Gynecol 21:881, 1978

Leppert P, Tisher CC, Cheng SC, Harlan WR: Antecedent renal disease and the outcome of pregnancy. Ann Intern Med 90:747, 1979

Pruyn SC, Phelan JP, Buchanan GC: Long-term propranolol therapy in pregnancy: Maternal and fetal outcome. Am J Obstet Gynecol 135:485, 1979

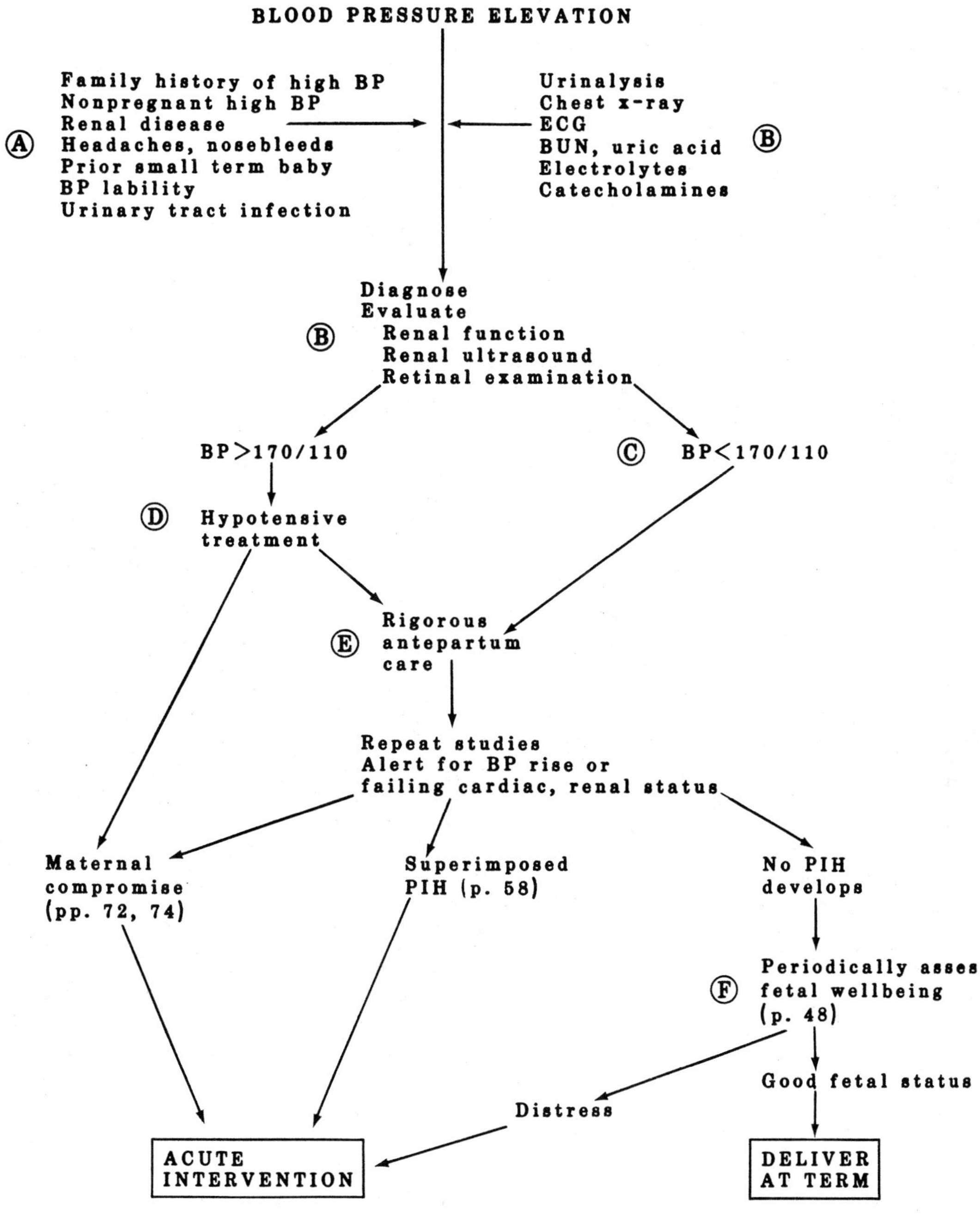
BLOOD PRESSURE ELEVATION
Ⓐ
Family history of high BP
Nonpregnant high BP
Renal disease
Headaches, nosebleeds
Prior small term baby
BP lability
Urinary tract infection
Ⓑ
Urinalysis
Chest x-ray
ECG
BUN, uric acid
Electrolytes
Catecholamines
Diagnose
Evaluate
Ⓑ
Renal function
Renal ultrasound
Retinal examination
BP>170/110
Ⓒ BP<170/110
Ⓓ Hypotensive treatment
Rigorous
Ⓔ antepartum
care
Repeat studies
Alert for BP rise or
failing cardiac, renal status
Maternal compromise (pp. 72, 74)
Superimposed PIH (p. 58)
No PIH develops
Periodically assess
Ⓕ fetal wellbeing
(p. 48)
Good fetal status
Distress
ACUTE INTERVENTION
DELIVER AT TERM

RENAL DISEASE

Balmookoot Balgobin, M.D.

COMMENTS

A. Renal disease should be suspected if symptoms are referable to the urinary tract of if there is a history of urinary tract disorders, diabetes, gout, hyperparathyroidism, heart failure, or collagen disease. Persistent bacteriuria (p. 118) is important also.

B. One should survey renal function bearing in mind that pregnancy normally increases renal blood flow and glomerular filtration. Blood urea nitrogen levels are quite low; concentrations considered normal in the nonpregnant state may reflect azotemia in pregnancy. Creatinine clearance is especially valuable. Urinary concentration or dye excretion is often unreliable. Uric acid may be falsely elevated after diuretic agents. Baseline studies should include serum electrolytes, blood urea nitrogen, serum creatinine and uric acid, as well as creatinine clearance. With heavy proteinuria, obtain 24-hour urinary protein, serum protein, and cholesterol tests.

C. Evidence of impaired or failing renal function is alarming. It signifies that the pregnancy is having an adverse effect on the mother. Interrupting the pregnancy may be in the best interest of the gravida, especially if her renal decompensation is progressive.

D. If possible, the specific underlying condition should be diagnosed, provided the diagnostic tests do not jeopardize fetus or mother. Unless strongly indicated, x-ray studies and renal biopsy are best avoided. Intravenous pyelography is not done without clear indication (although a single-film exposure may be acceptable). Past history, previous investigations, and course of disease state may help. General guidelines for care pertain to specific conditions. Acute glomerulonephritis can be expected to resolve if managed medically; consider interruption of the pregnancy only if there is no improvement after two weeks of treatment. Diabetic nephropathy demands strict control of the diabetes, recognizing the added risk to both mother and fetus. Renal calculi are treated expectantly with intervention reserved for unremitting ureteral obstruction. Such patients should be screened for hyperparathyroidism, gout, and cystinuria.

E. Optimal timing of the delivery depends on maternal and/or fetal risk. If the mother is in peril, one can justify interrupting the pregnancy at any gestational age. If the fetus shows evidence of compromise, however, interruption can be rationalized only if the infant is mature enough to survive.

REFERENCES

Davison JM, Lindheimer MD: Renal disease in pregnant women. Clin Obstet Gynecol 21:411, 1978

Knapp MS, Burden R: The recognition and management of renal failure in pregnancy. Clin Obstet Gynecol 4:717, 1977

Leppert P, Tisher CC, Cheng SCS, Harlan WR: Antecedent renal disease and the outcome of pregnancy. Ann Int Med 90:747, 1979

Strong DW, Murchison RJ, Lynch DF: Management of ureteral calculi during pregnancy. Surg Gynecol Obstet 146:604, 1978

Zachur HA, Mitch WE: Renal disease in pregnancy. Med Clin Am 61:89, 1977

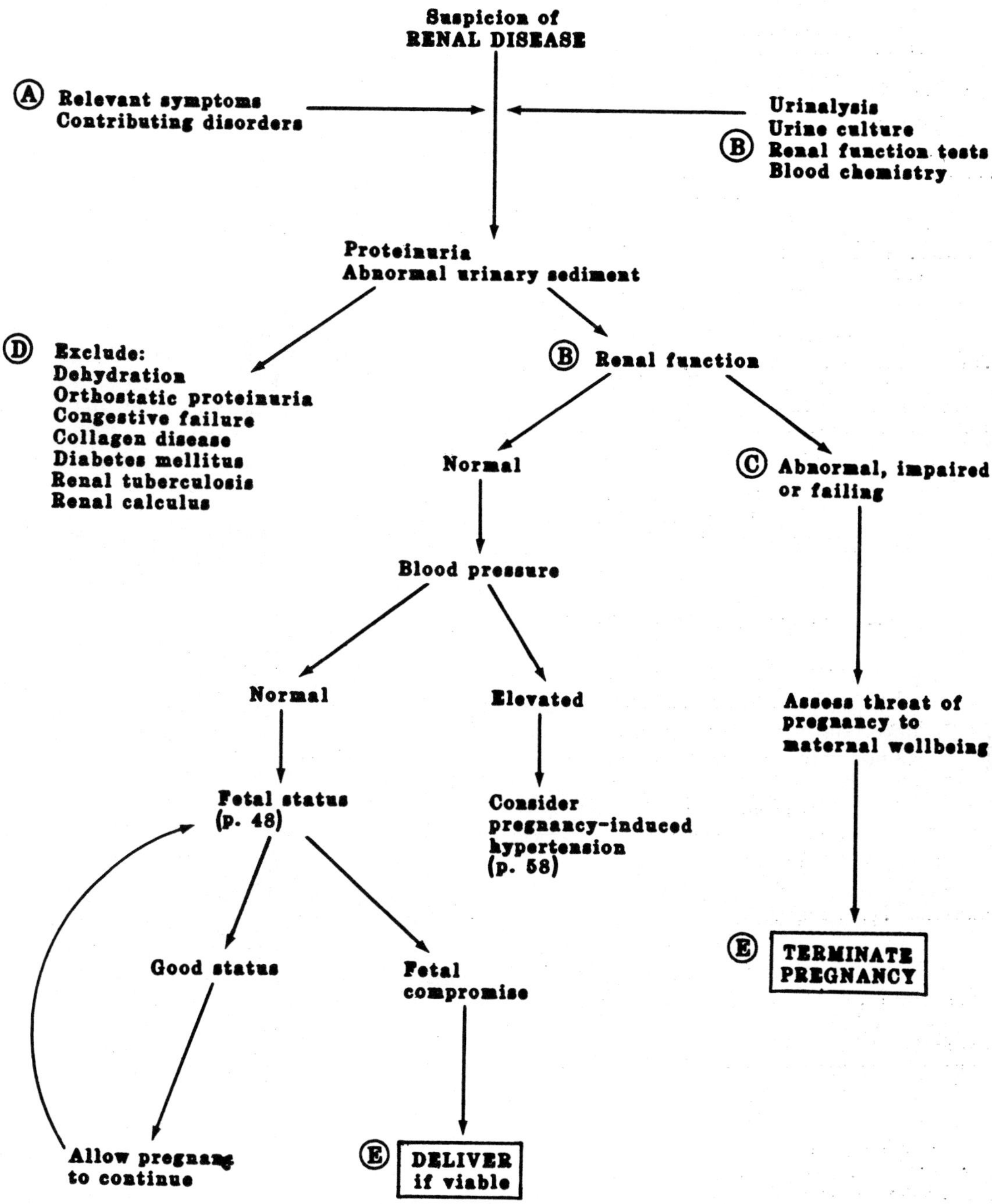
Suspicion of
RENAL DISEASE
(A) Relevant symptoms
Contributing disorders
Urinalysis
Urine culture
(B) Renal function tests
Blood chemistry
Proteinuria
Abnormal urinary sediment
(D) Exclude:
Dehydration
Orthostatic proteinuria
Congestive failure
Collagen disease
Diabetes mellitus
Renal tuberculosis
Renal calculus
(B) Renal function
Normal
(C) Abnormal, impaired
or failing
Blood pressure
Normal
Elevated
Assess threat of
pregnancy to
maternal wellbeing
Fetal status
(p. 48)
Consider
pregnancy-induced
hypertension
(p. 58)
Good status
Fetal
compromise
(E) TERMINATE
PREGNANCY
Allow pregnancy
to continue
(E) DELIVER
if viable

HEART DISEASE IN PREGNANCY

Henry Klapholz, M.D.

COMMENTS

A. Be alert for exertion-induced dyspnea, cyanosis, chest pain, palpitations, arrhythmia, and a background of rheumatic fever, limitation of activities, or heart murmur. Many pregnant women have widely split S_1 heart sounds, a third sound, and a systolic murmur at the left sternal border. Diagnose early and classify on a functional basis with special attention to marked limitation of activity.

B. Include periodic blood gas determinations, especially if cyanosis or dyspnea is present. Obtain chest x-rays at intervals for heart size and pulmonary edema. Serial chest auscultation will detect progressive left-sided failure; right-sided failure is reflected in pitting pretibial edema. Weigh the patient frequently. Electrocardiograms detect rhythm disturbances; normal cardiac displacement results from the enlarging uterus. Cardiac catheterization is not required except in the cyanotic patient; echocardiography is safe and may be useful.

C. Assess fetal growth and development, especially in cyanotic heart disease. Increasing cardiac failure diminishes placental perfusion. If there is significant fetal jeopardy, delivery should be pursued unless the fetus is previable.

D. Physical activity is reduced and daily rest enforced. Sodium intake is restricted to 2–4 g per day. Digitalis is given for congestive failure; diuretics may be required for failure unresponsive to rest alone. Give oxygen by controlled Venturi mask for cyanotic patients; it is especially indicated for pulmonary hypertension. Consider cardiac surgery for unresponsive critically ill patients, but this is rarely required. Limit weight gain to 15 pounds to minimize cardiac work load.

E. If fetal or maternal deterioration is evident, consider elective oxytocin induction. It has the advantage of orderly mobilization of specialists. Candidates should be easily inducible based on high Bishop scores.

F. Vaginal delivery under regional block anesthesia ensures circulatory stability better than cesarean section. Aim to relieve pain, avoid Valsalva maneuver, maintain stable blood volume by careful fluid administration and hemostasis, and deliver by elective low forceps. Balanced general anesthesia is used in cases of pulmonary congestion to control alveolar ventilation.

G. The critical postdelivery period requires that blood pressure be maintained and care taken to avoid blood loss from uterine atony or acute congestive failure from fluid overload. After successful delivery and recovery, attention should be given to appropriate counseling. A child born to parents with heart disease is at increased risk of heart disease.

REFERENCES

Conradsson TB, Werko L: Management of heart disease in pregnancy. Progr Cardiovasc Dis 16:407, 1974

Rowland TW: The pediatrician and congenital heart disease: 1979. Pediat 64:180, 1979

Szekely P, Julian DG: Heart disease and pregnancy. Curr Probl Cardiol 4:1, 1979

Ueland K: Intrapartum management of the cardiac patient. Clin Perinat 8:155, 1980

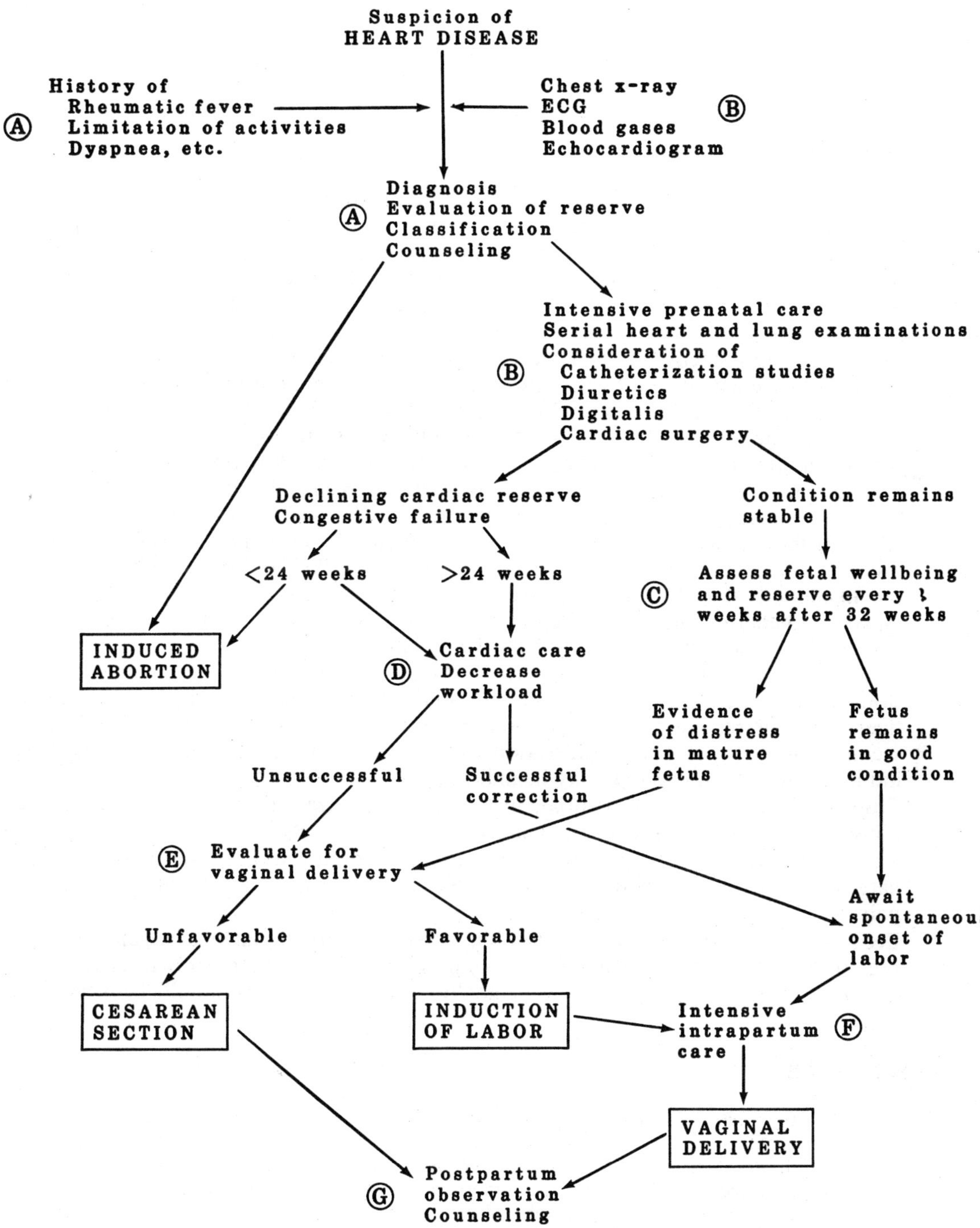
Suspicion of
HEART DISEASE
History of
Rheumatic fever
Limitation of activities
Dyspnea, etc.
Ⓐ
Chest x-ray
ECG
Blood gases
Echocardiogram
Ⓑ
Diagnosis
Evaluation of reserve
Classification
Counseling
Ⓐ
Intensive prenatal care
Serial heart and lung examinations
Consideration of
Catheterization studies
Diuretics
Digitalis
Cardiac surgery
Ⓑ
Declining cardiac reserve
Congestive failure
Condition remains stable
<24 weeks
>24 weeks
Assess fetal wellbeing and reserve every ½ weeks after 32 weeks
Ⓒ
INDUCED ABORTION
Cardiac care
Decrease workload
Ⓓ
Evidence of distress in mature fetus
Fetus remains in good condition
Unsuccessful
Successful correction
Evaluate for vaginal delivery
Ⓔ
Await spontaneous onset of labor
Unfavorable
Favorable
CESAREAN SECTION
INDUCTION OF LABOR
Intensive intrapartum care
Ⓕ
VAGINAL DELIVERY
Postpartum observation
Counseling
Ⓖ

SICKLE CELL DISEASE

Balmookoot Balgobin, M.D.

COMMENTS

A. Episodic crises, recurrent infection, and refractory or hemolytic anemia suggest the diagnosis. Both mother and fetus are at serious risk.

B. Positive sickle cell preparation test is useful for screening, but definitive diagnosis rests with hemoglobin electrophoresis. If the father also has sickle cell disease or trait, the infant is more likely to be affected. Prenatal diagnosis is possible in some centers by studying fetal erythrocytes or amniocytes obtained by fetoscopy.

C. Infection, severe anemia, and sickle cell crises pose a constant threat to mother and fetus. They are aggravated by the stress of pregnancy. Spontaneous abortion and stillbirth account for the 50 percent fetal loss. Intrauterine growth retardation and placental insufficiency are common. The patient can be offered the options of abortion or of continuing the pregnancy under rigorous prenatal care and close fetal surveillance.

D. Evaluate at least every 2 weeks. Give folic acid supplements with iron, if indicated. Screen periodically for infection, including urine for bacteriuria; if found, treat aggressively. If the hematocrit falls below 25 percent or the proportion of red cells that sickle exceeds 60 percent, give exchange transfusion with packed red blood cells to reduce the likelihood of crises and improve fetal salvage. There are transfusion hazards, especially hepatitis and late alloimmunization. Hospitalize the patient for severe anemia or an acute crisis, and prophylactically late in pregnancy.

E. Sickle cell crisis is a serious complication. Manage aggressively with exchange transfusion, intravenous fluids, oxygen, and sedation; treat acidosis, infections, and congestive heart failure; anticoagulate for pulmonary emboli. Acute crises in the first or second trimester warrant consideration of induced abortion; in the third trimester, induction or cesarean section may be indicated.

F. Close fetal surveillance is essential, including serial ultrasound, urinary estriols, and nonstress tests, as well as oxytocin challenge tests, if indicated.

G. Vaginal delivery is preferred, if feasible. Patients should be kept warm, well oxygenated, and not oversedated. Anesthesia consultation is useful to ensure appropriate pain relief while minimizing risk.

H. Because most of the infant's hemoglobin is fetal, hemolytic anemia is generally not present at birth. Hypoxia will cause sickling in an affected infant only after the fetal hemoglobin has been replaced by hemoglobin-S. Such infants should be kept well oxygenated.

REFERENCES

Carache S, Scott J, Niebyl J, Bonds D: Management of sickle cell disease in pregnant patients. Obstet Gynecol 55:407, 1980

Cunningham FG, Pritchard JA: Prophylactic transfusion of normal red blood cells during pregnancies complicated by sickle cell hemoglobinopathies. Am J Obstet Gynecol 135:994, 1979

Miller JM, Horger EO, Key TC Jr, Walker EM Jr: Management of sickle hemoglobinopathies in pregnant patients. Am J Obstet Gynecol 141:237, 1981

Morrison JC, Schneider JM, Whybrew WD, Bucovaz ET, Menzel DM: Prophylactic transfusion in pregnant patients with sickle hemoglobinopathies: Benefit versus risk. Obstet Gynecol 56:274, 1980

Philips JA, Kazazian HH, Bochm CD, Scott AF, Panny SR, Smith KD: Prenatal diagnosis of sickle cell anemia: Value of linked y-globin polymorphisms. Pediatr Res 14:526, 1980

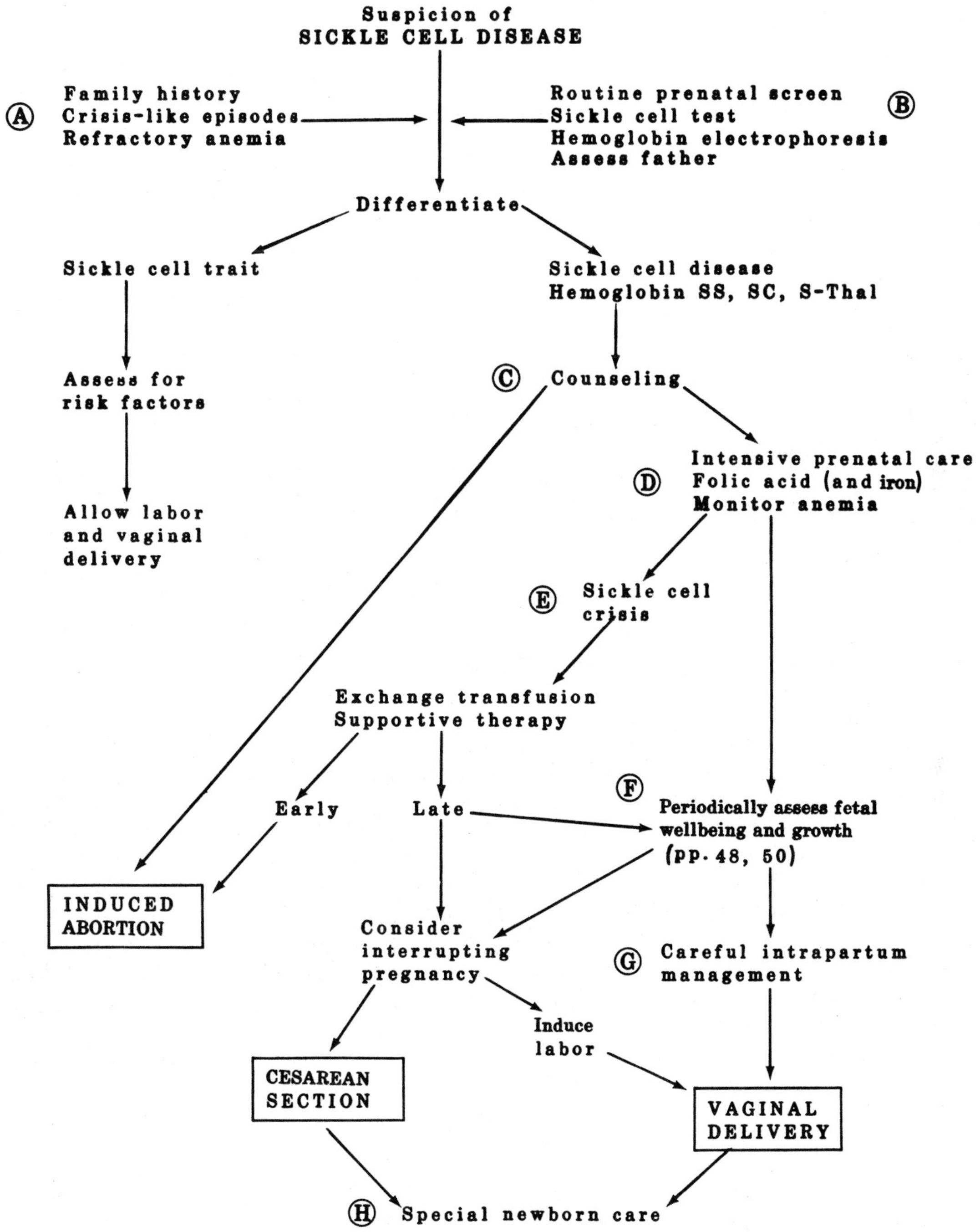
Suspicion of
SICKLE CELL DISEASE
(A)
Family history
Crisis-like episodes
Refractory anemia
Routine prenatal screen
Sickle cell test
Hemoglobin electrophoresis
Assess father
(B)
Differentiate
Sickle cell trait
Sickle cell disease
Hemoglobin SS, SC, S-Thal
Assess for
risk factors
Allow labor
and vaginal
delivery
(C)
Counseling
Intensive prenatal care
(D)
Folic acid (and iron)
Monitor anemia
(E)
Sickle cell
crisis
Exchange transfusion
Supportive therapy
Early
Late
(F)
Periodically assess fetal
wellbeing and growth
(pp. 48, 50)
INDUCED
ABORTION
Consider
interrupting
pregnancy
(G)
Careful intrapartum
management
Induce
labor
CESAREAN
SECTION
VAGINAL
DELIVERY
(H)
Special newborn care

THROMBOCYTOPENIC PURPURA

Balmookoot Balgobin, M.D.

COMMENTS

A. Autoimmune thrombocytopenic purpura (ATP) results from destruction of platelets by circulating IgG antibodies that attach themselves to platelet antigens. IgG may cross the placenta to cause fetal thrombocytopenia. Patients with ATP may be asymptomatic or suffer from easy bruising, petechiae, or mucosal bleeding.

B. Evaluation includes relevant laboratory studies to uncover thrombocytopenia (<100,000 per ml), increased capillary fragility, poor clot retraction, and increased (or normal) bleeding time.

C. Give prednisone (60–100 mg daily in divided doses) for bleeding or severe thrombocytopenia (platelets <50,000 per ml) to correct abnormal capillary fragility and increase the platelet count. Reduce it to the lowest dose needed to maintain hemostasis and the platelet count. Maternal prednisone may protect the fetus somewhat. To minimize the risk of fetal bleeding during labor and delivery, give 10–20 mg prednisone daily for 10–14 days before delivery.

D. Splenectomy is indicated if bleeding continues, but it should be avoided in pregnancy, if possible, because of the high associated maternal (9–10 percent) and fetal (25–30 percent) mortality rates.

E. If all else fails, platelet transfusion is given. If the mother's life is threatened, immunosuppressant therapy may be tried (e.g., cyclophosphamide, vincristine, or azathioprine), but they carry great fetal risk.

F. Fetal thrombocytopenia subjects the fetus to hemorrhagic complications during the course of labor, especially intracerebral bleeding. If the fetus is at risk, therefore, cesarean section is in order. This applies for the splenectomy patient with persistent IgG antibodies that may adversely affect the fetus. Assess the fetal platelet count by means of scalp blood sampling in labor. If the fetal platelet count is above 50,000 per ml, labor and vaginal delivery can be permitted. Supplementary intravenous steroids are indicated during labor and at delivery for patients who have previously been receiving them. Platelet transfusion may be necessary for hemostasis.

G. Thrombocytopenia in the newborn infant is self limiting, platelets returning to normal in 3–4 weeks. Lowest counts occur about the sixth day. Daily counts should be obtained during the first week of life. If petechiae or purpura develop, steroid therapy is given. Reduce dosage to the lowest amount to maintain the desired effect and continue for 3 weeks. Active bleeding requires platelet transfusion and exchange transfusion. Splenectomy is contraindicated.

REFERENCES

Carloss HW, McMillan R, Crosby WH: Management of pregnancy in women with immune thrombocytopenic purpura. JAMA 244:2756, 1980

Karpatkin M, Porges RF, Karpatkin S: Platelet counts in infants of women with autoimmune thrombocytopenia: Effect of steroid administration to the mother. New Engl J Med 305:937, 1981

Keleman E, Szalay F, Petefy M: Autoimmune (idiopathic) thrombocytopenic purpura in pregnancy and the newborn. Brit J Obstet Gynaecol 85:239, 1978

Scott JR, Cruikshank DP, Kochenour NK, Pitkin RM, Warenski JC: Fetal platelet counts in the obstetric management of immunologic thrombocytopenic purpura. Am J Obstet Gynecol 136: 495, 1980

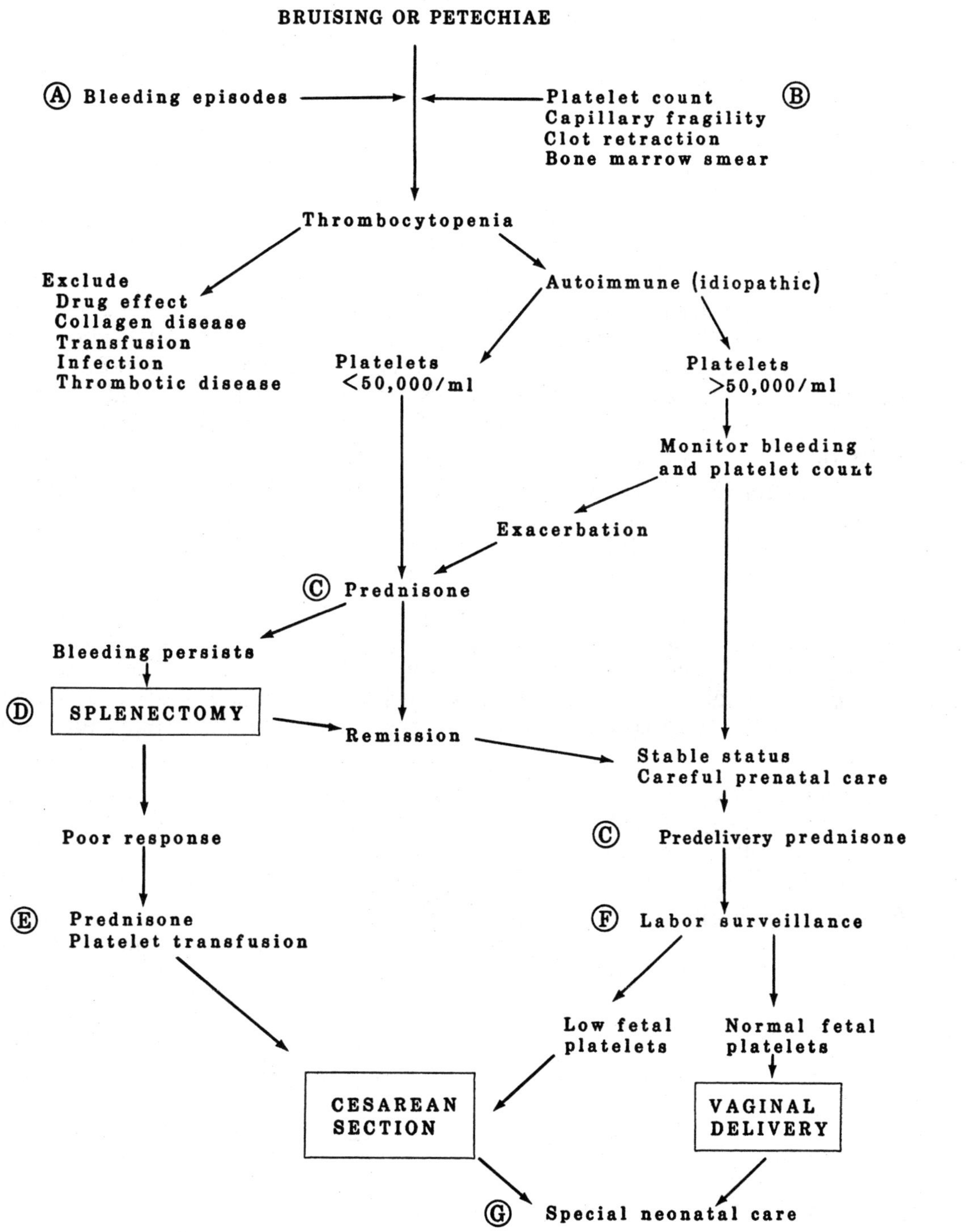
BRUISING OR PETECHIAE
(A) Bleeding episodes
Platelet count
Capillary fragility
Clot retraction
Bone marrow smear (B)
Thrombocytopenia
Exclude
Drug effect
Collagen disease
Transfusion
Infection
Thrombotic disease
Autoimmune (idiopathic)
Platelets
<50,000/ml
Platelets
>50,000/ml
Monitor bleeding
and platelet count
Exacerbation
(C) Prednisone
Bleeding persists
(D) SPLENECTOMY
Remission
Stable status
Careful prenatal care
Poor response
(C) Predelivery prednisone
(E) Prednisone
Platelet transfusion
(F) Labor surveillance
Low fetal
platelets
Normal fetal
platelets
CESAREAN
SECTION
VAGINAL
DELIVERY
(G) Special neonatal care

HEREDITARY HEMORRHAGIC DISORDERS

Balmookoot Balgobin, M.D.

COMMENTS

A. Any unusual bleeding or family history of a bleeding disorder requires careful investigation. Clotting and prothrombin times may be normal; partial thromboplastin time is a more sensitive indicator. Specific assays of coagulation factors should be done even if these tests are normal.

B. Von Willebrand's disease is manifested by easy bruising and bleeding, epistaxis, gastrointestinal bleeding, and menorrhagia. Reduced factor VIII activity and factor VIII-related antigen occurs with prolonged bleeding time, positive tourniquet test, and decreased platelet adhesiveness. Most cases are mild. Offspring are variably affected but seldom seriously unless the parents are homozygous.

C. Both hemophilia A (factor VIII deficiency) and hemophilia B (Christmas disease, factor IX deficiency) are sex-linked disorders. Male fetuses are most likely to manifest the disease. The carrier state for hemophilia A shows reduced ratio of factor VIII to factor VIII-related antigen (ratio of 1:2), but no comparable indicator exists for carriers of hemophilia B.

D. Males affected by hemophilia suffer life-threatening bleeding with resulting soft tissue and joint damage. Amniocentesis for chromosome analysis will identify fetal gender. A male fetus has a 50 percent chance of being affected. Carrier gravidas may elect to terminate such pregnancies. The newly developing technique of fetoscopy may identify the unaffected male fetus and avert abortion.

E. Serial factor assays should be done every 1–2 months. If persistently below 50 percent activity, consider transfusion of fresh frozen plasma or cryoprecipitate prior to surgery or if bleeding occurs. Note that cryoprecipitate lacks factor IX. Avoid aspirin because it interferes with platelet function.

F. Daily monitoring of coagulation factors is necessary after delivery. Maintain factor assays over 50 percent by transfusion, if necessary. The infant should be screened for evidence of disease.

REFERENCES

Bennett B, Ratnoff OD: Detection of the carrier state for classic hemophilia. New Engl J Med 288:342, 1973

Mibashan RS, Thumpston JK, Singer JD, Rodeck CH, Edwards RJ, White JM, Campbell S: Plasma assay of fetal factors VIIC and IX for prenatal diagnosis of hemophilia. Lancet 1:1309, 1979

Noller KL, Bowie W, Kempers RD, Owen CA: Von Willebrand's disease in pregnancy. Obstet Gynecol 41:865, 1973

Zimmerman TS, Ratnoff OD, Powell AE: Immunologic differentiation of classic hemophilia (factor VIII deficiency) and von Willebrand's disease. J Clin Invest 50:244, 1971

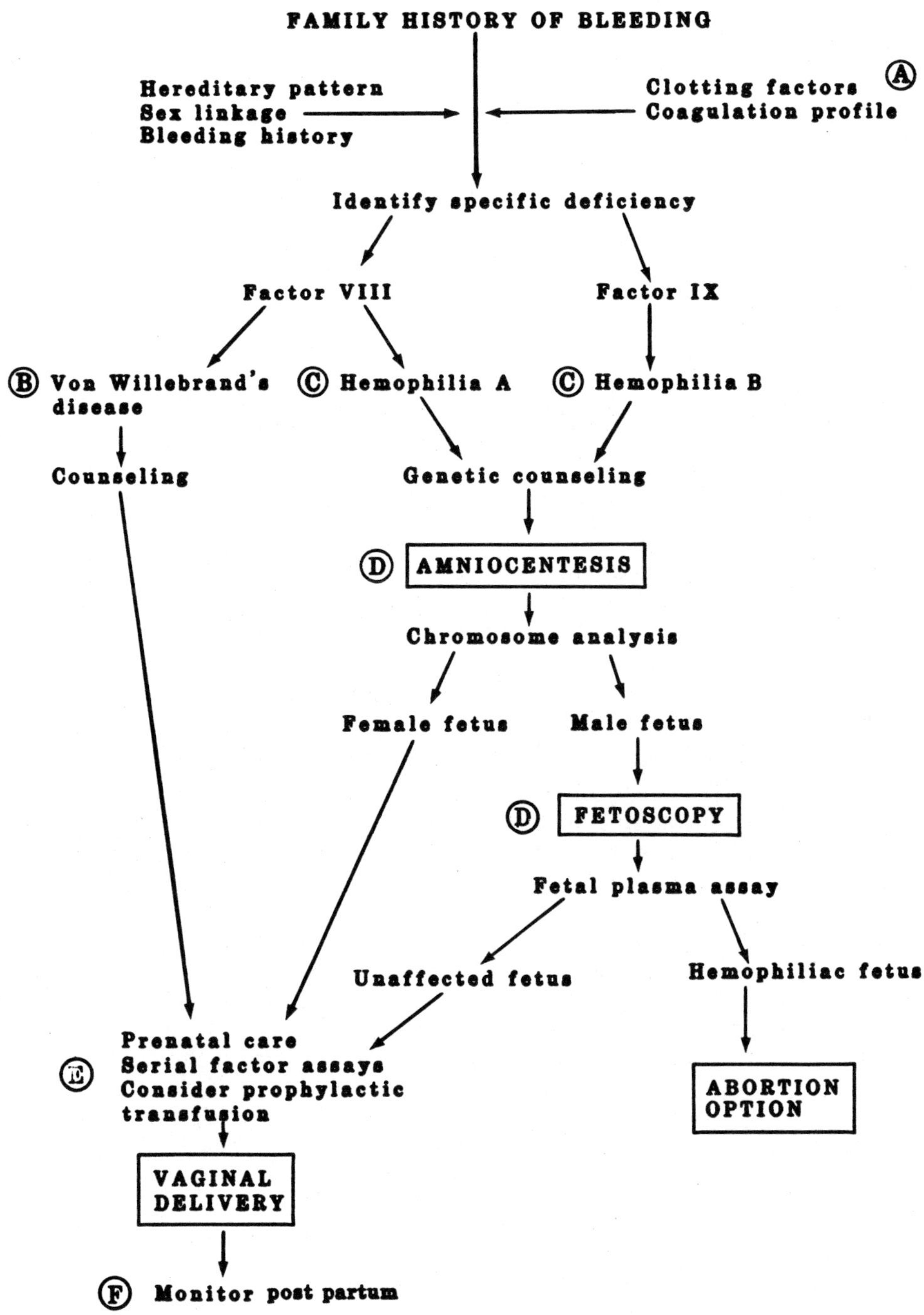
FAMILY HISTORY OF BLEEDING
Hereditary pattern
Sex linkage
Bleeding history
Clotting factors
Coagulation profile
A
Identify specific deficiency
Factor VIII
Factor IX
B Von Willebrand's disease
C Hemophilia A
C Hemophilia B
Counseling
Genetic counseling
D AMNIOCENTESIS
Chromosome analysis
Female fetus
Male fetus
D FETOSCOPY
Fetal plasma assay
Unaffected fetus
Hemophiliac fetus
E Prenatal care
Serial factor assays
Consider prophylactic transfusion
ABORTION OPTION
VAGINAL DELIVERY
F Monitor post partum

ANEMIA

Balmookoot Balgobin, M.D.

COMMENTS

A. Screening is done at the first visit, at 28–32, and at 36–38 weeks; it should include hemoglobin, hematocrit, red cell count, blood cell indices, and differential white count. Routine sickle cell preparation is useful in black women. Urinalysis will help reveal infection. If the serum is icteric, evaluate for liver disease and hemolytic anemia.

B. Iron and folic acid prophylaxis are warranted in all obstetric patients because of hemodilution and increased nutritional demands. Gravidas with hematocrit below 30 percent (or hemoglobin below 10 g percent) should be evaluated, along with those who are refractory to treatment. Search for noncompliance with recommended treatment, poor diet, vomiting, malabsorption, bleeding, chronic disease, and drug effect.

C. Study the peripheral blood smear, serum iron, total iron-binding capacity, percentage of iron saturation, serum and erythrocyte folate, and serum B_{12} levels. Red cell indices may be useful.

D. Iron deficiency anemia is common in pregnancy. Microcytosis precedes hypochromia. Clinical manifestations are rare. Typically, mean corpuscular volume (MCV) is <80, mean corpuscular hemoglobin concentration (MCHC) <30 percent, serum iron <50, and iron saturation less than 15 percent.

E. Folic acid deficiency is less common. Pancytopenia may be intense. The red cells are macrocytic; megaloblasts are seen in buffy coat smears of peripheral blood. MCV is >100, serum folate <3 ng percent, red cell folate <150 mg percent. Smears show more than 3 percent hypersegmented neutrophils.

F. Infection is a common cause of hypochromic microcytic anemia with low serum iron and total iron-binding capacity. Unless infection is identified and treated, the anemia will not respond to hematinic therapy.

G. Iron deficiency anemia is treated with good diet and oral iron (ferrous sulfate 300 mg 3 times daily), combined with prophylactic oral folic acid 1 mg daily. Response can be followed by reticulocyte count and peripheral blood smear. Intravenous or intramuscular iron has no real advantage except in patients with vomiting, intolerance to oral iron, or malabsorption syndromes. Folic acid deficiency is treated with oral folic acid 1–5 mg daily. Iron is given concurrently. Vitamin B_{12} deficiency should be ruled out first by assessing serum B_{12} levels even though such deficiency is rare; specific treatment consists of B_{12} injections. If blood transfusion is indicated, packed red blood cells are used; avoid cardiac failure by careful surveillance or exchange transfusion.

REFERENCES

McFee J: Anemia in pregnancy: A reappraisal. Obstet Gynecol Survey 28:11, 1973

Pritchard JA, Scott DE, Whalley PJ: Maternal folate deficiency and pregnancy wastage: IV. Effects of folic acid supplements, anticonvulsants and oral contraceptives. Am J Obstet Gynecol 110: 375, 1971

Wallerstein RO: Iron metabolism and iron deficiency during pregnancy. Clin Haematol 2:453, 1973

Willoughby MLN: Hematological disorders. Clin Obstet Gynecol 4:2, 1977

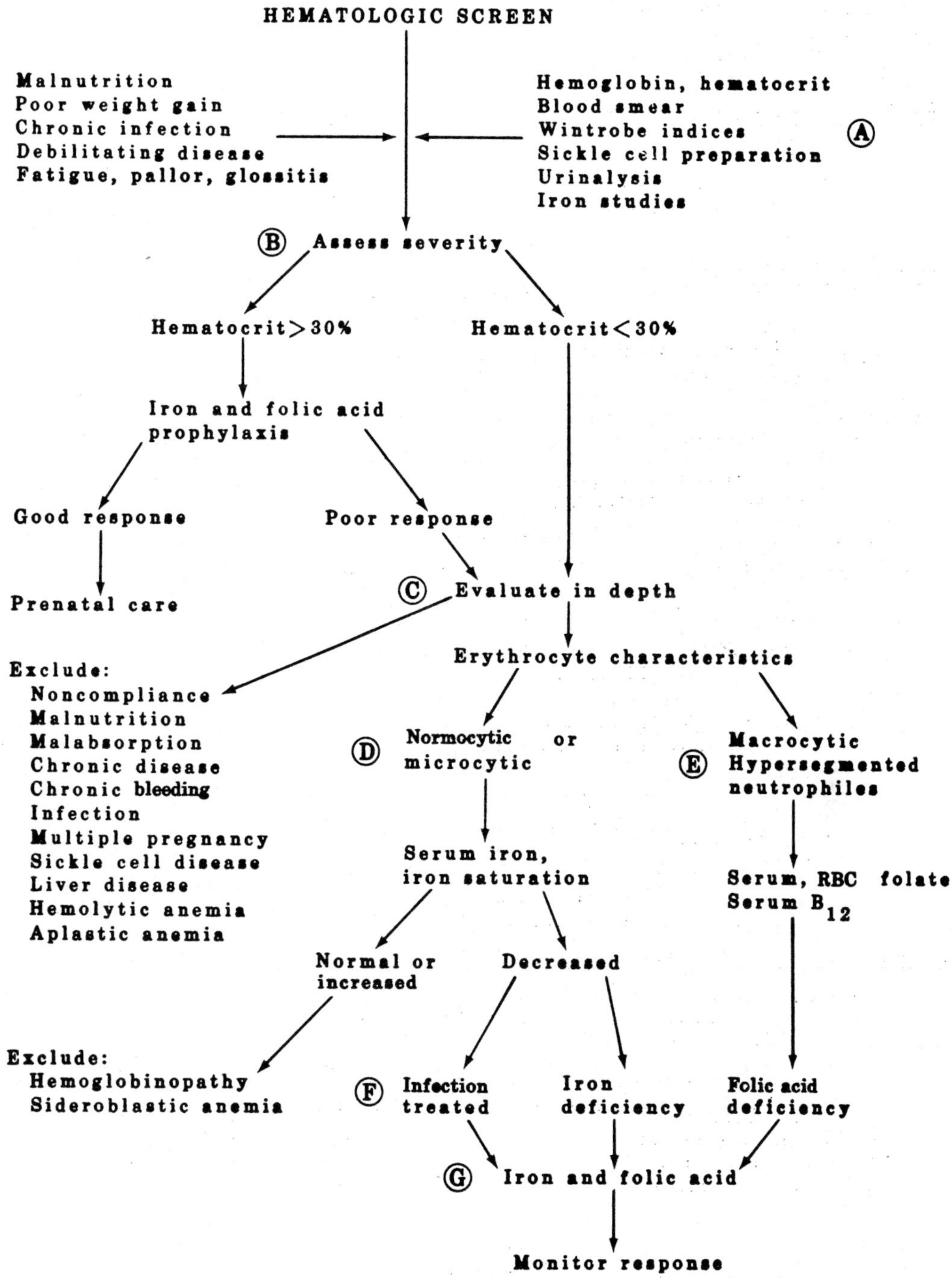
HEMATOLOGIC SCREEN
Malnutrition
Poor weight gain
Chronic infection
Debilitating disease
Fatigue, pallor, glossitis
Hemoglobin, hematocrit
Blood smear
Wintrobe indices
Sickle cell preparation
Urinalysis
Iron studies
A
B
Assess severity
Hematocrit > 30%
Hematocrit < 30%
Iron and folic acid prophylaxis
Good response
Poor response
Prenatal care
C
Evaluate in depth
Exclude:
Noncompliance
Malnutrition
Malabsorption
Chronic disease
Chronic bleeding
Infection
Multiple pregnancy
Sickle cell disease
Liver disease
Hemolytic anemia
Aplastic anemia
Erythrocyte characteristics
D
Normocytic or microcytic
E
Macrocytic
Hypersegmented neutrophiles
Serum iron, iron saturation
Serum, RBC folate
Serum B12
Normal or increased
Decreased
Exclude:
Hemoglobinopathy
Sideroblastic anemia
F
Infection treated
Iron deficiency
Folic acid deficiency
G
Iron and folic acid
Monitor response

COAGULOPATHY

Balmookoot Balgobin, M.D.

COMMENTS

A. Coagulopathy rarely develops spontaneously in pregnancy; more often it is associated with some apparent predisposing condition, such as prolonged retention of a dead fetus (p. 38), abruptio placentae (p. 64), septic abortion (p. 26), induced mid-trimester abortion with hypertonic saline (p. 30), or pregnancy-induced hypertension (p. 58). Survivors of catastrophic amniotic fluid embolism (p. 92) may also develop coagulopathy.

B. Observation of clot formation, retraction, and dissolution offers useful information concerning fibrinogen, platelets, and fibrin degradation products (the last reflecting fibrinolysis). Fibrinogen level, prothrombin time, and partial thromboplastin time are useful, along with peripheral blood smear and platelet count. Specific coagulation factors may be studied as well.

C. With retained dead fetus, consumption coagulopathy may develop slowly. This is reflected well in advance of clinical symptoms by falling fibrinogen levels.

D. Although heparin therapy is controversial, it may block the coagulation process in the patient with prolonged retention of a dead fetus, especially in the absence of any overt bleeding. Coagulation factors and platelet counts will improve spontaneously once the process has been arrested. After correction, steps can be taken to empty the uterus. One must avoid trauma and pay meticulous attention to hemostasis.

E. The patient with acute bleeding resulting from disseminated intravascular coagulation must be monitored carefully. Blood volume and tissue perfusion are maintained by replacing large volumes of blood and fluids while observing for congestive heart failure. The mainstay of therapy is to correct the underlying condition; if this cannot be done expeditiously, one may try to correct hypofibrinogenemia temporarily by giving fibrinogen (bearing in mind the risk of serum hepatitis). Fibrinogen (or fresh frozen plasma) may be useful to provide hemostasis for patients with coagulopathy who require surgery (e.g., cesarean section). Specific therapy for most pregnancy-related coagulopathies consists of uterine evacuation. Once the source of the underlying problem is corrected (by uterine evacuation or control of sepsis), the accelerated coagulation mechanism ceases. With intact liver function coagulation factors are synthesized rapidly, normal function resumes, and bleeding stops. In fulminant cases, when all other measures fail, continued fresh blood replacement in large volumes and surgical hemostasis (such as internal iliac ligations) may be in order.

REFERENCES

Hamilton PJ, Stalker AL, Douglas AS: Disseminated intravascular coagulation: A review. J Clin Pathol 31:609, 1978

Pritchard JA: Haematological problems associated with delivery, placental abruption, retained dead fetus and amniotic fluid embolism. Clin Haematol 2:563, 1973

Pritchard JA, Cunningham FG, Mason RA: Coagulation changes in eclampsia: Their frequency and pathogenesis. Am J Obstet Gynecol 124:855, 1976

Sharp AA: Diagnosis and management of disseminated intravascular coagulation. Brit Med Bull 33: 265, 1977

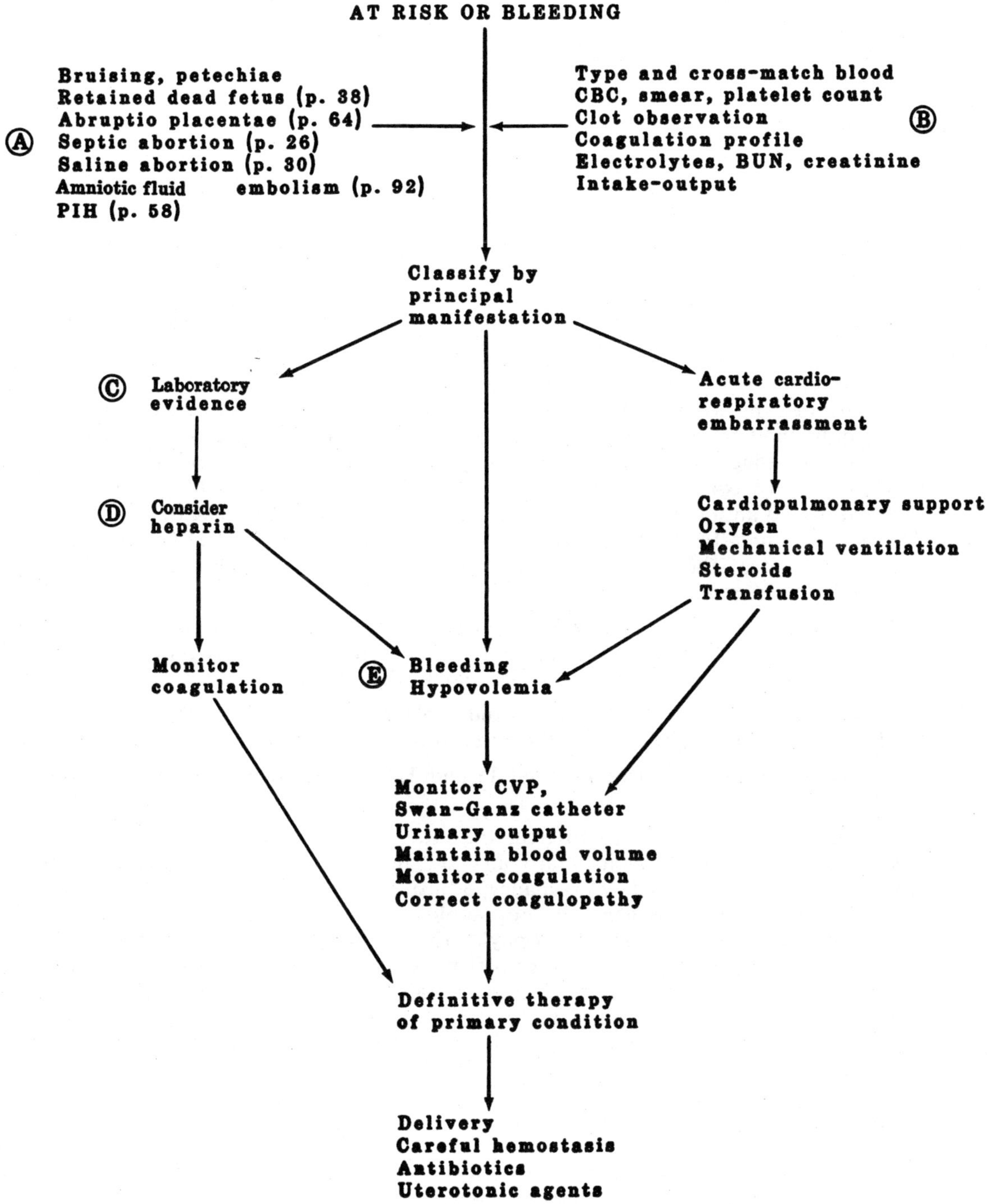
AT RISK OR BLEEDING
Ⓐ
Bruising, petechiae
Retained dead fetus (p. 38)
Abruptio placentae (p. 64)
Septic abortion (p. 26)
Saline abortion (p. 30)
Amniotic fluid embolism (p. 92)
PIH (p. 58)
Ⓑ
Type and cross-match blood
CBC, smear, platelet count
Clot observation
Coagulation profile
Electrolytes, BUN, creatinine
Intake-output
Classify by principal manifestation
Ⓒ Laboratory evidence
Ⓓ Consider heparin
Monitor coagulation
Acute cardio-respiratory embarrassment
Cardiopulmonary support
Oxygen
Mechanical ventilation
Steroids
Transfusion
Ⓔ Bleeding
Hypovolemia
Monitor CVP,
Swan-Ganz catheter
Urinary output
Maintain blood volume
Monitor coagulation
Correct coagulopathy
Definitive therapy of primary condition
Delivery
Careful hemostasis
Antibiotics
Uterotonic agents

THYROID DISORDER

Machelle M. Seibel, M.D.

COMMENTS

A. Pregnancy may obscure or mimic characteristic symptoms. Be alert for history of thyroid surgery or recurrent prematurity or fetal wastage.

B. Physical signs of pregnancy may resemble those of thyroid dysfunction, including thyroid bruit, fine tremor, widened pulse pressure, cardiac arrhythmias, and pretibial myxedema. More typical of thyroid disease are ocular signs (stare, lid lag, exophthalmos), onycholysis (separation of the distal nail from its bed), and profound hip and shoulder girdle myopathy.

C. Some laboratory tests are not useful because they cannot be interpreted in pregnancy. Basal metabolism normally rises to abnormal levels. Because radioiodine is readily taken up by the fetal thyroid from about 12–14 weeks, it cannot be used for diagnosis or treatment. Diagnosis is made with free thyroxine (T_4), total T_4 and T_3, T_3 resin uptake, and thyroxine-binding globulin (TBG). Thyroid-stimulating hormone (TSH) and antithyroid antibodies may also be useful. Pregnancy affects some of these tests: TBG rises; T_3 and T_4 levels increase, but they are mostly bound to TBG; T_3 uptake falls as a result of the excess unsaturated TBG binding sites. Biologically available free T_4, however, remains normal.

D. In hypothyroidism, free T_4 is diminished. A low T_3 uptake with a normal or low normal T_4 is indicative of hypothyroidism. Primary hypothyroidism is reflected in an elevated TSH level. Antithyroid antibodies may be demonstrable.

E. Treat primary hypothyroidism with thyroid replacement, adjusting dosage by serial TSH, T_3 uptake, and T_4 to about 150 mcg Synthroid daily.

F. Hyperthyroidism increases free T_4, total T_3 and T_4, and TBG, but T_3 uptake is typically normal.

G. Propylthiouracil (PTU) is used to treat the gravida with hyperthyroidism. Use the lowest possible dosage to avoid fetal goiter and hypothyroidism. Pre-existing thyrotoxicosis may be ameliorated by pregnancy; adjust therapy accordingly. Avoid iodides, especially for long-term usage. Give propranolol, if needed, with caution, because it can produce uterine tetany and a "floppy" baby. Serial T_3, T_4, and T_3 uptake help adjust treatment. Surgery is reserved for patients who are resistant or allergic to drugs. Life-threatening thyroid storm, often precipitated by labor or cesarean section, demands endocrinologic consultation for treatment with PTU, cortisol, fluids, and hypothermia, as well as propranolol and iodides, if indicated. Watch the newborn infant for signs of thyroid dysfunction.

REFERENCES

Cheron RG, Kaplan MM, Larsen PR, Selenkow HA, Crigler JF: Neonatal thyroid function after propylthiouracil therapy for maternal Graves' disease. New Engl J Med 304:525, 1981

Levy CA, Waite JH, Dickey R: Thyrotoxicosis and pregnancy: Use of preoperative propranolol for thyroidectomy. Am J Surg 133:319, 1977

Mestman JH: Management of thyroid disease in pregnancy. Clin Perinatol 7:371, 1980

Montoro M, Collea JV, Frasier SD, Mestman JH: Successful outcome of pregnancy in women with hypothyroidism. Ann Intern Med 94:31, 1981

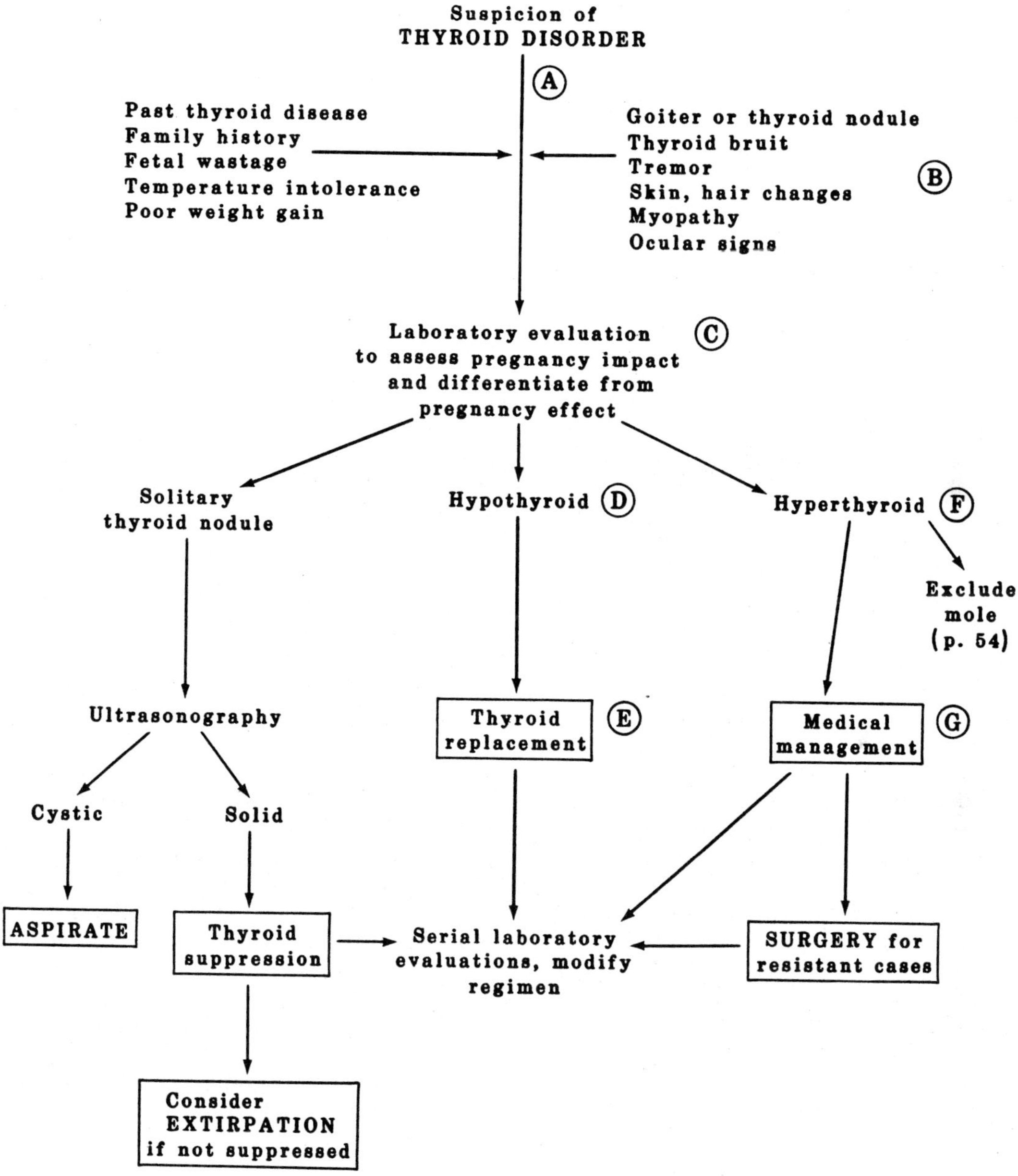
Suspicion of
THYROID DISORDER
A
Past thyroid disease
Family history
Fetal wastage
Temperature intolerance
Poor weight gain
Goiter or thyroid nodule
Thyroid bruit
Tremor
Skin, hair changes
Myopathy
Ocular signs
B
Laboratory evaluation
to assess pregnancy impact
and differentiate from
pregnancy effect
C
Solitary
thyroid nodule
Hypothyroid
D
Hyperthyroid
F
Exclude
mole
(p. 54)
Ultrasonography
Thyroid
replacement
E
Medical
management
G
Cystic
Solid
ASPIRATE
Thyroid
suppression
Serial laboratory
evaluations, modify
regimen
SURGERY for
resistant cases
Consider
EXTIRPATION
if not suppressed

EPILEPSY

Balmookoot Balgobin, M.D.

COMMENTS

A. The first diagnosis for a gravida who convulses is eclampsia (see p. 58). Absence of hypertension, proteinuria, hyperreflexia, and vasospasm makes other causes likely. Description of the seizure may be helpful (for example, if focalized), as are other manifestations, such as post-ictal state, paralysis, fever, headache, vomiting, and visual disturbances. Other causes include liver and renal disease, severe lung disease with anoxia or hypercarbia, hypoglycemia, hypocalcemia, and hyponatremia, encephalitis, cerebral abscess, drug usage (e.g., amphetamines) and withdrawal (from barbiturates, alcohol, and cerebral depressants), cerebrovascular accident, and intracranial neoplasm. Pseudoseizures are associated with syncope, hysteria, and hyperventilation.

B. Neurologic assessment is needed to diagnose idiopathic epilepsy and rule out other organic disorders. In addition to a thorough neurologic examination, lumbar puncture is needed to evaluate cerebrospinal fluid; other studies, such as electroencephalogram, skull x-rays, brain scan, CT scan, and cerebral angiography, may then be required.

C. Status epilepticus is a medical emergency to be treated aggressively. One must prevent aspiration, maintain a clear airway, give oxygen, and correct dehydration, electrolyte imbalance, and metabolic acidosis. Drugs that are used either singly or in combination include Valium, 5 to 15 mg, Dilantin, up to 1 gm, and phenobarbital, up to 500 mg, given by the intravenous route. One may also use paraldehyde, either intravenously or intramuscularly. If these measures fail, general anesthesia may have to be given. Therapy can cause respiratory depression and requires ventilatory support.

D. Once the acute phase is controlled, long-term therapy with Dilantin and phenobarbital should be instituted. Other agents, such as primidone or carbamazepine may be needed. Such agents tend to be most beneficial for grand mal or focal seizures. Petit mal is more effectively managed with ethosuximide, clonazepam, or Valium. Treatment objectives include seizure control with fewest side effects. Single drug therapy is preferable, although combinations may be required. Achieve and maintain a therapeutic level of drug by monitoring plasma concentrations monthly (or more often if indicated). Risks of teratogenicity are small but always present; cleft lip, cleft palate, and cardiac septal defects have been associated with Dilantin use. Trimethadione is best avoided in pregnancy because of its high teratogenic potential (dysmorphic changes and developmental delay). The hazard increases with multiple drug therapy. Maternal folic acid deficiency may result from drug use; patients should be screened and treated, if necessary. Delivery is undertaken only as indicated for obstetric reasons. The infant should be given vitamin K_1 at birth. One should continue to monitor drug levels post partum to ensure adequate therapy and to avoid overdose.

REFERENCES

Hansen JW, Smith DW: The fetal hydantoin syndrome. J Pediatr 87:285, 1975

Lander CM, Edwards VE, Eadie MJ, Tryer JH: Plasma anticonvulsant concentrates during pregnancy. Neurol 27:128, 1977

Montouris GD, Fenichel GM, McLain LW: The pregnant epileptic. Arch Neurol 36:601, 1979

Smith DW: Teratogenicity of anticonvulsant medications. Am J Dis Child 131:1337, 1977

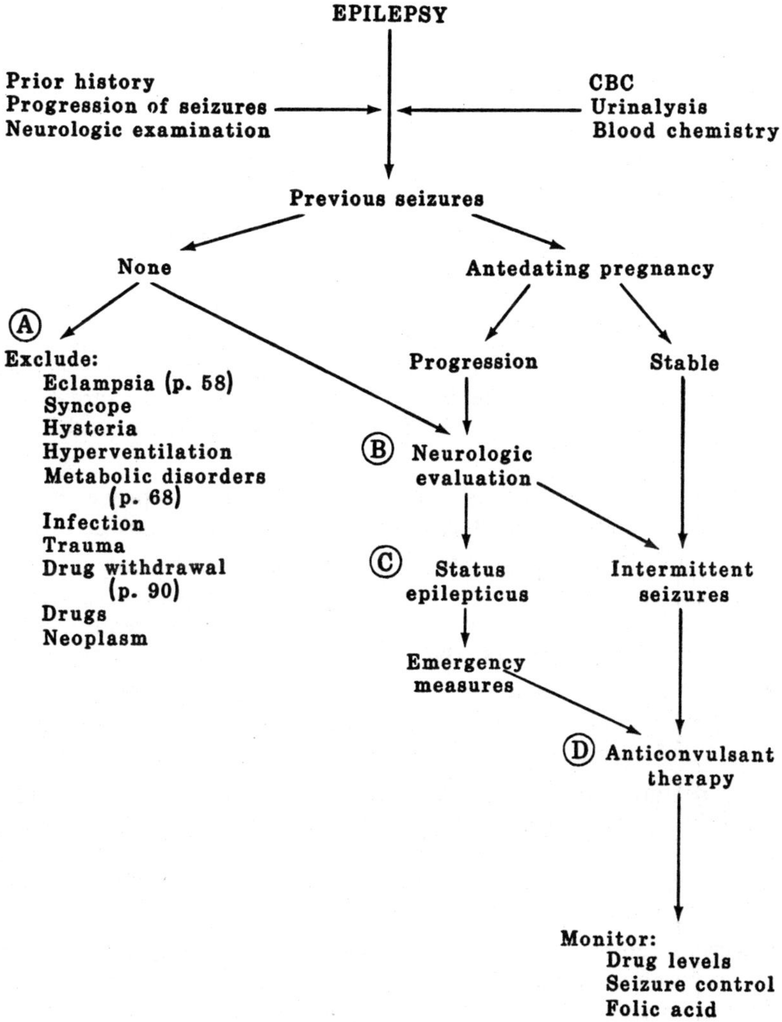
EPILEPSY
Prior history
Progression of seizures
Neurologic examination
CBC
Urinalysis
Blood chemistry
Previous seizures
None
Antedating pregnancy
Ⓐ
Exclude:
Eclampsia (p. 58)
Syncope
Hysteria
Hyperventilation
Metabolic disorders (p. 68)
Infection
Trauma
Drug withdrawal (p. 90)
Drugs
Neoplasm
Progression
Stable
Ⓑ Neurologic evaluation
Ⓒ Status epilepticus
Intermittent seizures
Emergency measures
Ⓓ Anticonvulsant therapy
Monitor:
Drug levels
Seizure control
Folic acid

PREGNANT ADDICT

Johanna F. Perlmutter, M.D.

COMMENTS

A. Gestational duration is difficult to determine because of amenorrhea and irregular menses. Assess nutritional status and use of multiple drugs, alcohol, and smoking; and investigate for infections, especially the venereal types.

B. Screen urine to uncover other drugs the patient is taking. Ultrasonography will help to date the pregnancy and disclose multiple gestation.

C. Investigate for medical illnesses, such as chronic pulmonary disease, malnutrition, hepatitis, and severe anemia.

D. Heroine addicts frequently use multiple drugs. Obtain periodic urine specimens for drug screens. Women in methadone maintenance programs tend to fare better than drug abusers. Their nutrition is improved, narcotic levels are stable, and infant outcome is better.

E. Whereas addicts on high-dose methadone maintenance tend to improve their general health, the withdrawal of the newborn from methadone addiction may be prolonged.

F. If methadone maintenance is not available for heroine addicts, the only options available are detoxification or continuation of drug abuse. Neither is ideal. Detoxification during pregnancy is not advised because it is associated with high fetal wastage. The best time is at 14–28 weeks, but serious adverse fetal effects have been reported.

G. The continued use of illicit drugs is inadvisable. Uncontrolled addicts get poor prenatal care and nutrition. As drug levels vary, the fetus may undergo withdrawal, resulting in hypoxia and even death.

H. Addicted gravidas require intensive prenatal care. About half the infants have low birth weight, both from intrauterine growth retardation and premature delivery. Follow fetal growth and maternal nutrition carefully. Watch for premature labor, abnormal presentations, pregnancy-induced hypertension, anemia, and urinary tract infections.

I. Give pain medication in labor with caution. Frequent doses may be necessary for adequate analgesia. Some narcotic antagonists can produce devastating effects in addicts by acute withdrawal. Because hypoxia may occur, continuous fetal monitoring is important. Consider peridural anesthesia.

J. The infant is at increased risk and deserves expert neonatal attention. Prematurity, low birth weight, and neonatal addiction are common. Signs of withdrawal appear as early as 72 hours or as late as 30 days following birth; if treated expeditiously, prognosis is good.

REFERENCES

Connaughton JF, Reeser D, Schut J, Finnegan LP: Perinatal addiction: Outcome and management. Am J Obstet Gynecol 129:679, 1977

Perlmutter J: Heroine addiction and pregnancy. Obstet Gynecol Survey 29:439, 1974

Rementeria JL, ed: *Drug Abuse in Pregnancy and Neonatal Effects.* St. Louis: CV Mosby Co, 1977

Zuspan FP, Gumpel JA, Mejia-Zelaya A, Madden J, Davis R: Fetal stress from methadone withdrawal. Am J Obstet Gynecol 122:43, 1975

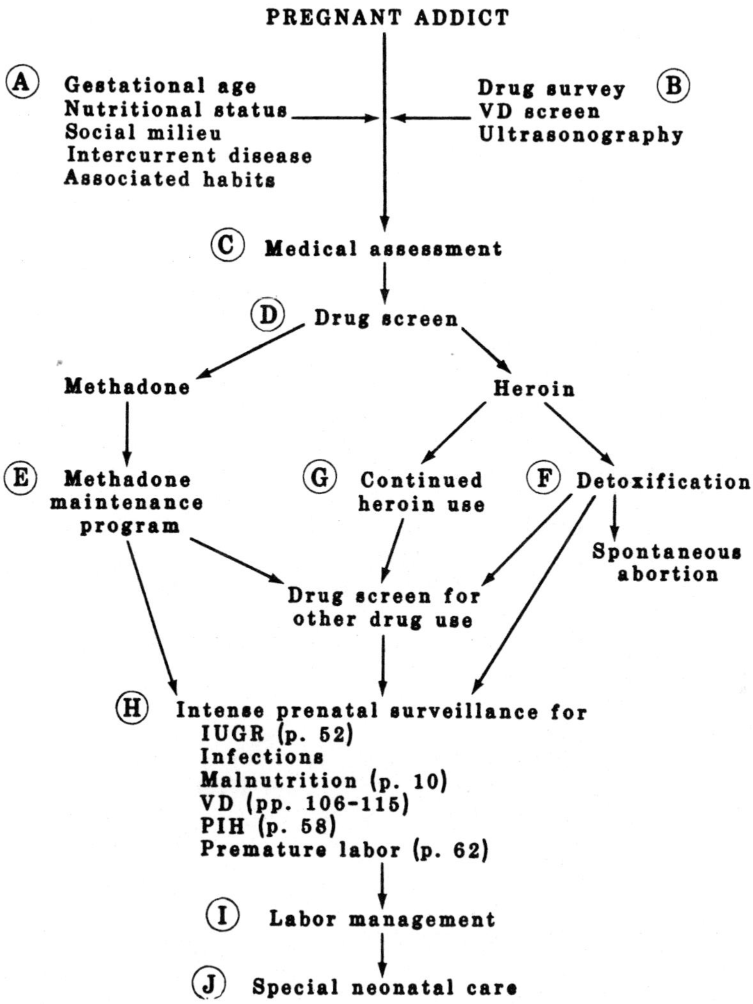
PREGNANT ADDICT
(A) Gestational age
Nutritional status
Social milieu
Intercurrent disease
Associated habits
Drug survey (B)
VD screen
Ultrasonography
(C) Medical assessment
(D) Drug screen
Methadone
Heroin
(E) Methadone maintenance program
(G) Continued heroin use
(F) Detoxification
Spontaneous abortion
Drug screen for other drug use
(H) Intense prenatal surveillance for
IUGR (p. 52)
Infections
Malnutrition (p. 10)
VD (pp. 106-115)
PIH (p. 58)
Premature labor (p. 62)
(I) Labor management
(J) Special neonatal care

PULMONARY EMBOLUS

Henry Klapholz, M.D.

COMMENTS

A. Patients at risk are those with prior peripheral venous disease, thrombophlebitis or pulmonary embolism, and those with pelvic infection, prolonged surgery, trauma, or protracted periods of immobilization or bedrest. Sudden precordial or substernal chest pain is seen with radiation to the neck or shoulder, plus pleuritic pain, shortness of breath, anxiety, agitation, and restlessness.

B. Physical findings include hypotension, tachycardia, and tachypnea. Peripheral and circumoral cyanosis also occur.

C. Transient electrocardiographic changes may be seen, reflecting acute cor pulmonale (typically $S_1Q_3T_3$ pattern, right axis deviation, or right bundle branch block). Serial electrocardiograms are sometimes helpful. Chest x-ray may show pulmonary infiltration, increased radiolucency, elevated diaphragm, or pleural effusion. Lung scan techniques are useful for screening, and especially for detecting lung perfusion defects with normal chest x-rays. Pulmonary function studies show increased ventilatory dead space, reduced alveolar pCO_2 and normal arterial pCO_2. Low arterial pO_2 (below 90 mm Hg) on room air with a positive lung scan establishes the diagnosis (with a good history and consistent physical examination). Although more hazardous than scanning, pulmonary angiography permits direct visualization of the pulmonary vessels and is, therefore, definitive for diagnosis of this condition. It should be done in doubtful cases before initiating treatment.

D. Immediate anticoagulant therapy is essential to prevent fatal complications. Heparin is the preferred treatment because it does not cross the placenta to affect the fetus adversely. Continuous intravenous infusion of about 1000 units of heparin per hour is effective. The partial thromboplastin time (PTT) is used to titrate the dosage; it should be adjusted until the PTT is twice the control. Bedrest, oxygen, analgesics, and antibiotics are needed; digitalis may be indicated for cardiac failure along with isoproterenol for hypotension and diuretics for pulmonary edema. After a few days, one can switch to intermittent subcutaneous heparin therapy, continuing to term.

E. At term, vaginal delivery is preferable to cesarean section. It is important to avoid a traumatic vaginal delivery. Delivery, even by cesarean section (if obstetrically indicated), can be safely carried out under full heparinization. If bleeding occurs, protamine counteracts the heparin effect.

F. Coumadin may be substituted for heparin post partum in an overlapping regimen. Warfarin is given daily in 10-15 mg doses for 2-3 days until prothrombin time is 2-3 times the control level. Then the heparin may be reduced and finally discontinued. Avoid breast feeding while on coumadin. Continue anticoagulants for 3-6 months.

REFERENCES

Coon WW: Epidemiology of venous thromboembolism. Ann Surg 186:149, 1977

Rosenow EC III, Osmundson PJ, Brown ML: Pulmonary embolism. Mayo Clin Proc 56:161, 1981

Sabiston DC Jr: Pathophysiology, diagnosis, and management of pulmonary embolism. Am J Surg 138:384, 1979

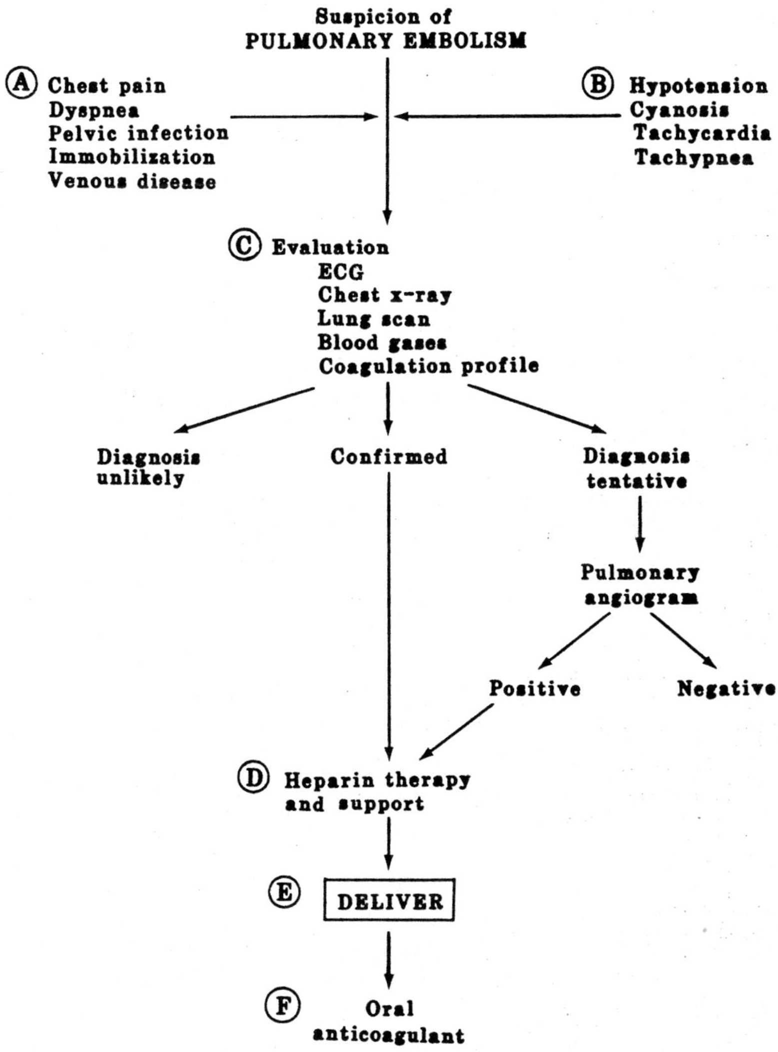
Suspicion of
PULMONARY EMBOLISM
A Chest pain
Dyspnea
Pelvic infection
Immobilization
Venous disease
B Hypotension
Cyanosis
Tachycardia
Tachypnea
C Evaluation
ECG
Chest x-ray
Lung scan
Blood gases
Coagulation profile
Diagnosis unlikely
Confirmed
Diagnosis tentative
Pulmonary angiogram
Positive
Negative
D Heparin therapy and support
E DELIVER
F Oral anticoagulant

Rh ISOIMMUNIZATION

Louis Burke, M.D.

COMMENTS

A. The risk of stillbirth in the first pregnancy is 8 percent. If the previous fetus was affected, the risk increases; if severely affected, the risk is more than 50 percent.

B. Anti-D antibody titer (indirect Coombs) is not a good index, although a level of 1:64 in albumin suggests Rh sensitization. A rising titer does, too, but titer level does not predict fetal outcome. Thus, antibody tests are used only for screening.

C. If the titer rises to 1:16 or more, or if the patient has a past history of serious fetal erythroblastosis, initiate amniocentesis. Beginning at about 18–20 weeks, repeat the taps every 2 weeks. If bilirubin peaks do not follow the expected downward slope, weekly taps are done.

D. Severity of isoimmunization is shown by measuring bilirubin level in amniotic fluid by spectrophotometric analysis. Low levels mean the infant is unaffected or, if affected, requires no treatment. Moderate levels (zone 2) occur with affected fetuses who have no hydrops. Values in zone 3 indicate infants with a grave prognosis, at risk for intrauterine death, hydrops, and severe hemolytic anemia.

E. The risks of intrauterine fetal transfusion are weighed against the risks of premature delivery. Prior to 32 weeks, give intrauterine transfusion to the severely affected fetus. Transfusions are repeated every two weeks. At 32 weeks, an L/S ratio is done (p. 124). If below 1.5:1, the fetus is transfused. Deliver if L/S is higher or after 34 weeks, regardless of the L/S ratio. Maternal plasmapheresis may be somewhat effective, especially for women with a history of early fetal loss.

F. Affected newborn infants need special attention, if possible in a tertiary center. Mild hyperbilirubinemia is treated with phototherapy. The more severe cases may need exchange transfusions and premature support resources.

G. Postpartum Rh prophylaxis by the administration of high-titer anti-D antigen (RhoGAM) should be given within 72 hours to an unsensitized Rh-negative woman who has just delivered an Rh-positive fetus. It is also indicated after abortion, ectopic pregnancy, and perhaps following amniocentesis or abruptio placentae. Prophylactic use in midpregnancy has also been suggested.

REFERENCES

Berkowitz RL, Hobbins JC: Current concepts in managing Rh incompatibility. Contemp Obstet Gynecol 9:125, 1977

Bowman J: Suppression of Rh isoimmunization: A review. Obstet Gynecol 52:385, 1978

Graham-Pole J, Barr W, Willoughby MLN: Continuous-flow plasmapheresis in management of severe rhesus isoimmunization. Brit Med J 1:1185, 1977

Liley AW: Liquor amnii analysis in management of pregnancy complicated by Rh sensitization. Am J Obstet Gynecol 82:1359, 1969

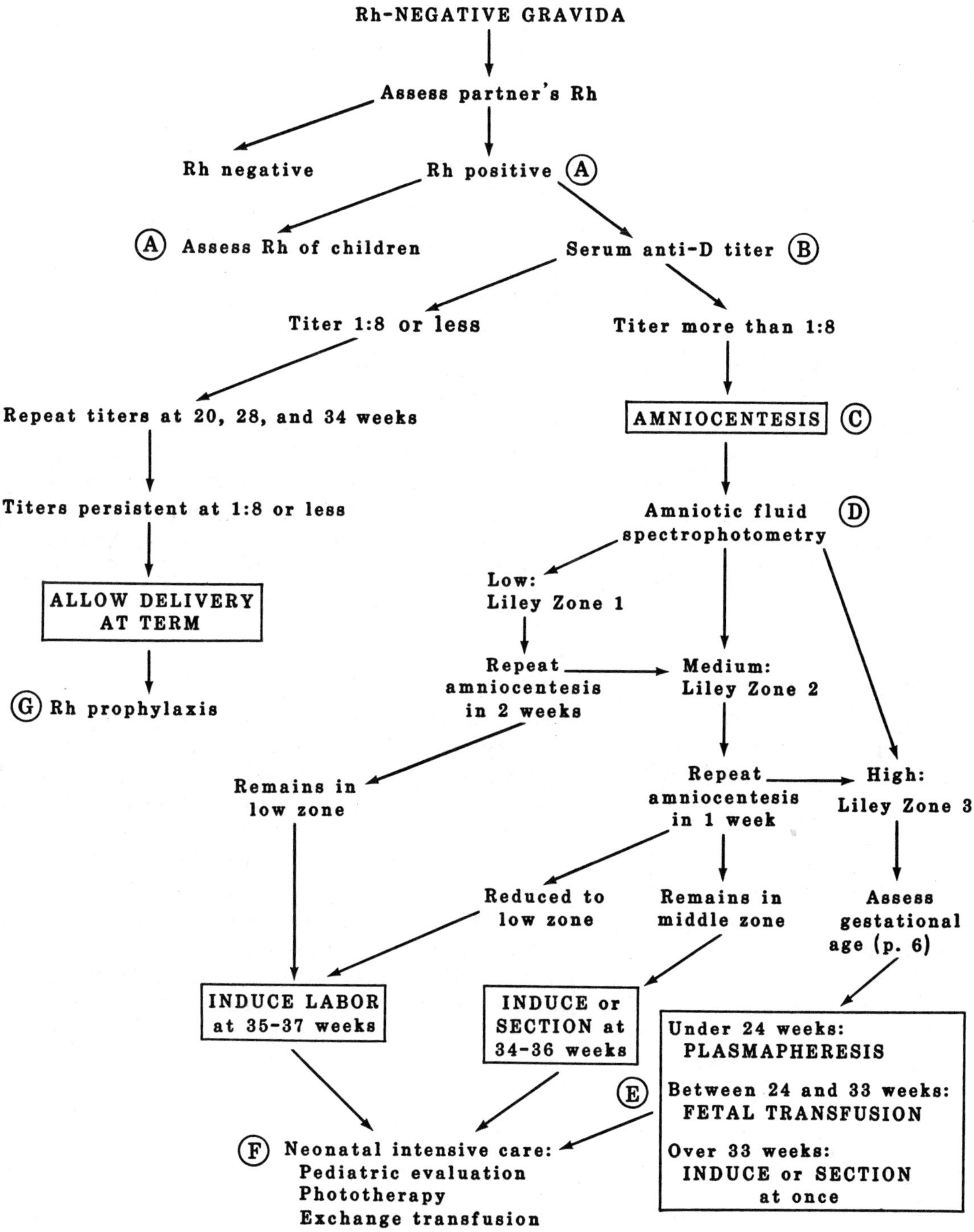
Rh-NEGATIVE GRAVIDA
Assess partner's Rh
Rh negative
Rh positive (A)
(A) Assess Rh of children
Serum anti-D titer (B)
Titer 1:8 or less
Titer more than 1:8
Repeat titers at 20, 28, and 34 weeks
AMNIOCENTESIS (C)
Titers persistent at 1:8 or less
Amniotic fluid spectrophotometry (D)
ALLOW DELIVERY AT TERM
Low: Liley Zone 1
(G) Rh prophylaxis
Repeat amniocentesis in 2 weeks
Medium: Liley Zone 2
Remains in low zone
Repeat amniocentesis in 1 week
High: Liley Zone 3
Reduced to low zone
Remains in middle zone
Assess gestational age (p. 6)
INDUCE LABOR at 35-37 weeks
INDUCE or SECTION at 34-36 weeks
Under 24 weeks: PLASMAPHERESIS
(E)
Between 24 and 33 weeks: FETAL TRANSFUSION
(F) Neonatal intensive care: Pediatric evaluation Phototherapy Exchange transfusion
Over 33 weeks: INDUCE or SECTION at once

OBSTRUCTIVE PULMONARY DISEASE

Henry Klapholz, M.D.

COMMENTS

A. Classify patients with obstructive pulmonary disease into those who have episodic attacks, those with chronic disorders that may or may not produce hypoxia, and the serious disorder of acute status asthmaticus.

B. Episodic attacks lend themselves to periodic treatment with bronchodilators (ephedrine 10 mg 4 times daily, theophylline tablets 100 mg 3 times daily, or epinephrine 0.5 mg as needed). These agents seem not to harm the fetus.

C. Women with uncomplicated episodic disease need routine care except at times of acute attacks. Cromolyn inhalation may help avoid allergic or exercise-induced attacks.

D. Patients with arterial pO_2 below 80 mm Hg should be tested periodically to check for secondary fetal hypoxia. Fetal growth is verified by ultrasound. Supplemental oxygen may be needed. Start assessing fetal status from 30 weeks.

E. Vigorous pulmonary toilet, including chest physical therapy, steam inhalation, and increased fluid intake, may prevent bronchopulmonary infection. Aerosol bronchodilators plus steroids (e.g., prednisone 30–40 mg per day for 3–5 days, slowly tapering by 5 mg per day to a maintenance dose of 10–15 mg per day) and antibiotics (ampicillin or penicillin), may be helpful. Avoid tetracycline because of its known fetal effects.

F. Acute status asthmaticus is a medical emergency requiring immediate hospitalization. The patient who fails to respond to a standard regimen (e.g., 0.1–0.2 ml 1:1000 epinephrine subcutaneously) is treated with intermittent positive pressure breathing, supplemental oxygen to maintain arterial pO_2 levels, and high-dose steroids (such as Solu-Cortef 250 mg intravenously every 4–6 hours). Mechanical ventilation should be considered if arterial pCO_2 rises above 40 mm Hg. Such patients may have to be maintained on a long-term program of bronchodilators and steroids.

G. Aim to deliver these patients under controlled conditions by elective induction of labor when conditions are optimal. Pain relief and hydration are essential. Bronchodilators, such as epinephrine and aminophylline, should be on hand. General anesthesia should be avoided unless status asthmaticus occurs; then, an agent such as halothane may be beneficial for relieving spasm. Even when conduction anesthesia is being used, due caution is necessary.

REFERENCES

Fishburne JI: Physiology and disease of the respiratory system in pregnancy: A review. J Reprod Med 22:177, 1979

Leontic EA: Respiratory disease in pregnancy. Med Clin North Am 61:111, 1977

Turner ES, Greenberger PA, Patterson R: Management of the pregnant asthmatic patient. Ann Intern Med 93:905, 1980

Weinberger SE, Weiss ST, Cohen WR, Weiss JW, Johnson TS: Pregnancy and the lung. Am Rev Resp Dis 121:559, 1980

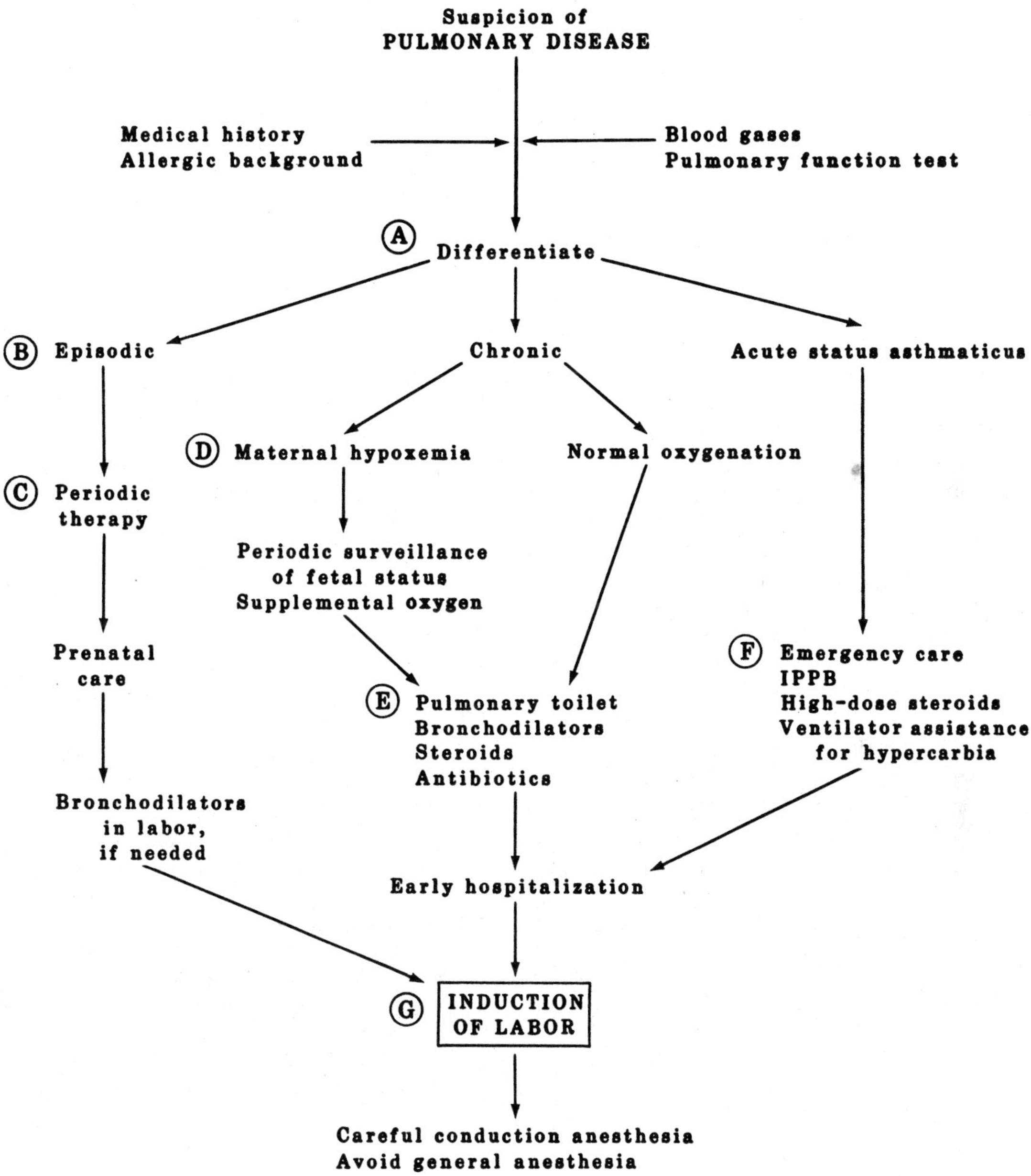
Suspicion of
PULMONARY DISEASE
Medical history
Allergic background
Blood gases
Pulmonary function test
(A) Differentiate
(B) Episodic
Chronic
Acute status asthmaticus
(D) Maternal hypoxemia
Normal oxygenation
(C) Periodic therapy
Periodic surveillance
of fetal status
Supplemental oxygen
Prenatal care
(F) Emergency care
IPPB
High-dose steroids
Ventilator assistance
for hypercarbia
(E) Pulmonary toilet
Bronchodilators
Steroids
Antibiotics
Bronchodilators
in labor,
if needed
Early hospitalization
(G) INDUCTION
OF LABOR
Careful conduction anesthesia
Avoid general anesthesia

ACUTE SURGICAL ABDOMEN

Louis Burke, M.D.

COMMENTS

A. Differentiating nonobstetrical surgical problems from purely obstetric and intercurrent medical illness is sometimes very difficult. Pain is common during pregnancy, but intense focal or generalized pain, particularly if persistent, deserves astute attention. Similarly, nausea and vomiting frequently occur early in pregnancy. Vomiting associated with pain or abdominal distention, especially when protracted, profuse, or projectile, demands evaluation. Rapidly developing or asymmetric abdominal distention is significant. Syncope is also common in pregnancy, but progressive cardiovascular instability in association with other manifestations of an intra-abdominal crisis strongly suggests a condition that may require surgical intervention.

B. A variety of nonsurgical conditions can mimic acute surgical problems. Pregnancy and salpingitis, for example, rarely coexist, but a flare-up of a pre-existing inflammatory process may occur. Past history, physical findings, and laboratory evidence of kidney, heart, gastrointestinal, or other concurrent illness help alert one to the proper diagnosis. Pregnancy-related problems tend to be far more common, of course. Those mimicking acute surgical crises, such as ectopic pregnancy, must be evaluated and managed as emergencies. The developing clinical picture, coupled with changing laboratory evidence, often clarifies the diagnosis.

C. True surgical emergencies are uncommon in pregnancy, but they can be devastating, particularly if intervention is unnecessarily delayed. Pregnancy may modify presenting manifestations somewhat. The focus of pain and tenderness in association with acute appendicitis, for example, may be moved cephalad by the growing uterus. Because manifestations may be atypical, a high index of suspicion is necessary.

D. One must weigh the risks of delaying surgical intervention for definitive care in terms of mortality against the risks of surgery in pregnancy. Nonsurgical approaches are preferable, of course, but patients who show evidence of progression of an acute surgical process demand such intervention. Similarly, the development of cardiovascular instability as a consequence of intraperitoneal bleeding, for example, makes surgery mandatory. Surgery is indicated for acute appendicitis, twisted ovarian cyst, intestinal obstruction, ruptured viscus, volvulus, and progressive peritonitis, among other conditions.

E. Temporization may be considered if the patient is in reasonably stable condition and her disease process is not progressive. This applies particularly to gall bladder disease, provided there is no increasing jaundice or suspicion of common duct stone. Acute pancreatitis may also be managed conservatively in most cases. If conservative management fails to resolve the problem, surgery can be reconsidered at any time.

REFERENCES

Crouch M: The acute abdomen in women. Practitioner 222:457, 1979

Cunningham FG, Coburn JH: Appendicitis complicating pregnancy. Obstet Gynecol 45:415, 1975

Devore GR: Acute abdominal pain in the pregnant patient due to pancreatitis, acute appendicitis, cholecystitis or peptic ulcer disease. Clin Perinatol 7:349, 1980

Hill LM, Symmonds RB: Small bowel obstruction in pregnancy. Obstet Gynecol 49:170, 1977

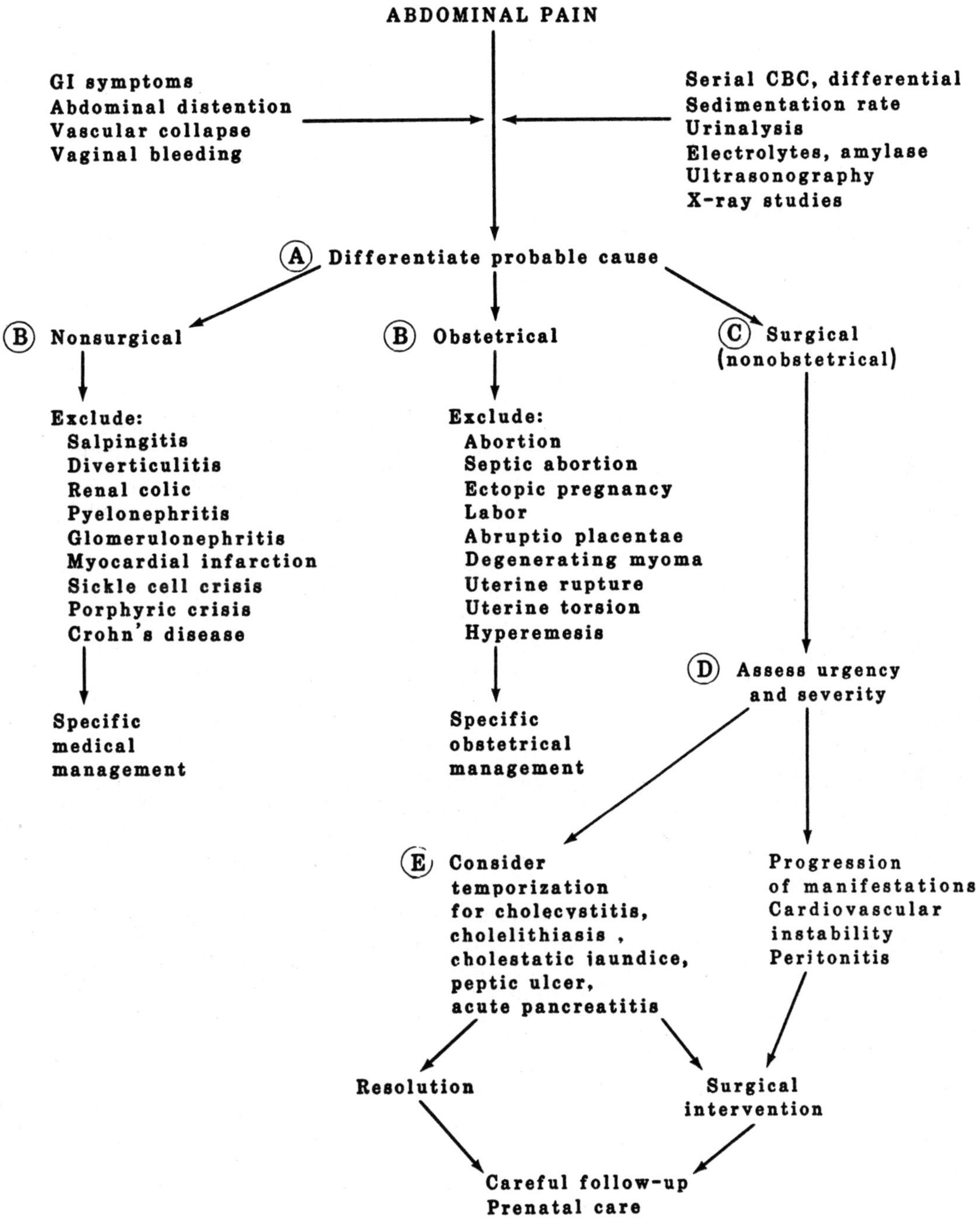
ABDOMINAL PAIN
GI symptoms
Abdominal distention
Vascular collapse
Vaginal bleeding
Serial CBC, differential
Sedimentation rate
Urinalysis
Electrolytes, amylase
Ultrasonography
X-ray studies
(A) Differentiate probable cause
(B) Nonsurgical
Exclude:
Salpingitis
Diverticulitis
Renal colic
Pyelonephritis
Glomerulonephritis
Myocardial infarction
Sickle cell crisis
Porphyric crisis
Crohn's disease
Specific medical management
(B) Obstetrical
Exclude:
Abortion
Septic abortion
Ectopic pregnancy
Labor
Abruptio placentae
Degenerating myoma
Uterine rupture
Uterine torsion
Hyperemesis
Specific obstetrical management
(C) Surgical (nonobstetrical)
(D) Assess urgency and severity
(E) Consider temporization for cholecystitis, cholelithiasis, cholestatic jaundice, peptic ulcer, acute pancreatitis
Progression of manifestations
Cardiovascular instability
Peritonitis
Resolution
Surgical intervention
Careful follow-up
Prenatal care

ABDOMINAL MASS

Selwyn P. Oskowitz, M.B.

COMMENTS

A. Differential diagnosis requires careful, methodical physical examination plus inquiry into history of acute or recurrent pain, fever, and gastrointestinal or urinary tract manifestations.

B. Growing abdominal tumors may mistakenly be assumed to be related to pregnancy, especially if accompanied by menstrual aberration. Attempt to verify that the patient is pregnant. Ultrasonography will show an intrauterine pregnancy, a blighted ovum, or molar degeneration.

C. One must ascertain whether the mass is intrinsic to the gravid uterus or distinct from it. If it is part of the uterus or intimately attached, adnexal pathology becomes unlikely. Asymptomatic uterine leiomyomata require no special care, but if acutely degenerating, symptomatic treatment may suffice. Surgical intervention for myomectomy is rarely indicated because of the risks of hemorrhage and abortion.

D. If uterine size is compatible with the gestational dates (p. 6), extrinsic neoplastic adnexal tumor is likely. If the uterus is too large, a pregnancy-related disorder must still be considered.

E. Although masses are most commonly ovarian in origin, they may represent such conditions as Crohn's disease, diverticulitis, and appendiceal abscess.

F. If the mass is hard, nodular, fixed, variegated in consistency, and bilateral, suspect malignancy especially if associated with ascites. By contrast, benign masses tend to be cystic, smooth, mobile, uniform in consistency, and unilateral.

G. If feasible, delay the surgery until the second trimester to avoid anesthesia or hypoxia during organogenesis and the risk of abortion. Functional or luteal cysts will subside spontaneously. Torsion, hemorrhage, and rupture of an ovarian cyst may necessitate surgical intervention. In early third trimester, delay may enhance fetal salvage. Measures to augment fetal maturity may be in order as well (p. 124).

H. Staging laparotomy requires a midline suprapubic incision. Ascites fluid should be collected for cell block; if there is no ascites, take peritoneal washings. The type and extent of the lesion should be determined, noting implants on the undersurface of diaphragm, omentum, mesentery, bowel, and paracolic gutters and obtaining biopsies from representative implants and aortic lymph nodes. Oncologic consultation is important for determining optimal surgery and subsequent adjunctive therapy.

REFERENCES

Bowes WA Jr, Halgrimson M, Simmons MH: Results of the intensive perinatal management of very-low-birth-weight infants (501–1000 grams). J Reprod Med 23:245, 1979

Creasman WT, Rutledge FH, Smith JP: Carcinoma of the ovary associated with pregnancy. Obstet Gynecol 38:111, 1971

White KC: Ovarian tumors in pregnancy: A private hospital 10 year survey. Am J Obstet Gynecol 116:544, 1973

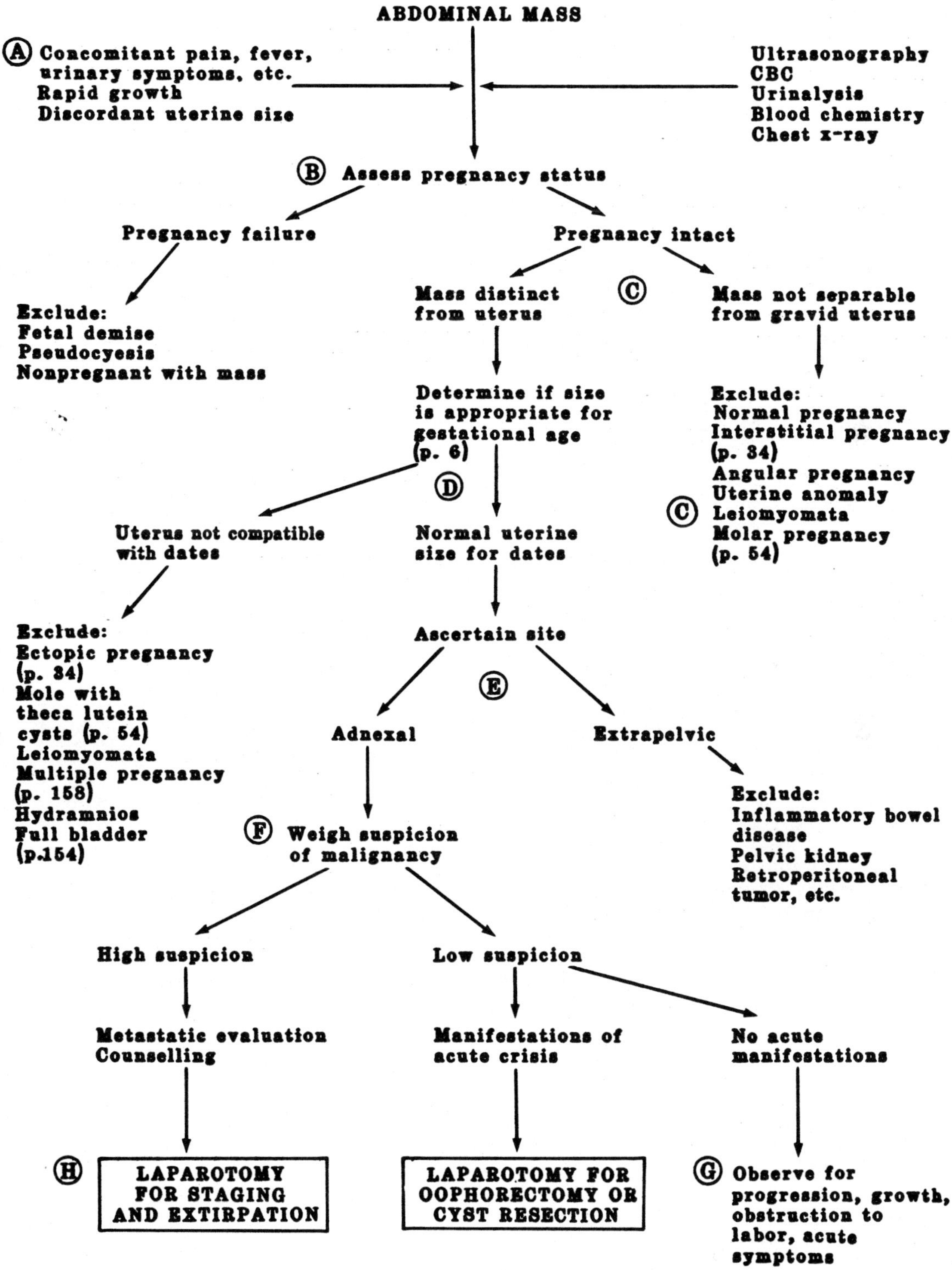
ABDOMINAL MASS
Ⓐ Concomitant pain, fever, urinary symptoms, etc.
Rapid growth
Discordant uterine size
Ultrasonography
CBC
Urinalysis
Blood chemistry
Chest x-ray
Ⓑ Assess pregnancy status
Pregnancy failure
Pregnancy intact
Exclude:
Fetal demise
Pseudocyesis
Nonpregnant with mass
Mass distinct from uterus
Ⓒ
Mass not separable from gravid uterus
Determine if size is appropriate for gestational age (p. 6)
Exclude:
Normal pregnancy
Interstitial pregnancy (p. 34)
Angular pregnancy
Uterine anomaly
Ⓒ
Leiomyomata
Molar pregnancy (p. 54)
Ⓓ
Uterus not compatible with dates
Normal uterine size for dates
Exclude:
Ectopic pregnancy (p. 34)
Mole with theca lutein cysts (p. 54)
Leiomyomata
Multiple pregnancy (p. 158)
Hydramnios
Full bladder (p.154)
Ascertain site
Ⓔ
Adnexal
Extrapelvic
Exclude:
Inflammatory bowel disease
Pelvic kidney
Retroperitoneal tumor, etc.
Ⓕ Weigh suspicion of malignancy
High suspicion
Low suspicion
Metastatic evaluation
Counselling
Manifestations of acute crisis
No acute manifestations
Ⓗ
LAPAROTOMY FOR STAGING AND EXTIRPATION
LAPAROTOMY FOR OOPHORECTOMY OR CYST RESECTION
Ⓖ Observe for progression, growth, obstruction to labor, acute symptoms

RUBELLA EXPOSURE

Selwyn P. Oskowitz, M.B.

COMMENTS

A. The level of hemagglutination inhibition (HI) titers that implies immunity against rubella will vary somewhat from laboratory to laboratory. Titers greater than 1:8 (or 1:10) are reassuring because they suggest foregoing disease with lasting immunity. Titers persistent at 1:8 (or 1:10) also imply immunity, provided one has ruled out the infrequent occurrence of a false positive or a titer that has not yet risen in response to a very recent infection.

B. If the HI titer remains at less than 1:8 for 5 weeks or more after exposure — or 3 weeks after a suspicious rash — one can be reassured that rubella infection is unlikely to have occurred.

C. Expeditious verification of a rubella infection is enhanced by properly timing the repeat HI titer according to the interval that has elapsed since the exposure. The titer rises rapidly to a plateau at or after 5 weeks. If the exposure occurred less than 1 week earlier, repeat the HI titer in 3–4 weeks; if exposure was 1–5 weeks earlier, repeat in 2 weeks.

D. After 5 weeks, HI titers less than 1:8 are very reassuring. Titers greater than 1:8 but less than 1:32 at this time make infection unlikely. About 99 percent of infected patients can be expected to reach a titer greater than 1:32 by 5 weeks and to maintain this level of titer for at least 6 months. Intermediate levels suggest prior immunity.

E. HI titers of 1:32 or more at this time, 5 weeks after exposure, indicate that a recent infection has probably taken place.

F. When the change in HI titer is unclear (that is, neither stable at a low level nor rising rapidly), one may resort to use of complement fixation (CF) testing. A fourfold rise in CF titer is good evidence that an infection has occurred within the preceding 5-week interval. If the CF test is merely positive at low titer levels, rubella-specific immunoglobulin-M (IgM) will be helpful in confirming a recent infection.

G. Considerations for pregnancy termination are based on the probability that rubella infection has occurred coupled with the recognized risks of such infections to the fetus, specifically the high frequencies of stillbirths and congenital rubella syndrome. Needless to say, the personal attitude and viewpoint of the patient with regard to abortion must prevail.

REFERENCES

Fulginiti VA, Alexander ER: Rubella in pregnancy: A guide to rational counseling. JAMA 245:1666, 1981

Mann JM, Preblud SR, Hoffman RE, Brandlins-Bennet RD, Hinman AR, Herrmann KL: Assessing risks of rubella infection during pregnancy: A standardized approach. JAMA 245:1647, 1981

Marks JS, Halpin TJ, Irvin JJ, Johnson DA, Keller JR: Risk factors associated with failure to receive vaccinations. Pediat 64:304, 1979

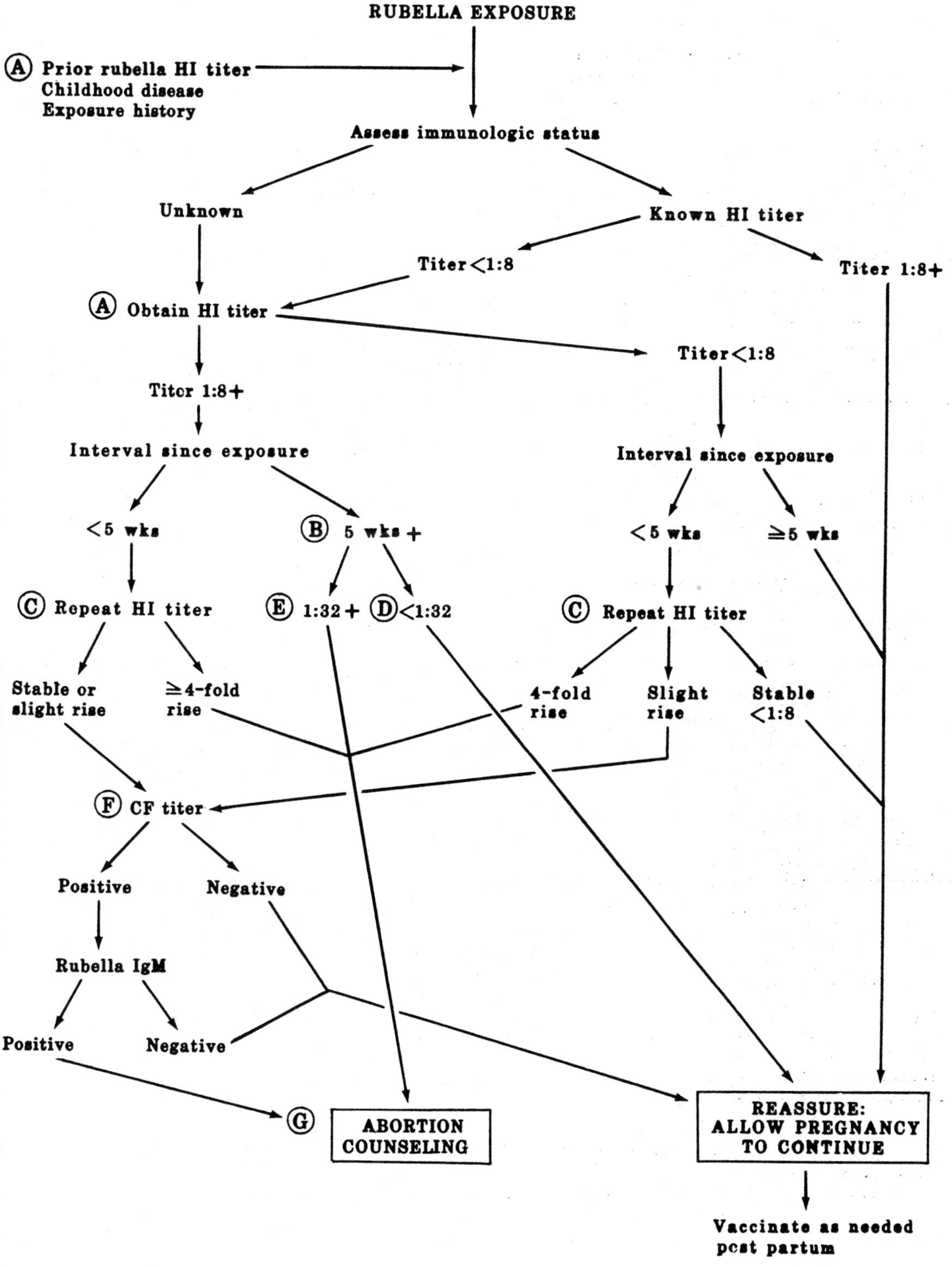
RUBELLA EXPOSURE
(A) Prior rubella HI titer
Childhood disease
Exposure history
Assess immunologic status
Unknown
Known HI titer
Titer <1:8
Titer 1:8+
(A) Obtain HI titer
Titer <1:8
Titer 1:8+
Interval since exposure
Interval since exposure
<5 wks
(B) 5 wks +
<5 wks
≧5 wks
(C) Repeat HI titer
(E) 1:32 +
(D) <1:32
(C) Repeat HI titer
Stable or slight rise
≧4-fold rise
4-fold rise
Slight rise
Stable <1:8
(F) CF titer
Positive
Negative
Rubella IgM
Positive
Negative
(G)
ABORTION COUNSELING
REASSURE: ALLOW PREGNANCY TO CONTINUE
Vaccinate as needed post partum

TOXOPLASMOSIS

Henry Klapholz, M.D.

COMMENTS

A. The primary source of toxoplasmosis infection in the United States is ingestion of raw meat. The parasite is very sensitive to heat, and even a small amount of cooking will prevent the disease. Adequate hand washing after handling raw meat must be emphasized to pregnant patients. The common house cat, if infected, can excrete millions of infectious oocysts in a single stool. These may survive for days. No other animal appears to excrete the parasite in feces.

B. Common screening tests use the hemagglutination-inhibition test (HI). They may yield false-positive results but are inexpensive. Routine prenatal screening can detect prior infection on the basis of elevated HI titers; a low level indicates susceptibility. If a woman has had an infected baby, she stands a negligible risk of ever having another such child, although repeated infestations are possible.

C. The usual presentation of the clinical disease in adults is a flulike illness, usually only a few days in duration with little or no fever. Lymphadenopathy is very common. Severe intrauterine infestation produces marked acute polyhydramnios. This should serve to alert the astute clinician.

D. A fourfold increase in HI titer (or more) over a period of 2 weeks is very suggestive of an acute infection. This should be verified by Sabin-Feldman dye test. There are no known false positives with this test. This is in sharp contrast to the HI screening tests, which yield elevated titers with many other diseases, including most collagen diseases.

E. If the Sabin-Feldman dye test is positive, one should consider pregnancy termination, if possible and agreeable to the patient. The likelihood is very high that the infant will be damaged. Early infection often results in spontaneous abortion; later infection, however, may produce congenital toxoplasmosis in the fetus. Major neurologic and developmental sequelae are associated with intracranial calcification, hydrocephalus, microcephaly, and chorioretinitis. Elevated toxoplasmosis-specific IgM also indicates recent infection.

F. If pregnancy termination is not a viable alternative, treatment may be undertaken. The treatment of choice is Spiromycin, which, regrettably, has not yet been formally approved for clinical use in this country (but is obtainable in Canada and Europe). Currently available agents include pyrimethamine and sulfapyrimidine, both of which are relatively toxic to the developing embryo.

REFERENCES

Desmonts G. Couvreur J: Congenital toxoplasmosis: A prospective study of 378 pregnancies. New Engl J Med 290:1110, 1974

Fuchs F, Kimball AC, Kean BH: The management of toxoplasmosis in pregnancy. Clin Perinatol 1: 407, 1974

Karim KA, Ludlam GB: Serological diagnosis of congenital toxoplasmosis. J Clin Pathol 28:383, 1975

Schoenbaum SC: Specific problems in diagnosis, prevention, and management of congenital infections. Clin Obstet Gynecol 22:321, 1979

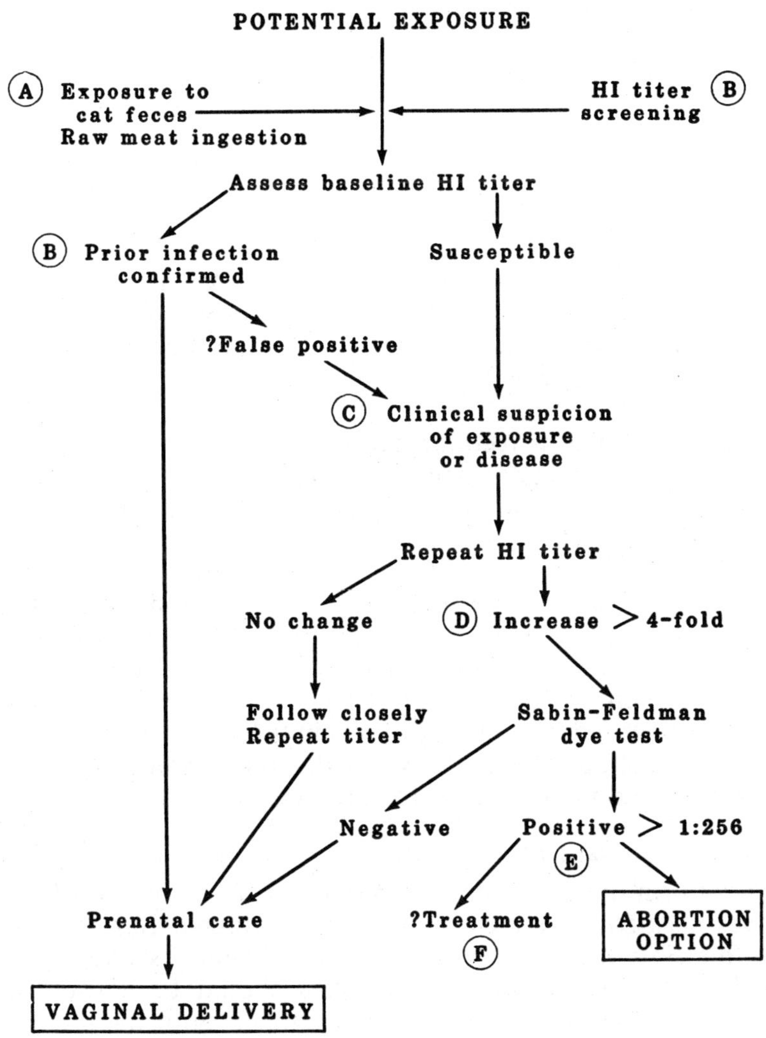
POTENTIAL EXPOSURE
A
Exposure to cat feces
Raw meat ingestion
HI titer screening
B
Assess baseline HI titer
B
Prior infection confirmed
Susceptible
?False positive
C
Clinical suspicion of exposure or disease
Repeat HI titer
No change
D
Increase > 4-fold
Follow closely
Repeat titer
Sabin-Feldman dye test
Negative
Positive > 1:256
E
Prenatal care
?Treatment
F
ABORTION OPTION
VAGINAL DELIVERY

SYPHILIS

Austin Wertheimer, M.D. and Carol London, R.N.

COMMENTS

A. RPR, Rapid Plasma Reagin test, substitutes effectively for the VDRL (Venereal Disease Research Laboratory) or the Hinton test.

B. FTA-ABS, Fluorescent Treponemal Antibody Absorption, is specific for syphilis, may be positive earlier than the RPR in a patient with recent infection, and remains positive after treatment. It should be repeated weekly for 3 weeks if it is persistently negative.

C. In pregnancy, treatment is recommended as soon as the diagnosis is suspected so as to avoid the sequelae of congenital syphilis. Treatment is the same as in the nonpregnant state with the exception that penicillin-allergic individuals should not be given tetracycline. Erythromycin is the drug of choice in this situation. The specific regimens are as follows: Primary and secondary syphilis is treated with benzathine penicillin-G, 2.4 million units intramuscularly, repeated in 7 days; or erythromycin 0.5 gm orally 4 times a day for 12 days (the estolate form is contraindicated because of liver toxicity). Latent and neurosyphilis require benzathine penicillin-G 2.4 million units intramuscularly at weekly intervals for 3 doses; or erythromycin 0.5 gm orally 4 times a day for 20 days. This protocol obviates the need for diagnostic spinal tap in patients with latent syphilis who do not have neurologic signs.

D. Investigations include RPR and FTA-ABS, if they have not already been drawn, to confirm the diagnosis and to rule out false-positive RPR. If the FTA-ABS proves negative, treatment may be discontinued. If syphilis is confirmed by a positive FTA-ABS, investigate and treat contacts and screen for other venereal diseases. Public health authorities should be consulted. Following treatment, RPR should be drawn every 3 months until the test becomes nonreactive. Patients with persistently reactive RPR may need a second course of therapy.

REFERENCES

McCormack WM: Management of sexually transmissible infections during pregnancy. Clin Obstet Gynecol 18:57, 1975

Fiumara NJ: *The Sexually Transmitted Diseases.* Boston: Commonwealth of Massachusetts Department of Public Health, 1978

Sexually transmitted diseases. American College of Obstetricians and Gynecologists Technical Bulletins Nos. 50 and 51, 1978

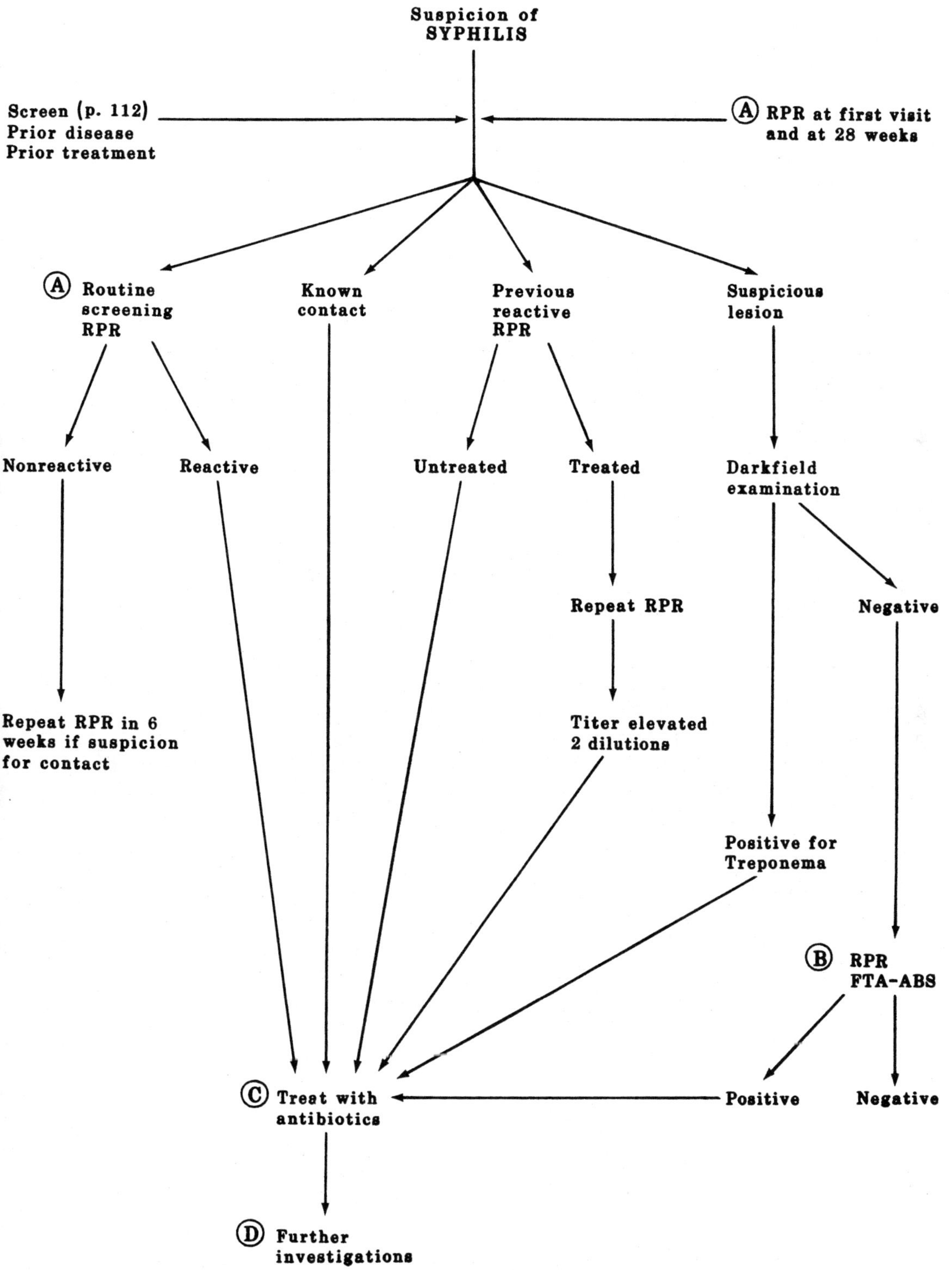
Suspicion of SYPHILIS
Screen (p. 112)
Prior disease
Prior treatment
(A) RPR at first visit and at 28 weeks
(A) Routine screening RPR
Known contact
Previous reactive RPR
Suspicious lesion
Nonreactive
Reactive
Untreated
Treated
Darkfield examination
Repeat RPR
Negative
Repeat RPR in 6 weeks if suspicion for contact
Titer elevated 2 dilutions
Positive for Treponema
(B) RPR FTA-ABS
(C) Treat with antibiotics
Positive
Negative
(D) Further investigations

GONORRHEA

Austin Wertheimer, M.D.

COMMENTS

A. The treatment for gonorrhea in pregnancy is the same as in the nonpregnant state, except that women who are allergic to penicillin should not be given tetracycline. Erythromycin or cefazolin should be substituted. Specific treatment regimens for uncomplicated gonorrhea include procaine penicillin, 4.8 million units intramuscularly (which will also cure incubating syphilis); or ampicillin, 3.5 gm orally with 1 gm probenecid (this is less effective and inadequate for treatment of incubating syphilis); or erythromycin, 1.5 gm orally followed by 0.5 gm 4 times a day for 4 days (the estolate form is contraindicated because of liver toxicity); or cefazolin, 2 gm intramuscularly with probenecid 1 gm orally.

B. A positive culture after treatment may indicate reinfection, noncompliance with an oral regimen, or a resistant organism. In cases in which resistance is likely, treat with spectinomycin, 2 gm intramuscularly and initiate tests for penicillinase-producing organisms. Do follow-up cultures about 1 week after treatment. This regimen is effective but does not cure incubating syphilis. In addition, its safety for the fetus has not been established.

REFERENCES

McCormack WM: Management of sexually transmissible infections during pregnancy. Clin Obstet Gynecol 18:57, 1975

Fiumara NJ: *The Sexually Transmitted Diseases.* Boston: Commonwealth of Massachusetts Department of Public Health, 1978

Sexually transmitted diseases. American College of Obstetricians and Gynecologists Technical Bulletins Nos. 50 and 51, 1978

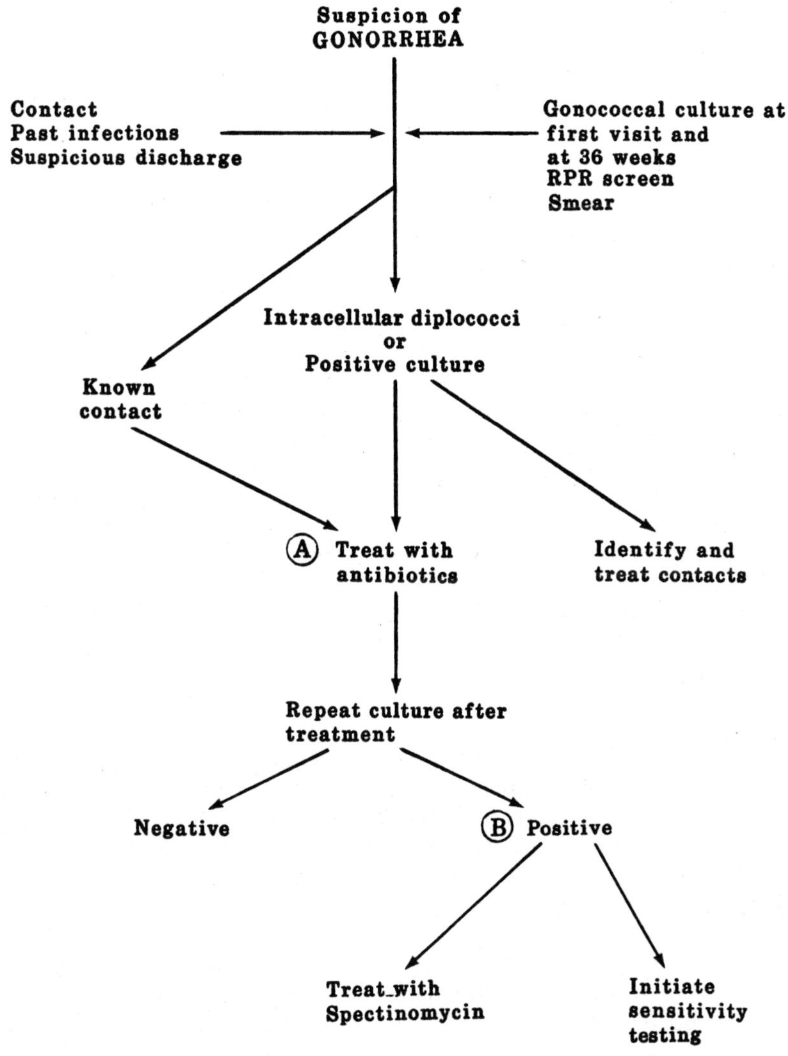
Suspicion of
GONORRHEA
Contact
Past infections
Suspicious discharge
Gonococcal culture at
first visit and
at 36 weeks
RPR screen
Smear
Intracellular diplococci
or
Positive culture
Known
contact
(A) Treat with
antibiotics
Identify and
treat contacts
Repeat culture after
treatment
Negative
(B) Positive
Treat with
Spectinomycin
Initiate
sensitivity
testing

TRICHOMONAS VAGINALIS VAGINITIS

Austin Wertheimer, M.D.

COMMENTS

A. Wet mount is a rapid and inexpensive way to detect *Trichomonas vaginalis*, although not as accurate as culture methods. A cotton-tipped applicator is used to collect a sample of discharge from the vaginal fornices and/or walls. It is placed in 1-2 cc normal saline in a small test tube and twirled to make a suspension. A few drops of the suspension are placed on a microscope slide and covered with a coverslip. Trichomonads appear as motile pear- or oblong-shaped cells with a cluster of rapidly undulating flagella at one end, slightly larger than white blood cells.

B. Treatment of the sexual partner is left up to the discretion of the physician. There are ethical concerns about prescribing medication for someone other than the patient. Condom usage should be encouraged to prevent reinfection. For reinfection, repeat treatment with metronidazole after ruling out leukopenia.

C. Although a teratogenic effect has not yet been shown in animals or humans, the data on metronidazole are not adequate to rule it out as a possibility. Therefore, it is recommended that the medication not be used in the first trimester of pregnancy. Supportive measures (vaginal creams or suppositories) may provide symptomatic relief; they should be tried initially before metronidazole.

D. If supportive measures have failed to give relief, metronidazole may be offered. *Trichomonas* infections are not associated with life-threatening maternal or neonatal complications. Isolated cases of neonatal infection have been reported with minimal sequelae. In mice, malignant lymphomas and pulmonary adenomas occur after prolonged high-level exposure to metronidazole. Mutagenic effects have also been demonstrated on bacteria. To apply these relationships to the human in clinical practice can only be considered conjectural. Metronidazole crosses the placenta and enters the fetal circulation rapidly. This provides tenuous support for a policy that interdicts use of this medication during pregnancy. If given, there are two accepted and effective dosage regimens: 250 mg orally three times daily for seven days, or a single 2 gm oral dose. The latter is less preferable in pregnancy because it results in higher serum levels in both maternal and fetal circulations. There is a low incidence of side effects, which include nausea, headache, dry mouth, vertigo, and diarrhea. Metronidazole is contraindicated with central nervous system disease or blood dyscrasia. Alcohol consumption should be avoided during administration, since this may evoke a disulfiram-like reaction.

REFERENCES

Al-Salihi FL, Curran JP, Wang J: Neonatal trichomonas vaginalis: Report of three cases and review of the literature. Pediat 53:196, 1974

Goldman P: Metronidazole: Proven benefits and potential risks. Johns Hopkins Med J 147:1, 1980

Haser WD, Brown ST, Kraus SJ, et al: Metronidazole for vaginal trichomoniasis: Seven-day vs. single-dose regimens. JAMA 244:1219, 1980

Lossick JG: Single-dose metronidazole treatment for vaginal trichomoniasis. Obstet Gynecol 56: 508, 1980

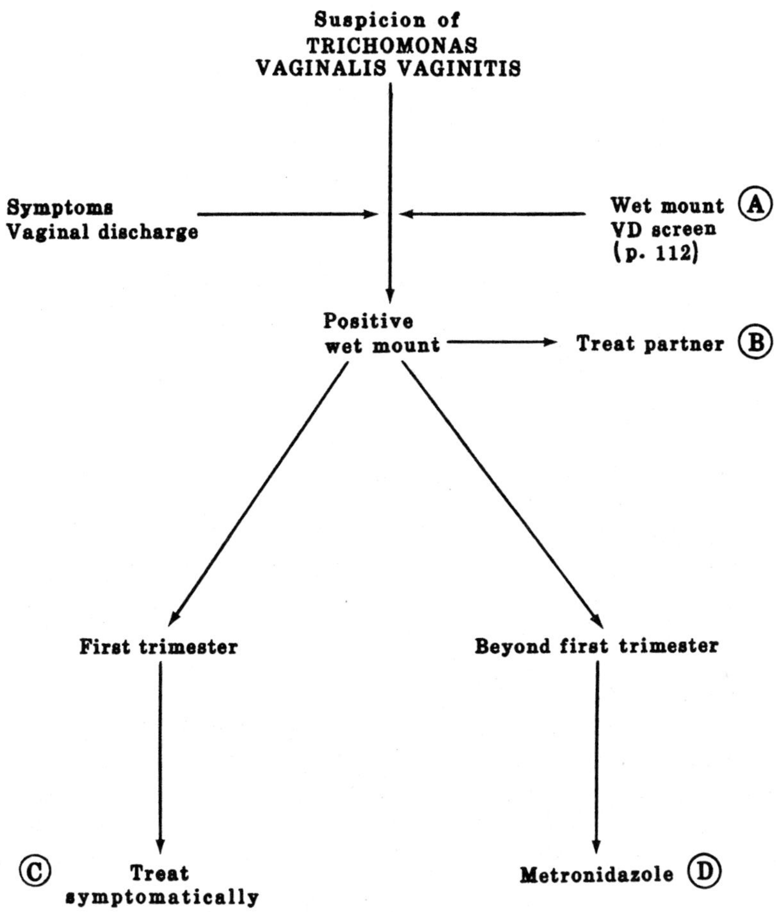
Suspicion of
TRICHOMONAS
VAGINALIS VAGINITIS
Symptoms
Vaginal discharge
Wet mount (A)
VD screen
(p. 112)
Positive
wet mount
Treat partner (B)
First trimester
Beyond first trimester
(C) Treat
symptomatically
Metronidazole (D)

CONDYLOMA ACUMINATA

Austin Wertheimer, M.D.

COMMENTS

A. Treatment options include cryotherapy, electrocautery, and laser beam ablation. Podophyllin is contraindicated in pregnancy.

B. Simple observation may be acceptable, since condylomata may regress spontaneously after pregnancy.

C. Cesarean section should be considered if multiple vaginal condylomata are present or if there is outlet obstruction by growths. This will minimize the risk of bleeding at the delivery or the development of laryngeal papillomas in the infant.

D. Routine screening for syphilis and gonorrhea is appropriate. Screening for the following is felt at present to be either impractical or controversial:
Chlamydia. Infants born to women who are colonized may develop inclusion conjunctivitis or pneumonitis.
Cytomegalovirus. Definite maternal infection in early pregnancy may warrant abortion because of the risk of mental retardation or central nervous system abnormalities. However, maternal infection is often asymptomatic.
Mycoplasma. This may be associated with spontaneous abortion, decreased birth weight, or postpartum fever. No major neonatal problems have been identified.
Group B Streptococcus. Twenty percent of pregnant women are colonized. Only a small percentage of their offspring develop streptococcal infection

REFERENCES

McCormack WM: Management of sexually transmissible infections during pregnancy. Clin Obstet Gynecol 18:57, 1975

Fiumara NJ: *The Sexually Transmitted Diseases.* Boston: Commonwealth of Massachusetts Department of Public Health, 1978

Sexually transmitted diseases. American College of Obstetricians and Gynecologists Technical Bulletins Nos. 50 and 51, 1978

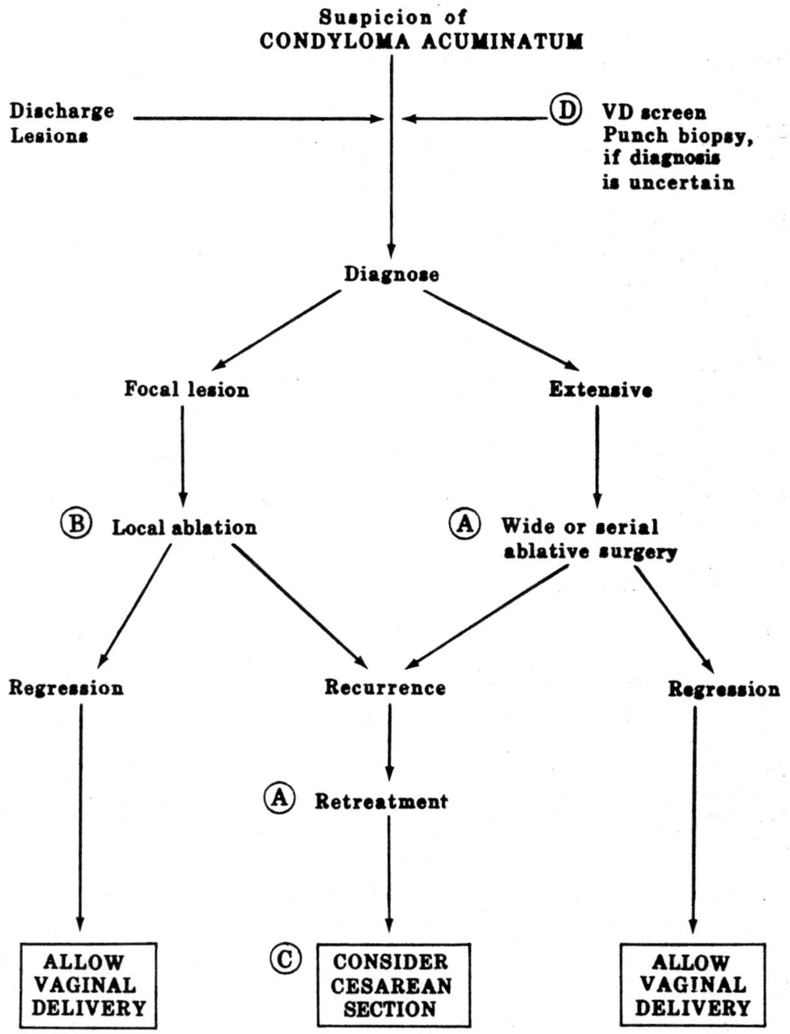
Suspicion of
CONDYLOMA ACUMINATUM
Discharge
Lesions
D VD screen
Punch biopsy,
if diagnosis
is uncertain
Diagnose
Focal lesion
Extensive
B Local ablation
A Wide or serial
ablative surgery
Regression
Recurrence
Regression
A Retreatment
ALLOW
VAGINAL
DELIVERY
C CONSIDER
CESAREAN
SECTION
ALLOW
VAGINAL
DELIVERY

HERPES VIRUS INFECTION

Austin Wertheimer, M.D. and John Modlin, M.D.

COMMENTS

A. Papanicolaou smear or Tzanck smear may be substituted to look for multinucleated giant cells if herpes culture is not available or rapid determination is necessary. However, there is a 20 to 40 percent false-negative rate with these methods.

B. There are a few reports in the literature of significant prenatal infection. If a primary maternal herpes infection is diagnosed in the first or second trimester, the option of amniocentesis with culture of amniotic fluid may be discussed. This is controversial, because virus has been found in amniotic fluid in cases in which the fetus was normal. Infection in utero following a recurrent episode is thought not to be of clinical significance because maternal antibodies prevent viremia.

C. Weekly screening from 32 weeks has been proposed, particularly for those at risk of premature labor. Fifty percent of infants who contract congenital herpes are born prematurely.

D. If recent cultures are positive, the option of scheduled cesarean section may be discussed with a patient who may not want to risk occult or prolonged rupture of membranes.

E. It is often recommended that vaginal delivery be considered if membranes are ruptured for more than 4 hours. It is the feeling at our institution, however, that if most recent cultures are positive or if an active lesion is present in labor, cesarean section should be performed regardless of membrane status. This is done to minimize direct contact between fetus and virus.

REFERENCES

Grossman JH, Wallen WC, Sever JL: Management of genital herpes simplex virus infection during pregnancy. Obstet Gynecol 58:1, 1981

Sever JL: Reducing the risk of congenital herpes. Contemporary Ob/Gyn 17:191, 1981

Stevenson RE: Herpes simplex virus. In *The Fetus and Newly Born Infant.* St. Louis: CV Mosby, 1977, pp 209–214

Whitley RJ, Nahmias AJ, Visintine AM, Fleming CL, Alford CA: The natural history of herpes simplex virus infection of mother and newborn. Obstet Gynecol Survey 36: 359, 1981

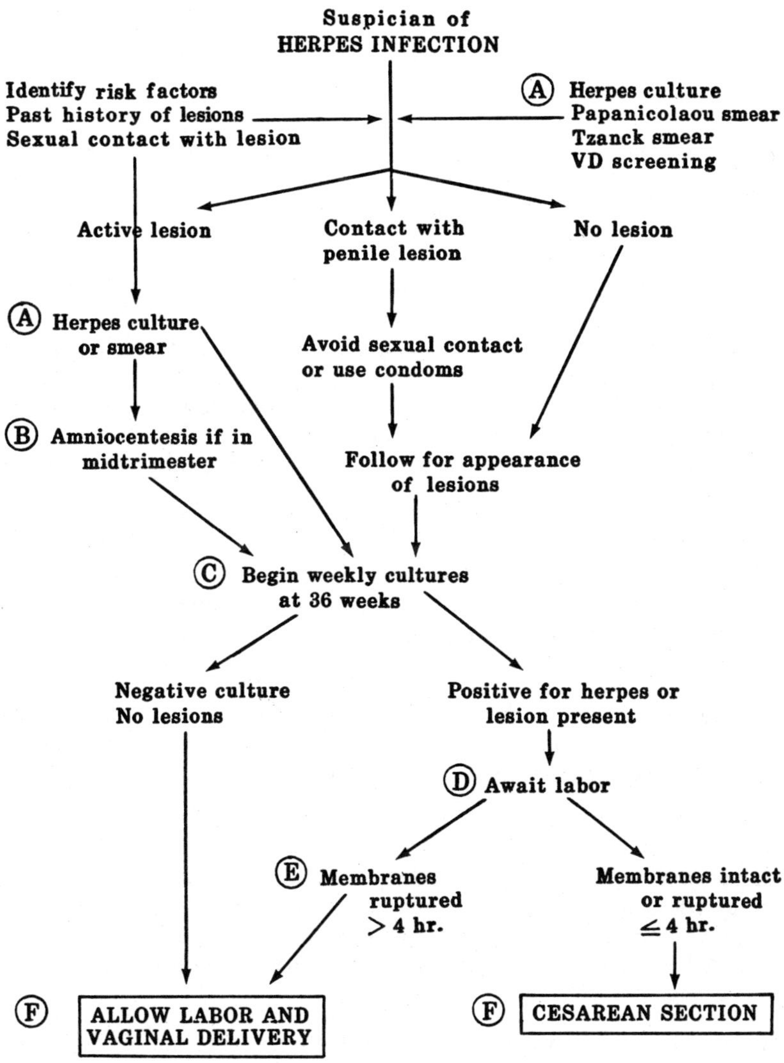
Suspician of
HERPES INFECTION
Identify risk factors
Past history of lesions
Sexual contact with lesion
(A) Herpes culture
Papanicolaou smear
Tzanck smear
VD screening
Active lesion
Contact with
penile lesion
No lesion
(A) Herpes culture
or smear
Avoid sexual contact
or use condoms
(B) Amniocentesis if in
midtrimester
Follow for appearance
of lesions
(C) Begin weekly cultures
at 36 weeks
Negative culture
No lesions
Positive for herpes or
lesion present
(D) Await labor
(E) Membranes
ruptured
> 4 hr.
Membranes intact
or ruptured
≤ 4 hr.
(F) ALLOW LABOR AND
VAGINAL DELIVERY
(F) CESAREAN SECTION

ABNORMAL CERVICAL CYTOLOGY

Louis Burke, M.D.

COMMENTS

A. Abnormal smears showing cervical intraepithelial neoplasia (CIN) can be expected in 40–50 asymptomatic women per 1000 screened; of these 40–50, only 2–3 will have invasive cancer. Among the younger population, a trend toward more CIN has been observed, reflected in an increased rate of detection of CIN during pregnancy. There is a 3–4 percent incidence of abnormal cytology associated with pregnancy.

B. Action is taken on the first smear showing dysplastic cells. Vaginal delivery is permissible in the presence of CIN, but invasive cancer must be aggressively attacked without delay. While ruling out the remote possibility of invasion, however, one must avoid injury to the fetus, premature labor, and harm to the mother. Colposcopy with directed biopsy has made it possible to evaluate these patients and, at the same time, avoid cervical conization in more than 90 percent (see F, below).

C. A satisfactory examination is one in which the entire lesion, squamous-columnar junction, and transformation zone can be clearly visualized, examined, and biopsied. Normal endocervical columnar epithelium must be seen cephalad to these areas.

D. An unsatisfactory examination is one that does not meet the aforementioned criteria (see C, above). Typically, the upper edge of the lesion is located within the cervical canal and is not accessible for examination and/or biopsy.

E. Lesions may be graded according to the method of Coppleson, based on color, surface texture, vascular atypia, and intercapillary distance. Invasive carcinoma is never associated with a grade I lesion (that is, one showing minimal colposcopic changes). Therefore, if the cytology suggests CIN 1 (mild dysplasia) only, it may not be necessary to biopsy the lesion. All other lesions are biopsied for histologic examination.

F. A principal objective here is to avoid cervical conization in pregnancy, if at all possible. If diagnosis cannot be made by any other means, conization may be done. However, it is important to weigh its risks, including severe hemorrhage, secondary infection, abortion, and incompetent cervix.

REFERENCES

Burke L, Mathews B: *Colposcopy in Clinical Practice.* Philadelphia: FA Davis, 1977

Feldman MJ, Linzey EM, Srebnik E, Kent DR, Goldstein AI, Nelson M: Abnormal cervical cytology in the teen-ager. Am J Obstet Gynecol 126:418, 1976

Kohan S, Beckman EM, Bigelow B, Klein SA, Douglas GW: Role of colposcopy in the management of CIN during pregnancy and post partum. J Reprod Med 25:279, 1980

Talebian F, Krumholz BA, Shayan A, Mann L: Colposcopic evaluation of patients with abnormal cytologic smears during pregnancy. Obstet Gynecol 47:693, 1976

ABNORMAL CERVICAL CYTOLOGY

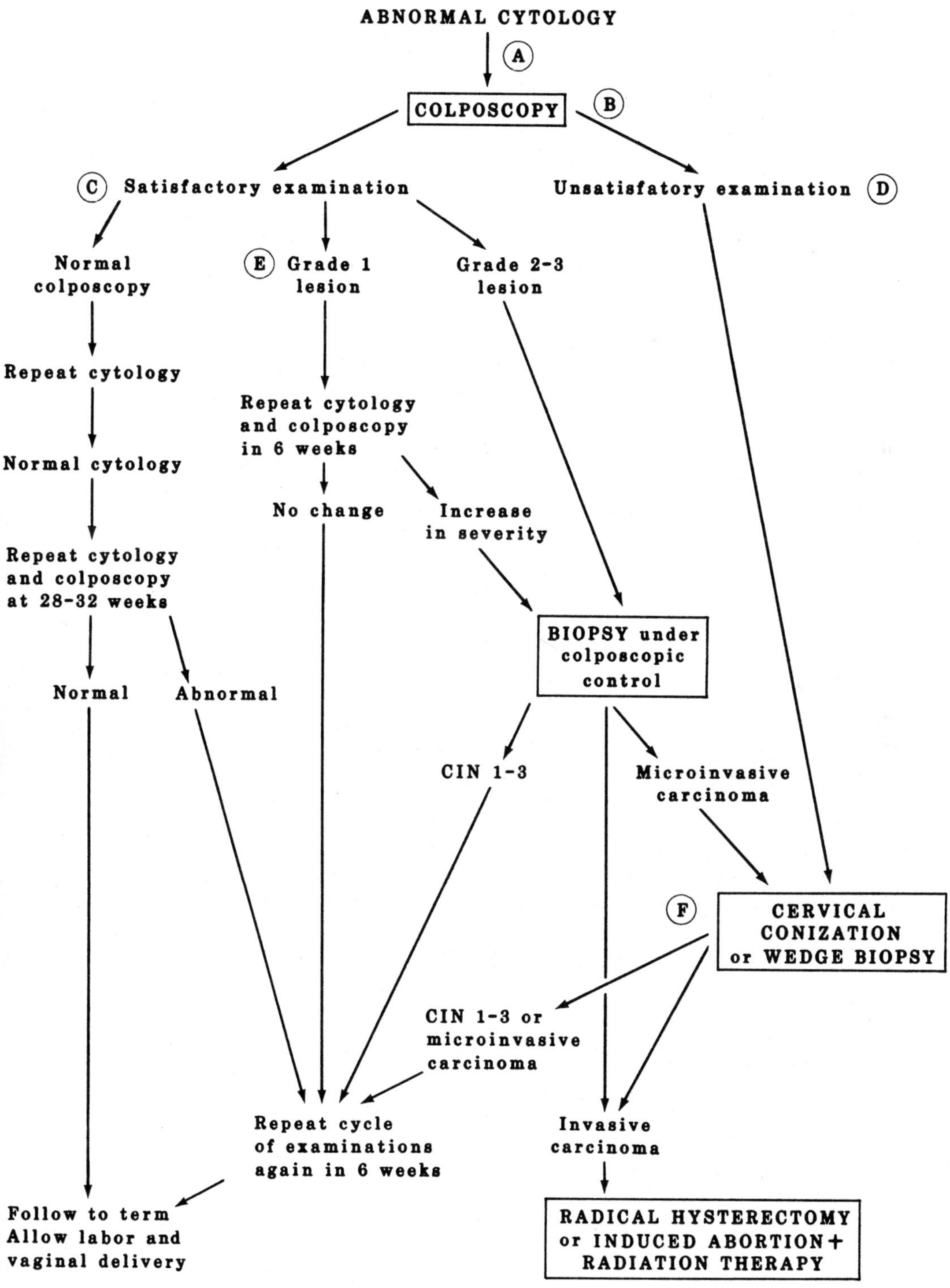

BACTERIURIA

Balmookoot Balgobin, M.D.

COMMENTS

A. Quantitative urine culture, using aerobic agar pour plate dilution technique to give the number of colonies per milliliter, is accurate but time-consuming and expensive. For reliable culture data, uncontaminated urine specimens are needed. The clean catch method is widely used. It avoids catheterization with its risk of infection. The patient washes her hands and cleanses the vulva. Then, separating the labia, she begins to void, collecting only the middle portion of the stream in a sterile container. The specimen is cultured immediately or refrigerated. Alternative techniques include catheterization or suprapubic aspiration. Colony counts exceeding 100,000 per ml indicate significant bacteriuria (especially if found in two consecutive specimens).

B. Antibiotic choice is guided by urinary Gram stain, culture, and sensitivity tests. Take care to avoid undesirable maternal and fetal effects. Suitable programs for asymptomatic bacteriuria or simple cystitis include ampicillin or Keflex (500 mg 4 times daily for 10–14 days) or sulfisoxazole (Gantrisin, 1 gm 4 times daily for 10–14 days).

C. Acute pyelonephritis may reduce glomerular filtration rate, making antibiotic choice difficult. Therefore, renal function should be evaluated with attention to intake and output, serum urea nitrogen, creatinine, and creatinine clearance.

D. Patients with acute pyelonephritis require hydration with intravenous fluids and vigorous antibiotic therapy, such as ampicillin or Keflin intravenously (1 g every 6 hours until afebrile for 48 hours, then 500 mg orally 4 times daily for 14 days). Gentamycin may also be used, but its ototoxicity must be borne in mind (it may be avoided by maintaining serum levels below 10 μg/ml). In life-threatening situations, kanamycin or gentamycin may be considered despite known toxicity; they may also be indicated in patients who are allergic to penicillin or who have infections with organisms that are resistant to penicillin and cephalosporin.

E. In unremitting cases, suspect obstructive disease or urinary tract abnormality. Ultrasonography may detect hydronephrosis. Renal calculi will pass spontaneously with conservative therapy in about half the cases. Reserve intravenous pyelography for such resistant cases. In severe symptomatic obstruction, manipulation via cystoscopy or retrograde ureteral catheterization may help provide drainage or dislodge the stone. Rarely, persistent obstruction may require surgical intervention. All patients with recurrent persistent urinary tract infections should be investigated post partum by intravenous pyelography.

REFERENCES

Harris RE: The significance of eradication of asymptomatic bacteriuria. Obstet Gynecol 52:71, 1979

Harris RE, Gilstrap LC: Prevention of recurrent pyelonephritis during pregnancy. Obstet Gynecol 44:637, 1974

Whalley PJ, Cunningham FG: Short term versus continuous antimicrobial therapy for asymptomatic bacteriuria in pregnancy. Obstet Gynecol 49:262, 1977

Whalley PJ, Cunningham FG, Martin FG: Transient renal dysfunction associated with acute pyelonephritis of pregnancy. Obstet Gynecol 46:174, 1974

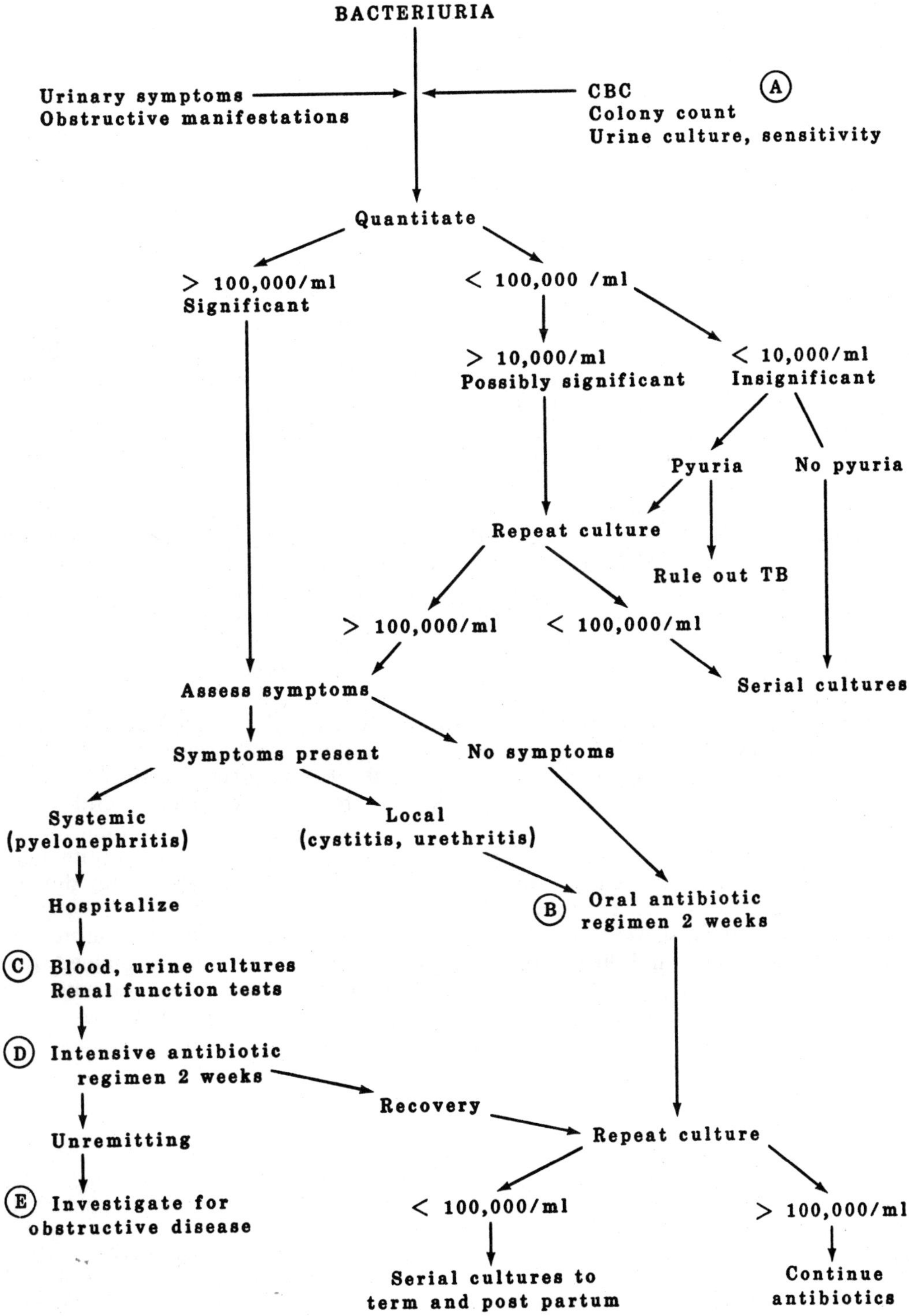
BACTERIURIA
Urinary symptoms
Obstructive manifestations
CBC
Colony count
Urine culture, sensitivity
A
Quantitate
> 100,000/ml
Significant
< 100,000 /ml
> 10,000/ml
Possibly significant
< 10,000/ml
Insignificant
Pyuria
No pyuria
Repeat culture
Rule out TB
> 100,000/ml
< 100,000/ml
Serial cultures
Assess symptoms
Symptoms present
No symptoms
Systemic
(pyelonephritis)
Local
(cystitis, urethritis)
Hospitalize
B
Oral antibiotic
regimen 2 weeks
C
Blood, urine cultures
Renal function tests
D
Intensive antibiotic
regimen 2 weeks
Recovery
Repeat culture
Unremitting
E
Investigate for
obstructive disease
< 100,000/ml
> 100,000/ml
Serial cultures to
term and post partum
Continue
antibiotics

PREMATURE RUPTURE OF MEMBRANES

Max Borten, M.D.

COMMENTS

A. Rupture of the membranes before labor carries a risk of infection. If managed conservatively with careful periodic assessment for the earliest appearance of amnionitis, these cases do well. Aggressive intervention is essential once infection develops.

B. In doubtful cases, confirm by sterile speculum examination and by testing the vaginal pool fluid pH with Nitrazine paper; if alkaline, it is probably amniotic fluid. Spread the specimen on a glass slide and allow it to dry in air to show characteristic ferning. Microscopically, one may see fetal squamous cells and lanugo. If volume is adequate, the glucose-fructose ratio may help. If the diagnosis is still in doubt, inject marker dye by amniocentesis (especially if also assessing fetal maturity); if the dye later appears in the vagina, it confirms rupture of the membranes.

C. Incipient or overt infection and fetal maturity should be investigated. Amniotic fluid is obtained vaginally (e.g., by sheathed sterile transcervical catheter) for smear and culture. The presence of bacteria and polymorphonuclear leukocytes does not prove overt amnionitis, but the clear absence of either bacteria or white cells is reassuring. If in doubt, examine a sample obtained by amniocentesis. Serum C-reactive protein may prove a useful early predictor of infection. Frequent observations of temperature, white blood count, and differential must be done, but may reflect only fully developed amnionitis.

D. The longer the membranes are ruptured before labor, the greater the risk of infection. Most patients will do well provided one has ruled out amnionitis, even in its preclinical form, from the outset. One has to weigh the risk of interference against the risk of infection. One may allow the preterm pregnancy to continue under careful surveillance in a hospital setting to avoid the risks of prematurity, failed or complicated induction, and the frequent need for cesarean section. At term, with more optimal conditions, the balance between risk and benefit is far less clear; induction may diminish the costs and inconveniences of a long hospital stay.

E. Manage by frequent surveillance of the hospitalized patient. Obtain temperature every 4 hours, white count and differential daily, and amniotic fluid smear (obtained transcervically under sterile conditions) for leukopedesis and bacteria on alternate days. Lacking evidence of infection, one need not intervene for ruptured membranes.

REFERENCES

Evans MI, Hajj SN, Devoe LD, Angerman NS, Moawad AH: C-reactive protein as a predictor of infectious morbidity with premature rupture of membranes. Am J Obstet Gynecol 138:648, 1980

Huff RW: Antibiotic prophylaxis for puerperal endometritis following premature rupture of the membranes. J Reprod Med 19:79, 1977

Kappy KA, Cetrulo CL, Knuppel RA, Ingardia CJ, Sbarra AJ, Scerbo JC, Mitchell GW: Premature rupture of the membranes: A conservative approach. Am J Obstet Gynecol 134:655, 1979

Stedman CM, Crawford S, Staten E, Cherny WB: Management of preterm premature rupture of membranes: Assessing amniotic fluid in the vagina for phosphatidylglycerol. Am J Obstet Gynecol 140:34, 1981

PREMATURE RUPTURE OF MEMBRANES

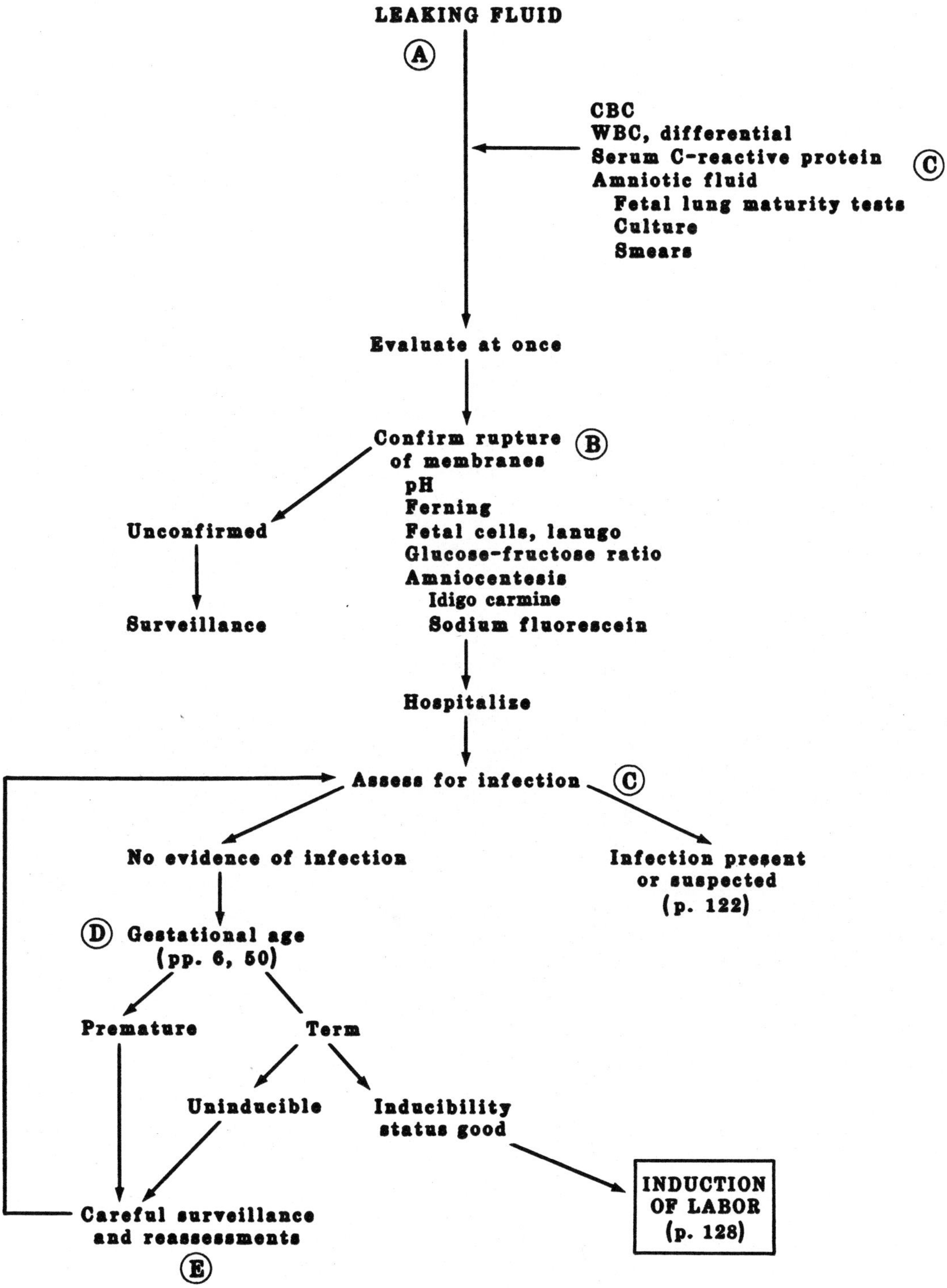

CHORIOAMNIONITIS

Max Borten, M.D.

COMMENTS

A. Chorioamnionitis is one of the most serious complications of the third trimester of pregnancy. It is associated with high fetal morbidity and mortality rates, and it threatens serious maternal sepsis with the risk of death from generalized septicemia. Once it develops, this life-threatening infection must be treated aggressively and decisively.

B. Chorioamnionitis is not limited to the third trimester, of course. Infection of amniotic fluid and membranes can occur, for example, as a result of transabdominal puncture in the course of amniocentesis, intrauterine transfusion, or fetoscopy. A difficult procedure with repeated punctures increases the likelihood of this complication.

C. Laboratory tests done for baseline evaluation and to confirm the diagnosis must be interpreted with caution. Pregnancy increases the erythrocyte sedimentation rate and white blood count. The presence of leukocytes and bacteria on a smear of amniotic fluid cannot be said to determine the diagnosis of chorioamnionitis; however, the absence of white blood cells or bacteria does suggest that the fever may originate from an extrauterine source.

D. Antibiotic therapy should be started as soon as the diagnosis has been made and after appropriate cultures have been obtained. If vaginal delivery is expected soon, one can delay administering antibiotics. This will enable one to obtain cultures from the newborn infant; such cultures can be interpreted reliably. It is important that the neonatologist be involved in the decision-making process and be present at the delivery. A brief delay in initiating antibiotic therapy does not appear to affect the mother adversely insofar as postpartum morbidity is concerned. Chorioamnionitis is frequently associated with premature labor, but use of steroid medication for purposes of enhancing pulmonary maturity is contraindicated.

E. Vaginal delivery is the route of choice for women with chorioamnionitis. Cesarean section should be limited to those requiring abdominal delivery for obstetric complications. If cesarean section should be indicated and undertaken, there is no clear evidence that the extraperitoneal approach will reduce postoperative morbidity as compared with the traditional transperitoneal technique.

REFERENCES

Bobbit RJ, Ledger WJ: Unrecognized amnionitis and prematurity: A preliminary report. J Reprod Med 19:8, 1977

Koh KS, Chan FH, Monfared AH, Ledger WS, Paul RH: The changing perinatal and maternal outcome in chorioamnionitis. Obstet Gynecol 53:730, 1979

Gibbs RS, Castillo MS, Rodgers PJ: Management of acute chorioamnionitis. Am J Obstet Gynecol 136:709, 1980

Shurin PA, Alpert S, Rosner B, Driscoll SG, Lee Y-H, McCormack WM, Santamarina BAG, Kass EH: Chorioamnionitis and colonization of the newborn infant with genital mycoplasmas. New Engl J Med 293:5, 1975

CHORIOAMNIONITIS

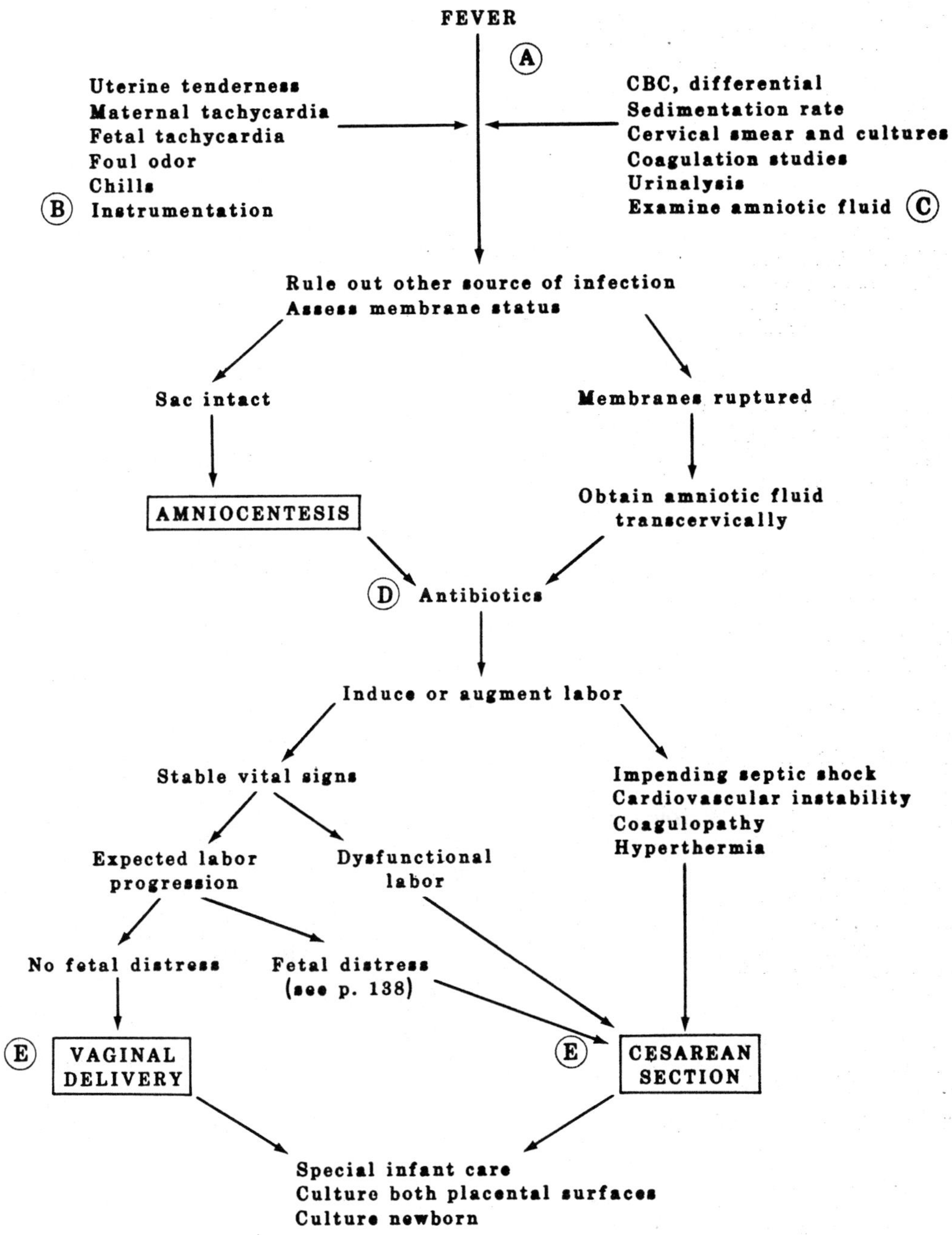

ARRESTING PREMATURE LABOR

Wayne R. Cohen, M.D.

COMMENTS

A. The diagnosis of premature labor requires that there be objective evidence of changing dilatation or effacement accompanying regular uterine contractions.

B. Bedrest and hydration may have some value in suppressing premature labor. Moreover, prompt treatment of a urinary tract infection, if present, may improve the likelihood of successful tocolysis.

C. Assessment of gestational age (p. 6) is important. Because neonatal mortality rates are very low after 34 complete weeks of gestation, labour can be allowed to evolve in such cases. However, if expert pediatric care is not available, 35–36 weeks might be considered a more appropriate threshold.

D. Absolute contraindications to arresting labor include amnionitis, nonremediable fetal distress, and maternal conditions that render the intrauterine environment progressively more hostile. Relative contraindications are rupture of membranes, cervical dilatation greater than 4 cm, and abruptio placentae. If the fetal lung is known to be mature, it is prudent to allow labor. Beta-mimetic agents should be used with caution in women with cardiopulmonary disease, thyrotoxicosis hypertension or diabetes.

E. Pulmonary maturity should be assessed by amniotic fluid lecithin/sphingomyelin (L/S) ratio or other measures of surfactant production (e.g., disaturated phosphatidylcholine). A shake test is useful while awaiting more definitive studies. In some marginal situations (e.g., ruptured membranes or suspicious fetal heart rate pattern), L/S ratio near maturity (greater than 1.5) may be acceptable because the risk of severe respiratory distress in the newborn is relatively low, while the risk of expectancy is somewhat increased.

F. High doses of corticosteroids given to the mother may reduce the frequency and severity of the respiratory distress syndrome in the newborn. Among tocolytic agents, only ritodrine, a beta-mimetic agent, is approved for use in the United States. It should be given initially by intravenous infusion (50 μg/min, increasing if needed to stop contractions to 300 μg/min). During administration, the mother should be well hydrated and in the lateral recumbent position. The concomitant use of steroids and beta-mimetic agents may cause maternal pulmonary edema; therefore, use these agents with caution, carefully monitoring both mother and fetus.

G. Corticosteroids appear to exert their maximum effect on the fetal lung in 48 hours. Ritodrine may therefore be continued begining 12 hr. after contractions stop (10 mg orally 4 times daily); repeat infusions are given if labor recurs, especially in cases with extreme prematurity and no developing contraindications to tocolysis.

REFERENCES

Alper M, Cohen WR: Pulmonary edema associated with ritodrine and corticosteroid therapy of threatened premature labor. Obstet Gynecol, in press

Cohen WR, Friedman EA: Etiology and management of premature labor. Curr Probl Obstet Gynecol 1:1, 1978

Liggins GC, Howie MD: A controlled trial of antepartum glucocorticoid treatment for prevention of respiratory distress syndrome in premature infants. Pediat 50:515, 1972

Merkatz IR, Peter JB, Barden TP: Ritodrine hydrochloride: Betamimetic agent for use in preterm labor: II. Evidence of efficacy. Obstet Gynecol 56:7, 1980

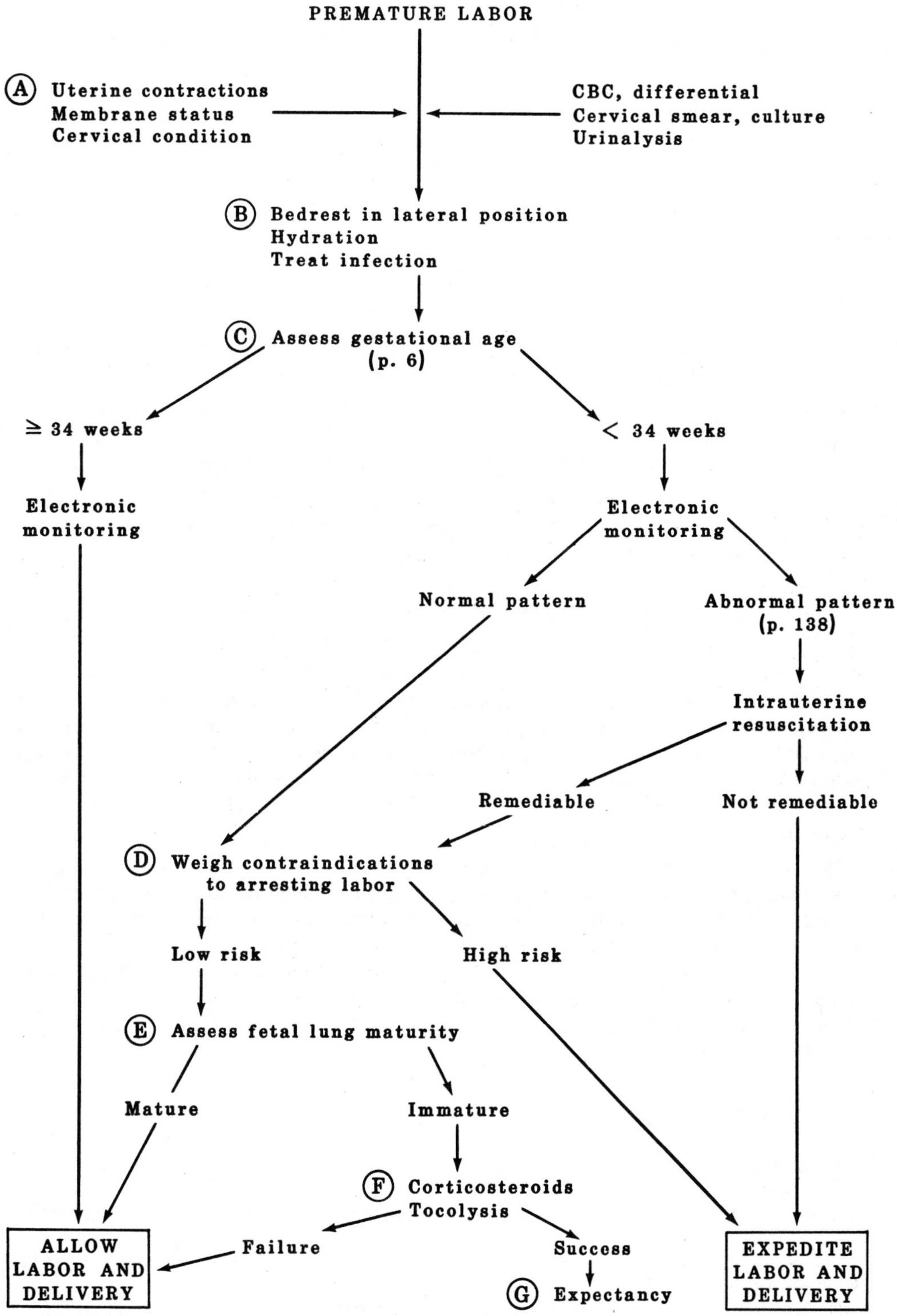
PREMATURE LABOR
A Uterine contractions
Membrane status
Cervical condition
CBC, differential
Cervical smear, culture
Urinalysis
B Bedrest in lateral position
Hydration
Treat infection
C Assess gestational age
(p. 6)
≥ 34 weeks
< 34 weeks
Electronic monitoring
Electronic monitoring
Normal pattern
Abnormal pattern
(p. 138)
Intrauterine resuscitation
Remediable
Not remediable
D Weigh contraindications to arresting labor
Low risk
High risk
E Assess fetal lung maturity
Mature
Immature
F Corticosteroids
Tocolysis
Failure
Success
G Expectancy
ALLOW LABOR AND DELIVERY
EXPEDITE LABOR AND DELIVERY

MANAGING PREMATURE LABOR AND DELIVERY

Wayne R. Cohen, M.D.

COMMENTS

A. The diagnosis of premature labor is made on the basis of observing objective changes in the cervix in response to uterine contractions.

B. The use of continuous electronic fetal heart rate (FHR) monitoring is important for maximizing the chance of a good outcome for a premature baby.

C. Information from FHR monitoring and fetal scalp blood sampling should be interpreted in the same way as for term fetuses. Severe hypoxemia may increase the risk and severity of respiratory distress syndrome of the newborn infant.

D. There is a bimodal distribution of premature labor patterns. That is, there are two kinds of labors characteristically seen: labors are often rapid, but an unexpectedly high frequency of abnormal labors occur as well.

E. Maternal analgesic medications should be used in minimally effective doses because premature newborn infants are particularly susceptible to their respiratory depressant effects. Epidural anesthesia is the preferred technique if pain relief is required.

F. Potential trauma to the fragile premature infant should be minimized. Using a generous episiotomy and avoiding forceps are important in this regard. There is no convincing evidence that forceps delivery provides protection for the premature fetal head. When cesarean section is indicated, an adequate uterine incision must be used to avoid excessive fetal head compression at delivery. When the lower uterine segment is narrow and not well developed, a vertical Kroenig or a classic incision is recommended.

G. If the baby requires resuscitation, the cord should be clamped and divided immediately so that appropriate resuscitative measures can be taken expeditiously. If the baby is vigorous, 30–45 seconds of passive placental transfusion provide the potential benefits of increased blood volume and red cell mass with minimal risks of severe circulatory overload or hyperbilirubinemia. All necessary equipment and personnel for neonatal resuscitation must always be present in the delivery room when anticipating the birth of a premature infant. The placenta should be studied pathologically to search for possible explanations for the premature labor.

REFERENCES

Cohen WR, Friedman EA: Etiology and management of premature labor. Curr Probl Obstet Gynecol 1:1, 1978

Epstein M: Resuscitation of the newborn. In Cohen WR, Friedman EA (eds): *Management of Labor.* Baltimore: University Park Press, 1983

Fanaroff AA, Merkatz IR: Modern obstetrical management of the low birth weight infant. Clin Perinat 4:215, 1977

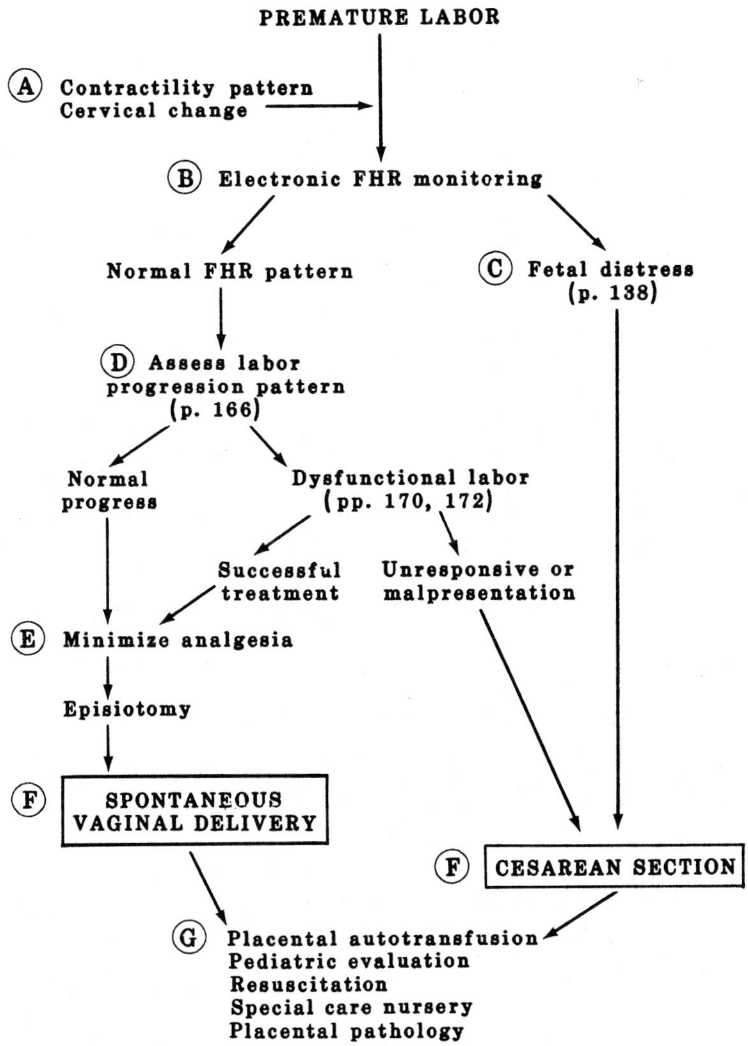
PREMATURE LABOR
(A) Contractility pattern
Cervical change
(B) Electronic FHR monitoring
Normal FHR pattern
(C) Fetal distress
(p. 138)
(D) Assess labor progression pattern
(p. 166)
Normal progress
Dysfunctional labor
(pp. 170, 172)
Successful treatment
Unresponsive or malpresentation
(E) Minimize analgesia
Episiotomy
(F) SPONTANEOUS VAGINAL DELIVERY
(F) CESAREAN SECTION
(G) Placental autotransfusion
Pediatric evaluation
Resuscitation
Special care nursery
Placental pathology

INDUCTION OF LABOR

Emanuel A. Friedman, M.D.

COMMENTS

A. Elective induction is no longer condoned. Indications are conditions that place mother or fetus in jeopardy greater than that of the induction. These include pregnancy-induced hypertension, diabetes mellitus, erythroblastosis fetalis, amnionitis, and abruptio placentae.

B. Selection criteria are fetal maturity (verified by amniotic fluid L/S ratio), cervical condition, fetal presentation, pelvic adequacy, and uterine integrity. Malpresentation, cephalopelvic disproportion, fetal distress, uterine overdistention, and cesarean section or myomectomy scar are contraindications. Prerequisites are personnel and facility suitability, patient's acceptance, and physician presence.

C. The Bishop score assesses inducibility. Points are tallied for each of 5 factors:
  (1) cervical dilatation (closed = 0, 1–2 cm = 1, 3–4 cm = 2, 5+ cm = 3);
  (2) effacement (0–30% = 0, 40–50% = 1, 60–70% = 2, 80+ percent = 3);
  (3) fetal station (−3 = 0, −2 = 1, −1 or 0 = 2, +1 or +2 = 3);
  (4) cervical consistency (firm = 0, medium = 1, soft = 2); and
  (5) cervical position (posterior = 0, midposition = 1, anterior = 2).

  Scores of 9 or more are expected to be readily inducible; scores of 0 to 4 indicate a 20 percent failure rate.

D. Amniotomy will often initiate labor within 6 hours with a high Bishop score. If successful induction is in doubt or if the indications are too weak to warrant cesarean section in the event the induction fails, the membranes should be left intact. If the fetus is at risk, electronic fetal heart rate monitoring is in order (see p. 136).

E. Oxytocin is administered in dilute solutions (10 IU in 1000 ml 5 percent aqueous dextrose) by carefully titrated infusion beginning at 6–8 drops/min increasing by 4 drops/min every 15–30 minutes until strong clinical labor is produced. Use of an infusion pump is preferable. Frequent monitoring of uterine contractions, vital signs, and fetal status is essential until they are stabilized and then at intervals of 15 minutes. Reduce drip rate if contractions become excessive or an adverse reaction develops.

F. Weighing possible benefits against risk is critical if the Bishop score is low because the chance of failure is great. If the indication is strong, one can proceed with both amniotomy and oxytocin infusion, recognizing that cesarean section will be needed if the induction fails. If the indication is weak, consider desisting altogether or giving a trial of oxytocin only.

G. "Priming" the cervix, not yet recommended for clinical practice, involves use of laminaria, cervical balloon, or prostaglandins (not an approved use). All require time for an effect. Once the cervix is favorable, induction by oxytocin infusion may be successful.

H. Cesarean section is done for failed induction if the maternal or fetal condition warrants delivery at that time or if the membranes have been ruptured unduly long and vaginal delivery within a few hours is unlikely.

REFERENCES

Bishop EH: Pelvic scoring for elective induction. Obstet Gynecol 24:266, 1964

Cross WG, Pitkin RM: Laminaria as an adjunct in induction of labor. Obstet Gynecol 51:606, 1978

Friedman EA, Niswander KR, Bayonet-Rivera NP, Sachtleben MR: Relation of prelabor evaluation to inducibility and the course of labor. Obstet Gynecol 28:495, 1966

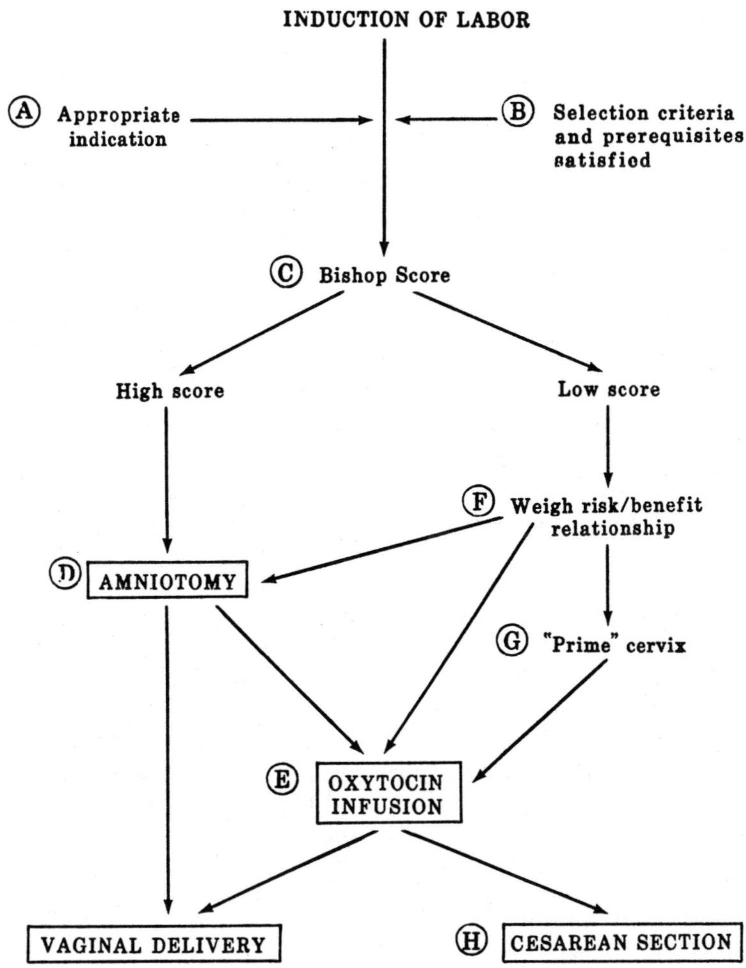
INDUCTION OF LABOR
Ⓐ Appropriate indication
Ⓑ Selection criteria and prerequisites satisfied
Ⓒ Bishop Score
High score
Low score
Ⓕ Weigh risk/benefit relationship
Ⓓ AMNIOTOMY
Ⓖ "Prime" cervix
Ⓔ OXYTOCIN INFUSION
VAGINAL DELIVERY
Ⓗ CESAREAN SECTION

POST-TERM PREGNANCY

Selwyn P. Oskowitz, M.B.

COMMENTS

A. Conditions associated with pregnancy prolonged beyond 42 weeks include an abnormal fetus (particularly anencephaly) and the use of certain drugs (such as aspirin and other inhibitors of prostaglandin synthesis). Post-term pregnancy is also seen with large fetuses and in elderly gravidas.

B. Patients with poorly documented dates are frequently those who seek obstetric care late in the pregnancy. Their gestational milestones may be inappropriate, for example, the fetal heart may not have been heard by 20 weeks or the uterine fundal height may not have been consistent with dates. They may not be able to recall the date of their last menstrual period or they may have conceived while breast feeding, while on oral contraceptives, or while amenorrheic. Assessment of dates is further complicated in women who are poorly compliant in regard to recommendations given to them to improve their care and reduce their risk.

C. Fetal dysmaturity is the condition of intrauterine malnutrition resulting from fetoplacental insufficiency; it may be associated with growth retardation if severe and present for a long time. It is difficult to diagnose before birth, but it may be associated with oligohydramnios and thick meconium staining of the amniotic fluid. Ultrasonography may show the presence of oligohydramnios; growth retardation, however, is difficult to ascertain in the post-term pregnancy without prior serial examinations. Decreased fetal movement and maternal weight loss are suggestive worrisome features. Some use transcervical amnioscopy to determine if meconium is present in the amniotic fluid; amniocentesis may also be done for this purpose.

D. The current controversy in management of post-term pregnancy centers on whether or not active intervention is indicated in the absence of objective evidence of fetoplacental insufficiency. Elective induction of labor with oxytocin is no longer acceptable (p. 128); whether induction can be justified as indicated on the basis of anticipated problems is questionable. As long as the fetus can be documented to be in good condition, allowing the pregnancy to continue is appropriate, with frequent periodic reassessments as in any other high-risk situation.

E. In those cases in which expeditious delivery is desirable and vaginal delivery preferred, it may be possible to alter an uninducible cervix so that induction of labor becomes more feasible. Priming techniques, including use of laminaria or a Foley catheter in the cervix, carry risks of infection.

REFERENCES

Boyce A, Mayaux MJ, Schwartz O: Classical and true gestational postmaturity. Am J Obstet Gynecol 125:911, 1976

Hertz RH, Sokol RJ, Knoke JD, Rosen MG, Chik L, Hirsch VJ: Clinical estimation of gestational age: Rules for avoiding preterm delivery. Am J Obstet Gynecol 131:395, 1978

Klapholz H, Friedman EA: The incidence of intrapartum fetal distress with advancing gestational age. Am J Obstet Gynecol 127:405, 1977

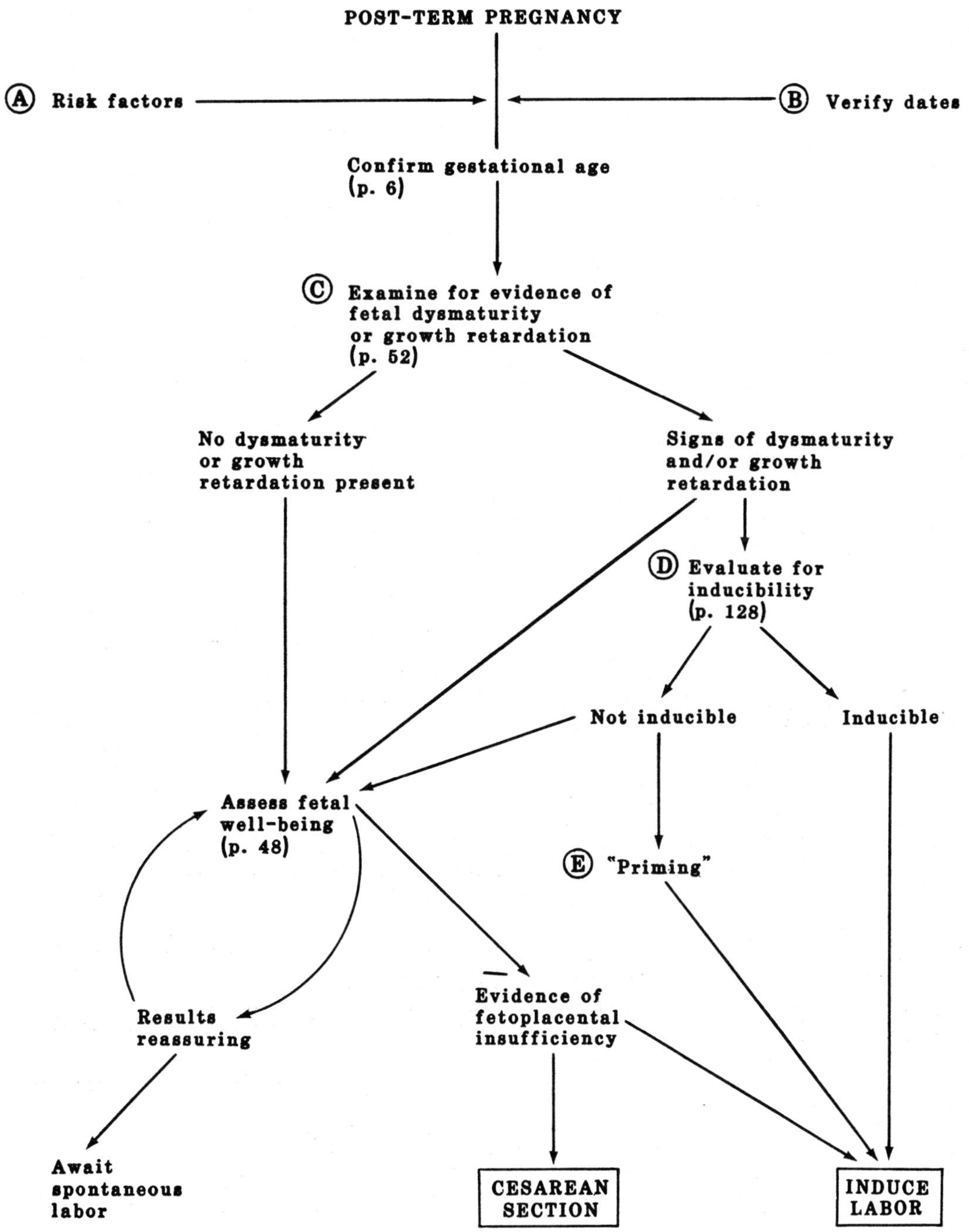
POST-TERM PREGNANCY
Ⓐ Risk factors
Ⓑ Verify dates
Confirm gestational age (p. 6)
Ⓒ Examine for evidence of fetal dysmaturity or growth retardation (p. 52)
No dysmaturity or growth retardation present
Signs of dysmaturity and/or growth retardation
Ⓓ Evaluate for inducibility (p. 128)
Not inducible
Inducible
Assess fetal well-being (p. 48)
Ⓔ "Priming"
Evidence of fetoplacental insufficiency
Results reassuring
Await spontaneous labor
CESAREAN SECTION
INDUCE LABOR

ANALGESIA IN LABOR

David J. Snyder, M.D.

COMMENTS

A. The analgesia regimen should be designed to minimize risk and ensure safety. It should not adversely affect the labor process or impact unfavorably on the fetus. Choice of analgesia depends not only on the patient's emotional condition and desires regarding pain relief and state of awareness during labor and at delivery, but must take into account a number of other relevant factors. Her medical condition is of obvious importance. Chronic obstructive pulmonary disease, for example, will dictate avoidance of agents that potentially depress respiratory function and recommend the use of a continuous regional block to minimize the stresses on an already compromised respiratory state (p. 96). Prior obstetric history can be helpful; a previous rapid labor suggests reliance on short-acting agents that are unlikely to depress the newborn infant if it should be delivered quickly. The status of the fetus is also critical (p. 136), as is the nature of the labor process (p. 166).

B. The latent phase is readily inhibited by use of narcotic analgesic agents, especially if given in large doses. Regional block anesthesia is likewise to be avoided for the same reason. Barbiturates, by contrast, are less inhibitory. Nonetheless, the use in labor of short- and medium-acting barbiturates, such as secobarbital, has been discouraged in view of their prolonged neonatal depressant effects, with somnolence, hypoventilation, hypotonia, and diminished attention span for up to 2 to 4 days. These sedative-hypnotic drugs have no analgesic effect for the patient in labor and may induce paradoxical excitement and disorientation in the presence of pain. Their use is suggested only during the very early latent phase, 12 to 24 hours before the expected time of delivery. Tranquilizers are useful, including promethazine, propiomazine, hydroxyzine, and diazepam, especially because they potentiate the analgesic effects of narcotic agents, which can then be given in much smaller doses. Narcolept-analgesia (with Innovar, for example) may be effective as well, both late in the latent phase and in the early active phase of labor.

C. The mainstay of pharmacologic pain relief in labor is narcotic analgesia. Narcotic analgesics are administered during the active phase of labor to reduce rather than to eliminate pain; their concomitant effects of respiratory depression, peripheral vasodilatation with postural hypotension, and diminished gastric motility must be recognized. They result in neonatal respiratory depression if given 2-3 hours before delivery. The choice and route of administration of a narcotic should be based on the desired onset and duration of action of the particular drug. The principal agents in current use are meperidine, pentazocine, and fentanyl. Their use should be minimized if labor is unduly rapid or abnormally slow or if one anticipates that regional block will be given (p. 134).

REFERENCES

Brackbill Y, Kane J, Mannielo RL: Obstetric meperidine usage and assessment of neonatal status. Anesthesiol 40:116, 1974

Irving FC: Advantages and disadvantages of barbiturates in obstetrics. R I Med J 28:493, 1945

Ovadia L, Halbrecht I: Neuroleptanalgesia: A new method of anesthesia for normal childbirth. Harefuah 72:143, 1967

Scott JR, Rose NB: Effects of psychoprophylaxis (Lamaze preparation) on labor and delivery in primiparas. New Engl J Med 294:1205, 1976

Yeh SY, Paul RH, Cordero L, Hon EH: A study of diazepam during labor. Obstet Gynecol 43· 363, 1974

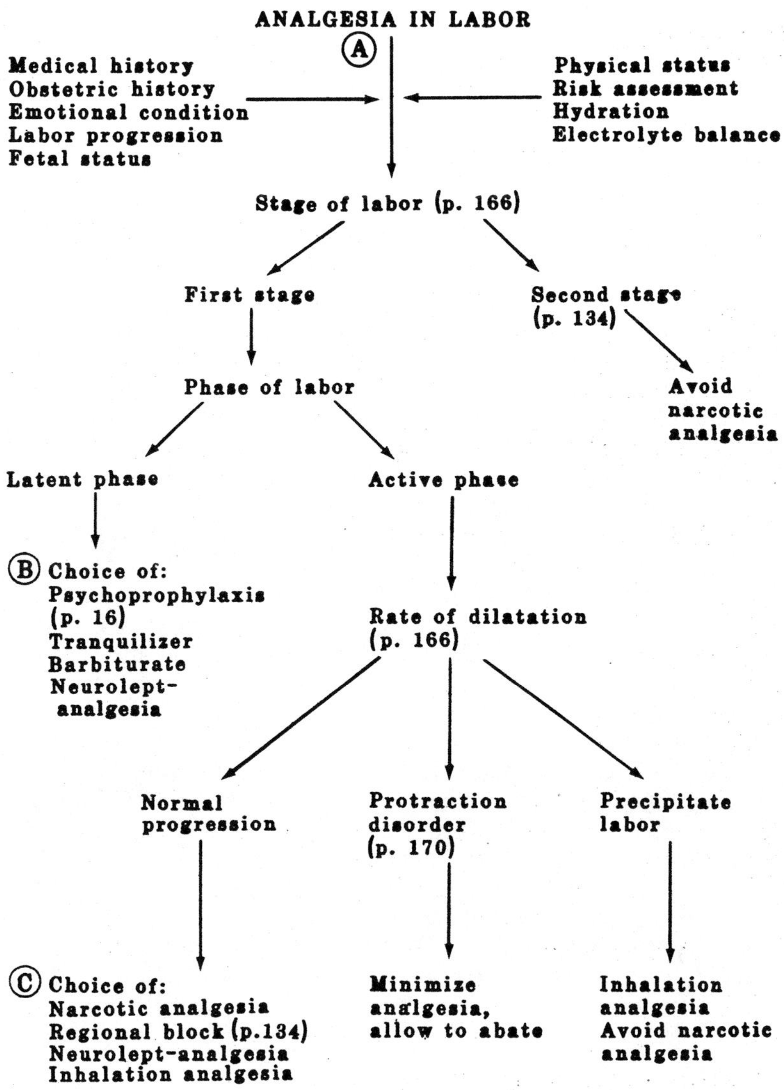
ANALGESIA IN LABOR
(A)
Medical history
Obstetric history
Emotional condition
Labor progression
Fetal status
Physical status
Risk assessment
Hydration
Electrolyte balance
Stage of labor (p. 166)
First stage
Second stage
(p. 134)
Avoid
narcotic
analgesia
Phase of labor
Latent phase
Active phase
(B) Choice of:
Psychoprophylaxis
(p. 16)
Tranquilizer
Barbiturate
Neurolept-
analgesia
Rate of dilatation
(p. 166)
Normal
progression
Protraction
disorder
(p. 170)
Precipitate
labor
(C) Choice of:
Narcotic analgesia
Regional block (p.134)
Neurolept-analgesia
Inhalation analgesia
Minimize
analgesia,
allow to abate
Inhalation
analgesia
Avoid narcotic
analgesia

ANESTHESIA FOR DELIVERY

David J. Snyder, M.D.

COMMENTS

A. Choice of anesthesia for delivery is based on the skills and capabilities of available personnel, the mother's general state of health, and her desire to be awake or asleep for delivery.

B. Anesthesia requirements differ for vaginal delivery versus cesarean section. One may have to modify the type, depth or level of anesthesia to accommodate to changing needs.

C. The patient who wishes to remain awake benefits from psychoprophylactic preparation (p. 16). If local or pudendal block anesthesia is used for the episiotomy and repair, avoid toxic dosages of the agent. Paracervical block anesthesia may be associated with fetal complications.

D. Supplement analgesics, if needed, by low dose ketamine, nitrous oxide-oxygen or methoxyflurane (Penthrane). Pregnancy decreases functional residual capacity, increases alveolar ventilation, and decreases anesthetic minimum alveolar concentration, thus facilitating induction of anesthesia. Inadvertent loss of consciousness may risk aspiration.

E. Forceps procedures require more than local infiltration or pudendal block. Uterine relaxation, if needed, cannot be accomplished with regional block anesthesia. The necessary depth of general anesthesia increases the risks. Halothane is effective, but it risks hemorrhage from uterine atony post partum.

F. Emergencies requiring cesarean section are common. Thus, a facility with suitable personnel and equipment for expeditiously dealing with critical problems is essential. Delay must be avoided. General anesthesia is preferable for emergencies. Assume the stomach to be full. Endotracheal intubation with an occlusive cuff will prevent gastric acid aspiration. Apply cricoid pressure to occlude the esophagus and then induce anesthesia rapidly with intravenous thiopental. Maintain anesthesia with nitrous oxide (50% with oxygen) and a muscle relaxant (D-tubocurarine).

G. Peridural anesthesia requires constant attendance and skill to deal with hypotension and drug reactions. Pudendal block, local infiltration or saddle block is effective for vaginal delivery, but a fuller block (spinal anesthesia to T-4) is required for cesarean section. Prophylactic vasopressors are commonly used to avert hypotension that may compound hypovolemia from blood loss. General anesthesia is preferable if acute hemorrhage is anticipated.

REFERENCES

Asling JK, Shnider SM, Margolis AJ, Way EL, Wilkinson GL: Paracervical block anesthesia in obstetrics: II. Etiology of fetal bradycardia following paracervical block anesthesia. Am J Obstet Gynecol 107:626, 1970

Coleman AJ, Downing JW: Enflurane anesthesia for cesarean section. Anesthesiol 43:354, 1975

Crawford JS: Patient management during extradural anaesthesia for obstetrics. Brit J Anaesth 47: 273, 1975

Galloon S: Ketamine for obstetric delivery. Anesthesiol 44:522, 1976

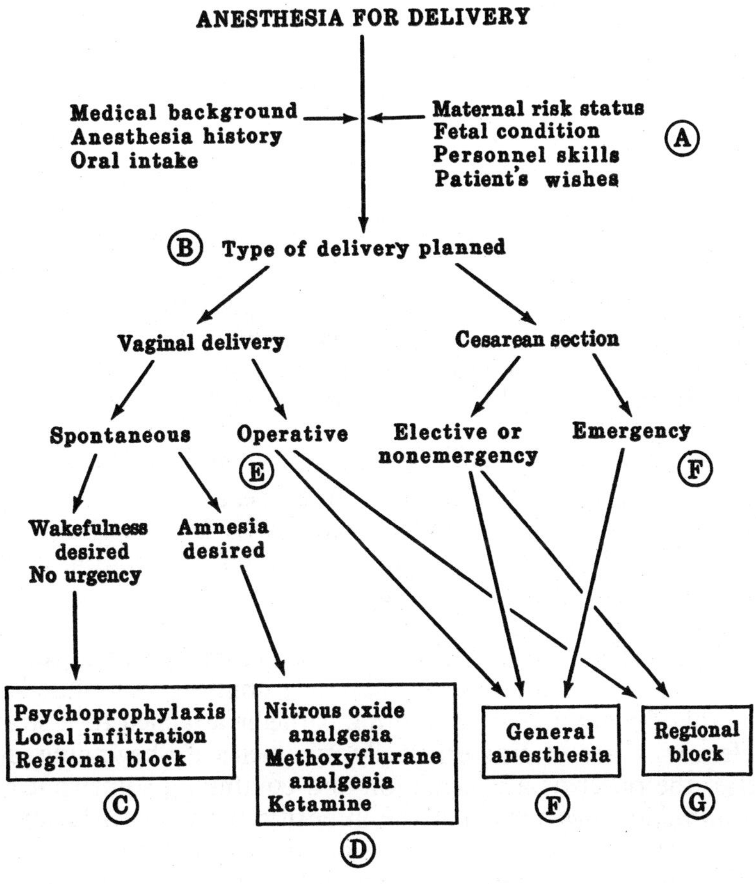
ANESTHESIA FOR DELIVERY
Medical background
Anesthesia history
Oral intake
Maternal risk status
Fetal condition
Personnel skills
Patient's wishes
A
B
Type of delivery planned
Vaginal delivery
Cesarean section
Spontaneous
Operative
E
Elective or nonemergency
Emergency
F
Wakefulness desired
No urgency
Amnesia desired
Psychoprophylaxis
Local infiltration
Regional block
C
Nitrous oxide analgesia
Methoxyflurane analgesia
Ketamine
D
General anesthesia
F
Regional block
G

FETAL MONITORING IN LABOR

Henry Klapholz, M.D.

COMMENTS

A. The absence of periodic heart rate changes (that is, decelerations from the baseline) and the presence of good reactivity (accelerations with fetal movement) are sufficient to assure fetal well-being. External monitors that utilize ultrasound transducers display artifactually increased variability owing to the uncertainty in the timing of the reflected fetal signals from the heart. Abdominal wall electrocardiography will display variability more accurately, but it is operable (that is, it gives a usable signal) in only 50 percent of the cases. Obesity and prematurity tend to reduce effectiveness of this technique.

B. Internal fetal heart rate monitoring provides a reliable electrocardiographic signal via a fetal scalp electrode. Continuous beat-to-beat rates are recorded and displayed, thus depicting variability accurately. It is relatively free of complications. Variability is difficult to quantitate, but a variation of 4–10 beats per minute from beat to beat is acceptable.

C. When periodic decelerations from the baseline are encountered, they should be related temporally to the uterine contractions (monitored simultaneously either by external tokodynamometer or internal catheter attached to a strain gauge). Late decelerations are characteristically symmetrical, beginning at least 20 seconds after the onset of a contraction and continuing somewhat beyond the time the contraction has subsided; the intensity of the deceleration is proportional to the amplitude of the contraction. Late decelerations, diagnostic of placental insufficiency, are repetitive. Variable decelerations rise and fall rapidly; they have variable shape, variable onset, and variable ending; they may even occur between contractions. Variable decelerations signify compression of the umbilical cord. Beat-to-beat variability (see A and B, above) is a function of the arousal state of the fetal central nervous system; it is absent in chronic hypoxia, after anesthesia or drug depression, and with some cardiac arrhythmias.

REFERENCES

Goodlin RC: Fetal cardiovascular responses to distress: A review. Obstet Gynecol 49:371, 1977

Hobbins JC, Freeman R, Queenan JT: The fetal monitoring debate. Pediatr 63:942, 1979

Hon EH, Petrie RH: Clinical value of fetal heart rate monitoring. Clin Obstet Gynecol 18: 1, 1975

Klapholz H: Techniques of fetal heart rate monitoring. Sem Perinatol 2:119, 1978

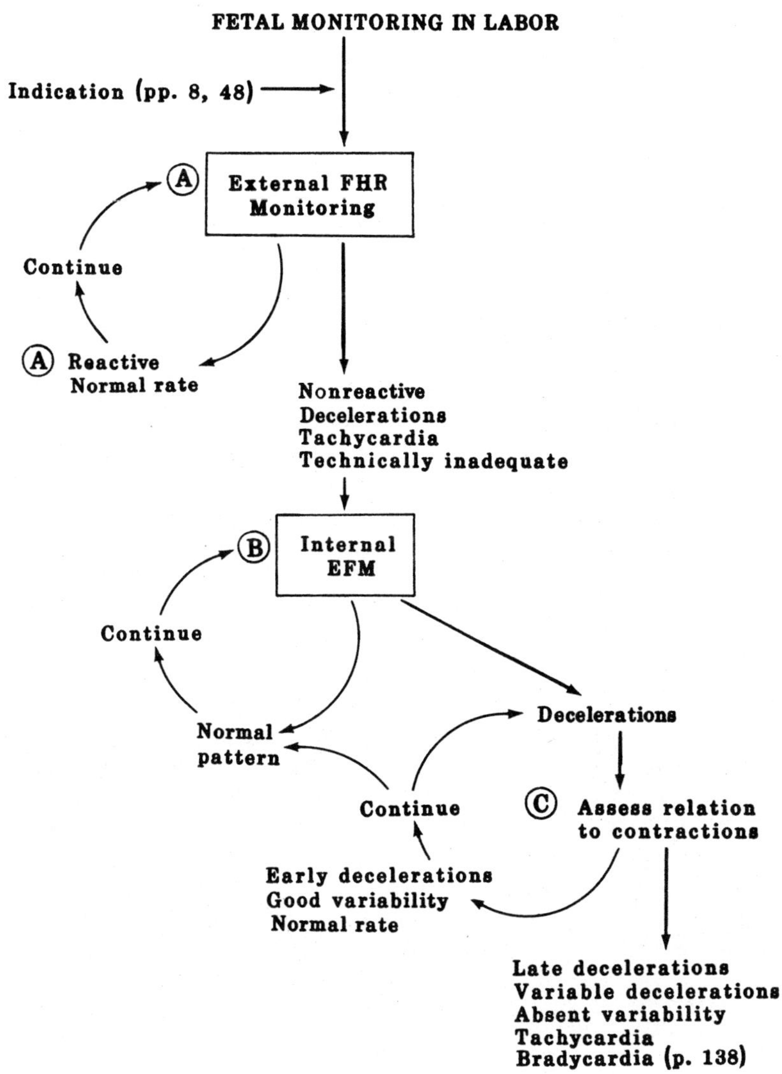
FETAL MONITORING IN LABOR
Indication (pp. 8, 48)
(A) External FHR Monitoring
Continue
(A) Reactive
Normal rate
Nonreactive
Decelerations
Tachycardia
Technically inadequate
(B) Internal EFM
Continue
Normal pattern
Decelerations
Continue
(C) Assess relation to contractions
Early decelerations
Good variability
Normal rate
Late decelerations
Variable decelerations
Absent variability
Tachycardia
Bradycardia (p. 138)

FETAL DISTRESS

Wayne R. Cohen, M.D.

COMMENTS

A. Fetal distress as it refers to fetal asphyxia is diagnosed only by electronic fetal heart rate (FHR) monitoring used in conjunction with fetal scalp blood sampling, when indicated. Abnormal FHR patterns can be divided into (1) suspicious, (2) threatening, (3) ominous signs, depending on the likelihood that severe fetal asphyxia will be associated with them. Suspicious patterns include those with an abnormal baseline FHR (tachycardia, bradycardia, or one with decreased beat-to-beat variability) and no periodic decelerations. Threatening patterns have a normal baseline rate and normal variability but are associated with recurrent decelerations (late or variable). Ominous patterns have both recurrent periodic decelerations and an abnormal baseline.

B. Obstetric intervention for evidence fetal asphyxia can be justified only when all attempts at correction have failed. The primary goal of intrauterine resuscitation is to maximize uterine and umbilical blood flow. Its success is best assessed by demonstrating improvements in the FHR pattern and/or scalp blood pH. Uterine blood flow is enhanced by placing the gravida in the lateral position, increasing her hydration by means of rapid infusion of fluid, and decreasing uterine contractility (e.g., by stopping oxytocin infusion). Cord entrapment may be alleviated at times by changing maternal position (side-to-side, Trendelenburg, or knee-chest). Improve oxygenation by administering 100 percent oxygen.

C. Continual reassessment of the FHR pattern will indicate whether resuscitation attempts are successful. Continuing ominous patterns demand intervention. A threatening pattern requires confirmation by determining fetal scalp blood pH. A suspicious pattern that had previously been normal can be followed carefully; if the prior pattern is unknown or showed recurrent late or variable decelerations, scalp blood pH is in order. If intrauterine resuscitation completely corrects the problem, only continuing surveillance is required.

D. Documentation of fetal acidosis is possible by means of scalp blood pH determination. Normal values (>7.24) are reassuring, while clearly abnormal values (<7.20) confirm asphyxia. Intermediate values (between 7.20 and 7.24) should be repeated to determine the trend.

E. Deliver by the least traumatic and most expeditious route possible. Cesarean section, if it can be accomplished promptly, is preferred over midforceps operations because of the possible synergistic effects of mechanical forceps trauma and brain asphyxia. Intervention is indicated by fetal asphyxia that is not remediable.

REFERENCES

Cohen WR, Schifrin BS: Diagnosis and management of fetal distress during labor. Sem Perinatol 2: 155, 1978

Cohen WR: Intrapartum evaluation. In Ostheimer G (ed): *Manual of Obstetric Anesthesia.* London: Churchill Livingstone, 1982

Saling E, Schneider D: Biochemical supervision of the fetus during labour. J Obstet Gynaecol Brit Comm 74:799, 1967

Wood C: Scalp blood pH in assessing fetal well-being. Contemp Ob Gyn 5:87, 1975

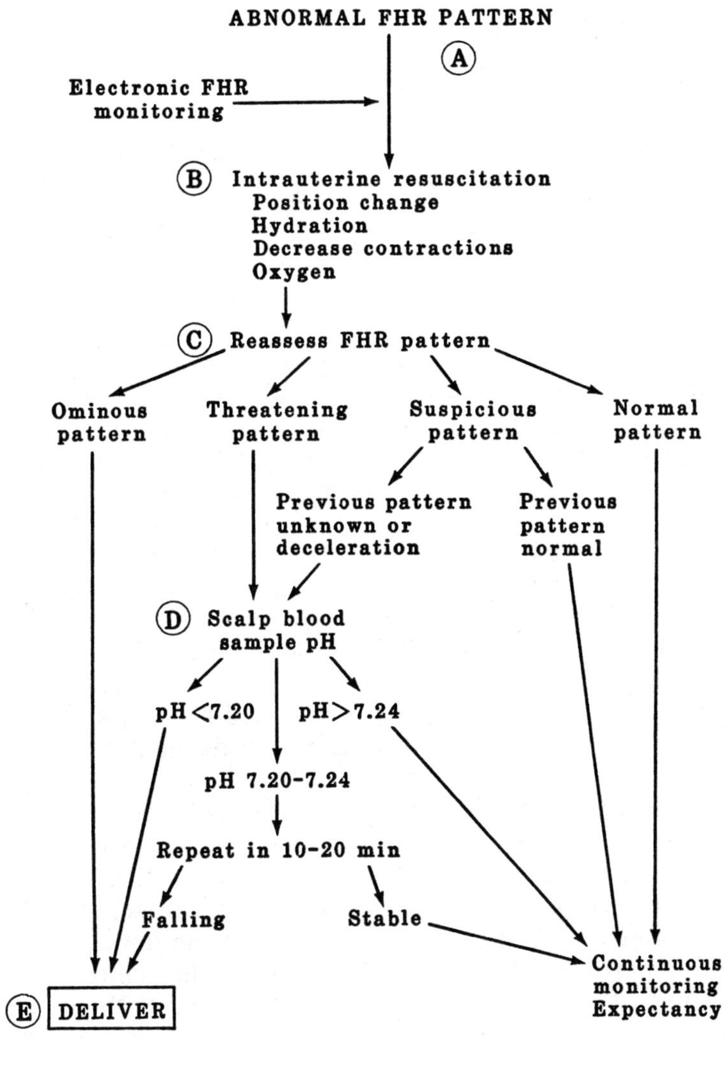
ABNORMAL FHR PATTERN
A
Electronic FHR monitoring
B Intrauterine resuscitation
Position change
Hydration
Decrease contractions
Oxygen
C Reassess FHR pattern
Ominous pattern
Threatening pattern
Suspicious pattern
Normal pattern
Previous pattern unknown or deceleration
Previous pattern normal
D Scalp blood sample pH
pH<7.20
pH>7.24
pH 7.20-7.24
Repeat in 10-20 min
Falling
Stable
E DELIVER
Continuous monitoring Expectancy

MALPRESENTATION DIAGNOSIS

Louis Burke, M.D.

COMMENTS

A. Factors to alert one to the possibility of a malpresentation include previous surgery, uterine malformation, grand multiparity, diabetes mellitus, prematurity, multiple pregnancy, hydramnios, fetal death, placenta previa, a small pelvis, and past difficult labors.

B. Abdominal palpation is useful for purposes of ascertaining the fetal axis (whether longitudinal, transverse, or oblique) and orientation (cephalic or breech). Location of the fetal heart may provide helpful information: e.g., if it is in the upper uterus, breech is likely. Vaginal examination is especially valuable in doubtful cases, particularly if obesity makes palpation difficult.

C. Insinuating the extended examining hands suprapubically into the pelvic inlet on either side of the fetal head will give information concerning the cephalic prominence and its relationship to the fetal back. In a well-flexed head in vertex presentation, the cephalic prominence will be opposite the fetal back. The somewhat deflexed head of a brow presentation will be reflected in bilaterally equal cephalic prominences. By contrast, the extended head of a face presentation will yield a cephalic prominence on the same side as the fetal back.

D. Vaginal assessment of cranial fontanelles and sutures is necessary for confirming a brow presentation. The large, diamond-shaped anterior fontanelle should be identifiable; if there is much caput formation, palpation for an ear may be necessary. In face presentation, one may feel the orbital ridge, eyes, bridge of nose, nostrils, lips, gums, and firm alveolar process of the jaws. The irregularity of the presenting part is characteristic, as is the straight-line relationship between the projection of zygomas and nose (as contrasted with the triangular relationship between ischial tuberosities and coccyx in breech presentation). In brow presentation, one should easily palpate both fontanelles and the orbital ridge.

E. If the cervix is dilated, one should be able to palpate the ischial tuberosities, genitals, and anus. If the membranes are ruptured, meconium can be obtained by inserting the finger into the fetal anus. If a limb is encountered, ensure that it is a foot by determining that the toes form a straight line (as opposed to the curved line formed by the fingers).

F. If the pelvis is empty and the uterus forms a transverse ovoid, the diagnosis of transverse lie is almost certain. Ultrasonography is necessary for confirmation only in doubtful cases.

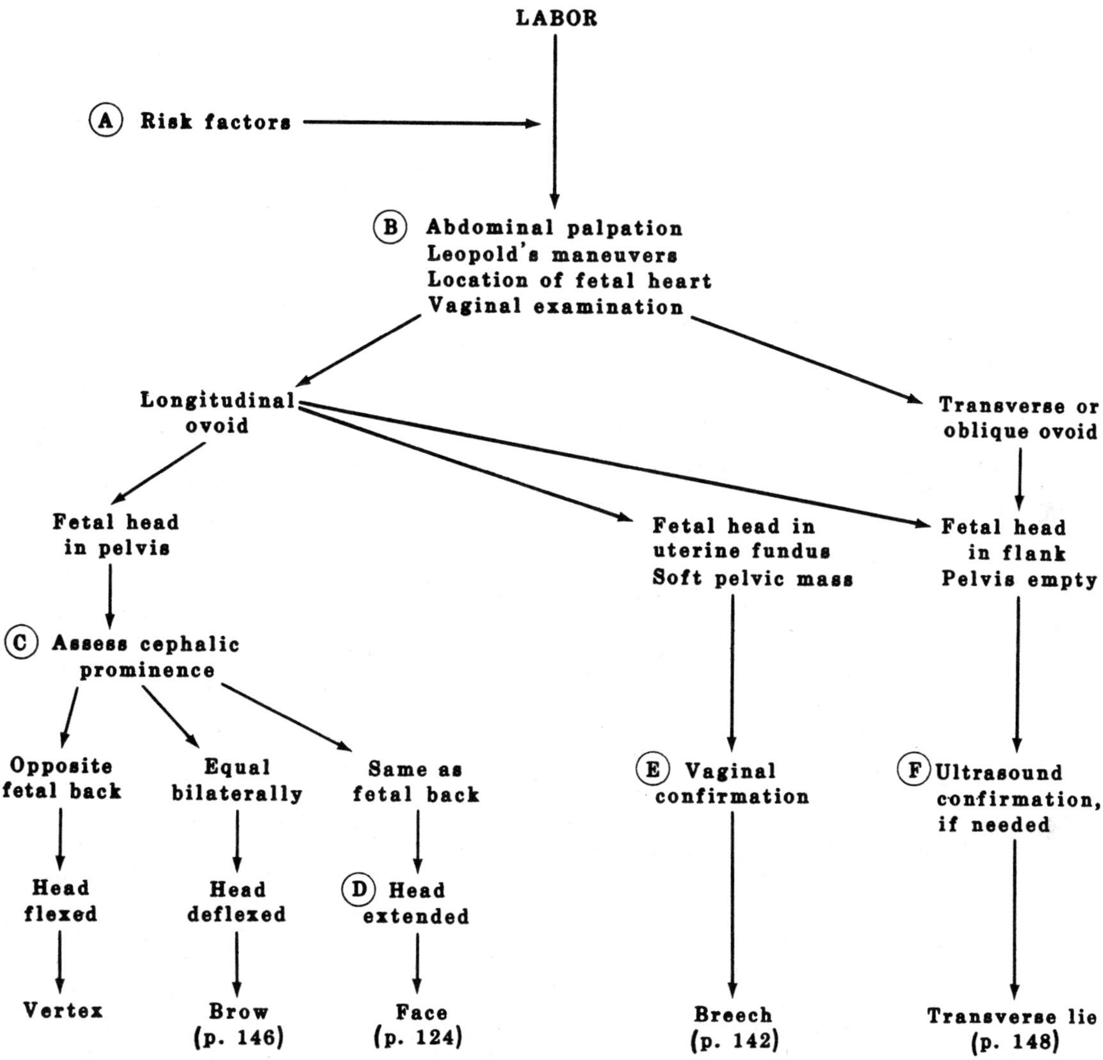
LABOR
(A) Risk factors
(B) Abdominal palpation
Leopold's maneuvers
Location of fetal heart
Vaginal examination
Longitudinal ovoid
Transverse or oblique ovoid
Fetal head in pelvis
Fetal head in uterine fundus
Soft pelvic mass
Fetal head in flank
Pelvis empty
(C) Assess cephalic prominence
Opposite fetal back
Equal bilaterally
Same as fetal back
(E) Vaginal confirmation
(F) Ultrasound confirmation, if needed
Head flexed
Head deflexed
(D) Head extended
Vertex
Brow (p. 146)
Face (p. 124)
Breech (p. 142)
Transverse lie (p. 148)

BREECH PRESENTATION

Max Borten, M.D.

COMMENTS

A. Fetal malpresentations may correct themselves spontaneously as term approaches, prior to the onset of labor. Leiomyomata, uterine anomaly, and placenta previa should alert one to the possibility that a malpresentation exists. Intervention prior to labor is debatable; there may be advantages to external cephalic version to counterbalance its potential risks (including abruptio placentae and cord complications). If undertaken, version should be done after administering a tocolytic agent (p. 124) with continuous external electronic fetal heart rate monitoring to ensure both uterine relaxation and fetal well-being.

B. The head of a premature fetus is relatively larger than its body; moreover, it is more vulnerable than a term-sized fetal head to intracranial damage from rapid transit through the birth canal. It is recommended that women in labor with small fetuses (<2000 gm) in breech presentation be delivered by cesarean section. An exception to this recommendation is the anomalous infant; vaginal delivery may be acceptable for such an infant. Ultrasonographic B-mode or real-time scanning is essential both at term and in premature labor. Ultrasound examination helps in determining fetal head dimensions and in uncovering some gross fetal anomalies.

C. Vaginal delivery in association with hyperextension of the fetal head in breech presentation may result in a devastating transverse section of cervical spinal cord. It is critical to rule out this problem before proceeding. Ultrasonography may be useful, but roentgenographic examination is a more definitive study. Hyperextension greater than 90° is significant and warrants cesarean section. Care should be taken during the course of the cesarean section to ensure that hyperextension (and subsequent damage) does not occur while extracting the baby through the uterine incision; a large incision is essential under these circumstances.

D. In order to allow labor to evolve in a patient with breech presentation, one must be reasonably certain that the pelvic capacity is ample to accommodate that particular fetal head (not just a hypothetical fetal head). X-ray pelvimetry is helpful in this regard, but only if the technique used is capable of measuring both maternal pelvic and fetal head dimensions (p. 18).

E. Whereas normal labor progress does not guarantee that a fetus in breech presentation will deliver vaginally without serious problems, an abnormal labor pattern is a strong indicator that vaginal delivery may be complicated. Protraction and arrest disorders with vertex presentation (pp. 170, 172) are indicators of fetopelvic disproportion; they may serve as comparable indices for labors with breech presentation. Sensitive periodic assessment of labor is critical in detecting such abnormal progression patterns as they arise (p. 166).

REFERENCES

Ballas S, Toaff R: Hyperextension of the fetal head in breech presentation: Radiological evaluation and significance. Brit J Obstet Gynaecol 83:201, 1976

Braun FHT, Jones KL, Smith DW: Breech presentation as an indicator of fetal abnormality. J Pediat 86:419, 1975

Fall D, Nilsson BA: External cephalic version in breech presentation under tocolysis. Obstet Gynecol 53:712, 1979

Goldenberg RL, Nelson KG: The premature breech. Am J Obstet Gynecol 127:240, 1977

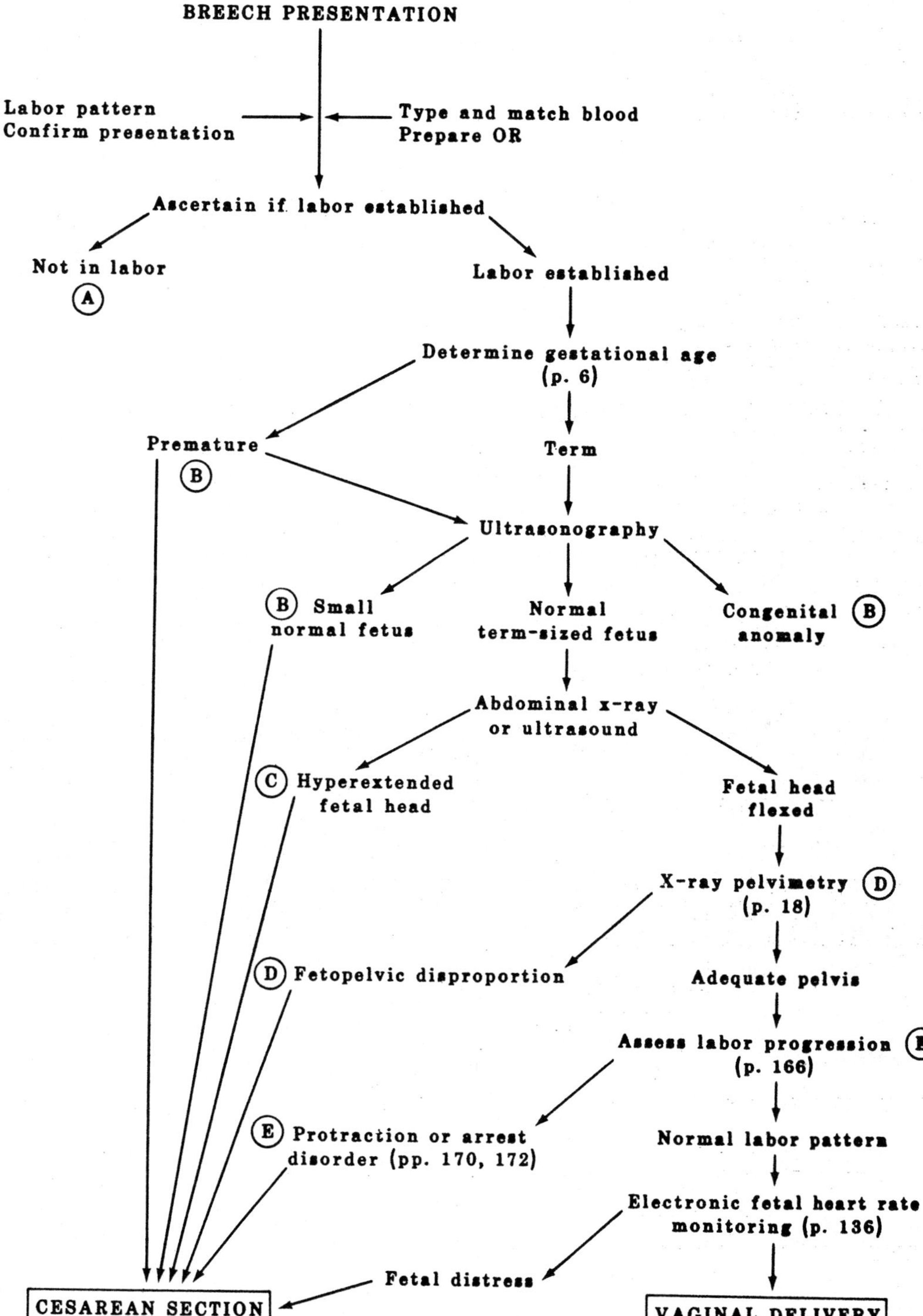
BREECH PRESENTATION
Labor pattern
Confirm presentation
Type and match blood
Prepare OR
Ascertain if labor established
Not in labor
A
Labor established
Determine gestational age
(p. 6)
Premature
B
Term
Ultrasonography
B Small
normal fetus
Normal
term-sized fetus
Congenital
anomaly
B
Abdominal x-ray
or ultrasound
C Hyperextended
fetal head
Fetal head
flexed
X-ray pelvimetry
D
(p. 18)
D Fetopelvic disproportion
Adequate pelvis
Assess labor progression
E
(p. 166)
E Protraction or arrest
disorder (pp. 170, 172)
Normal labor pattern
Electronic fetal heart rate
monitoring (p. 136)
Fetal distress
CESAREAN SECTION
VAGINAL DELIVERY

FACE PRESENTATION

Lenard R. Simon, M.D.

COMMENTS

A. The predisposing factors for face presentation are essentially the same as for brow (p. 146). Fetal anomalies are perhaps somewhat more common here. Therefore they should be looked for, perhaps with real-time or B-scan ultrasound.

B. Fetal weight assessment is alluded to in the comments on brow presentation (p. 146).

C. Cephalopelvimetry is essential with a face presentation (p. 18). Only if it can be shown that the pelvis is adequate to accommodate the fetal head in a face presentation should labor be allowed to continue.

D. The graphic recording of the labor pattern is valuable for detecting abnormal progression indicative of disproportion (pp. 170 and 172). While oxytocin will shorten the labor somewhat, its use is not recommended and its value is unproved with a face presentation.

E. A mentum posterior fetal head position cannot deliver vaginally without considerable trauma. This is so because the head is already maximally extended (deflexed) and delivery over the perineum requires additional extension, a physiologically impossible achievement. Cesarean section must be done to avoid fetal trauma. Manipulation to rotate to a mentum anterior is often traumatic, and is therefore of dubious value.

REFERENCES

Dede JA, Friedman EA: Face presentation. Am J Obstet Gynecol 87:515, 1963

Posner AC, Friedman S, Posner LB: Modern trends in the management of face and brow presentations. Surg Gynecol Obstet 104:485, 1957

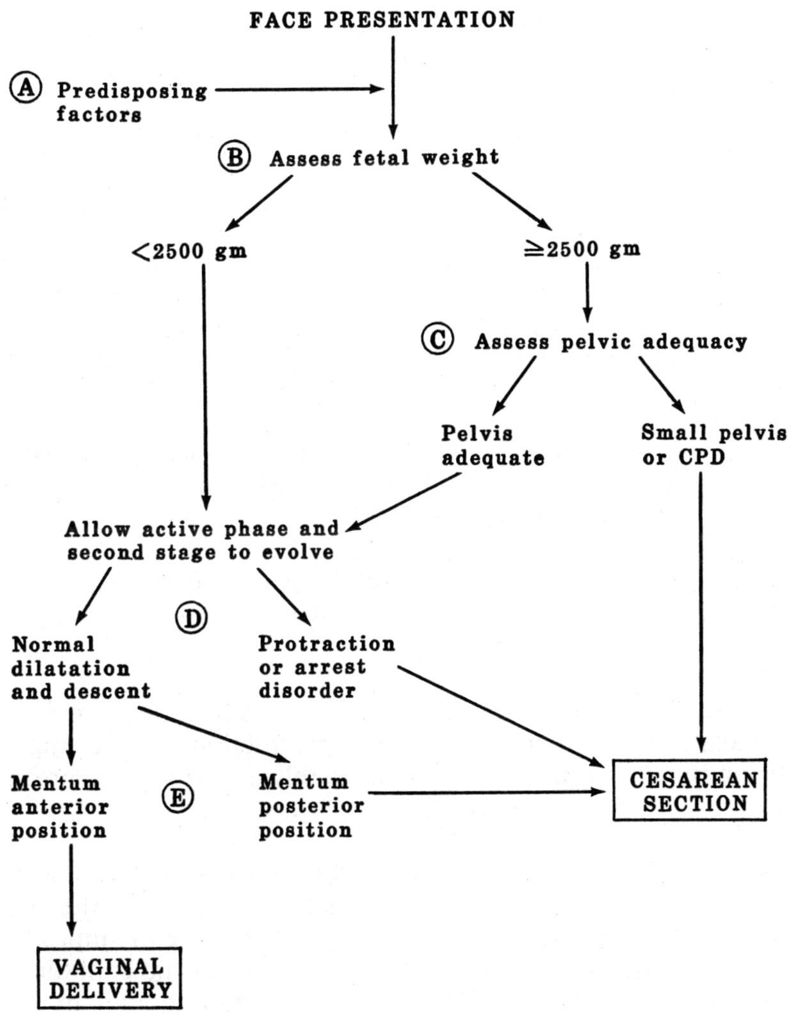
FACE PRESENTATION
Ⓐ Predisposing factors
Ⓑ Assess fetal weight
<2500 gm
≥2500 gm
Ⓒ Assess pelvic adequacy
Pelvis adequate
Small pelvis or CPD
Allow active phase and second stage to evolve
Ⓓ
Normal dilatation and descent
Protraction or arrest disorder
Ⓔ
Mentum anterior position
Mentum posterior position
CESAREAN SECTION
VAGINAL DELIVERY

BROW PRESENTATION

Lenard R. Simon, M.D.

COMMENTS

A. Predisposing factors include any condition that promotes extension or prevents flexion of the fetal skull. Some degree of pelvic contracture is frequently seen. Low implantation of the placenta may contribute to this condition. Exceptionally large infants with a resultant degree of relative disproportion may develop brow presentation. Secondary enlargement of the neck or thorax from growths or deformities as well as structural shortening of the cervical muscles will also effectively prevent flexion of the fetal head. Certain congenital anomalies, such as microcephaly and anencephaly are frequently associated with various degrees of deflexion.

B. Methods for assessing fetal weight include x-ray pelvimetry (especially by the Ball technique), B-mode or real-time ultrasonography, and, least reliably, clinical evaluation (pp. 18 and 50).

C. Cephalopelvic relationships must be carefully evaluated in this condition (p. 18) because of the aforementioned common association of brow presentations with large fetuses and/or small pelves.

D. Follow the course of labor assiduously to detect abnormal progress early (p. 166). The appearance of either an arrest or a protraction disorder (pp. 170 and 172) is a strong signal that disproportion probably exists; here cesarean section is warranted.

E. Spontaneous conversion to face or vertex will frequently occur under these circumstances, obviating any of the dubious maneuvers used in the past to attempt to convert brow presentations. Such maneuvers are of unproven value, are potentially traumatic, and are best avoided. If there is no spontaneous conversion in the second stage, descent will not occur, although molding may delude the observer into believing that descent is actually taking place. Therefore, one should always verify descent with suprapubic palpation (p. 176) under these circumstances.

REFERENCES

Cruikshank DP, White CA: Obstetric malpresentations: Twenty years' experience. Am J Obstet Gynecol 116:1097, 1973

Meltzer RM, Sachtleben MR, Friedman EA: Brow presentation. Am J Obstet Gynecol 100:255, 1968

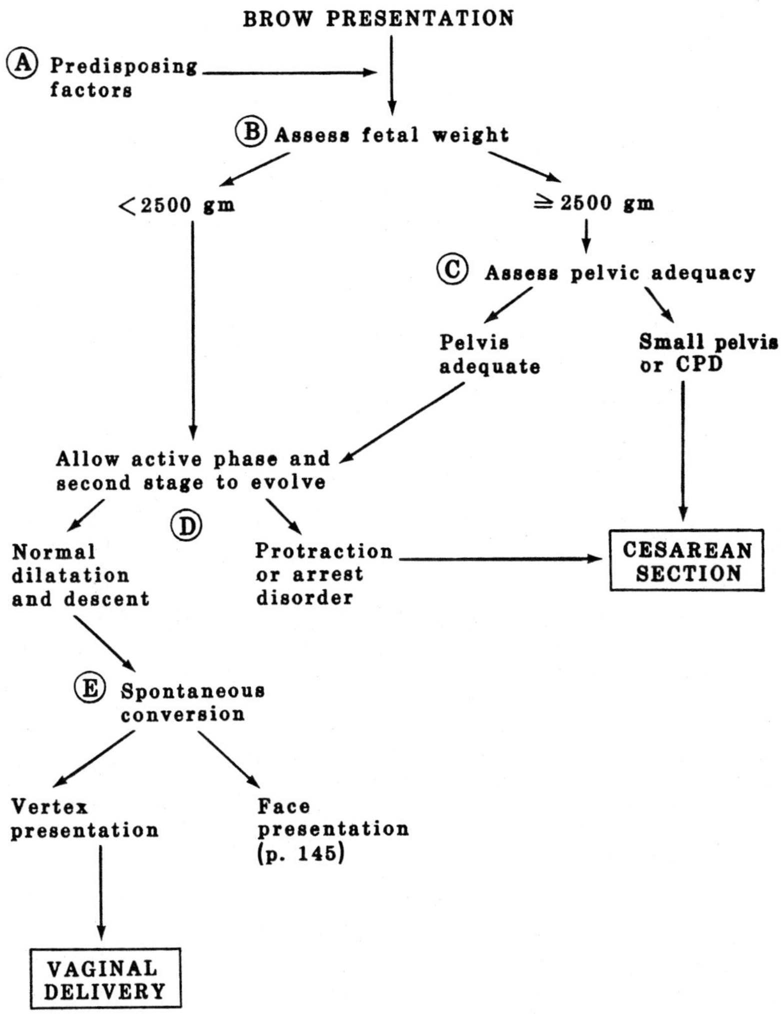
BROW PRESENTATION
(A) Predisposing factors
(B) Assess fetal weight
< 2500 gm
≥ 2500 gm
(C) Assess pelvic adequacy
Pelvis adequate
Small pelvis or CPD
Allow active phase and second stage to evolve
(D)
Normal dilatation and descent
Protraction or arrest disorder
CESAREAN SECTION
(E) Spontaneous conversion
Vertex presentation
Face presentation (p. 145)
VAGINAL DELIVERY

TRANSVERSE LIE

Lenard R. Simon, M.D.

COMMENTS

A. The diagnosis of transverse lie (p. 140) is generally made by abdominal palpation, which will reveal a transversely oriented uterus and neither fetal pole in the pelvis. The fetal head is generally found in one iliac fossa and the breech in the other. The pelvis is generally devoid of fetal parts unless the shoulder has become impacted in the inlet. Vaginal examination may encounter the gridiron sensation of the rib cage. Abnormal relaxation of the abdominal wall, such as is commonly seen in grand multiparas, pelvic contracture, and placenta previa or other soft tissue mass filling the pelvis may prevent either fetal pole from entering the pelvis.

B. Delivery of a living, viable infant invariably requires operative intervention by cesarean section. If a transverse lie is encountered in the course of labor, attempts at manipulation should be scrupulously avoided because of the inherent risks of serious harm to both mother and fetus, particularly if labor is advanced and/or the membranes are ruptured. External cephalic version has been practiced in some areas for transverse lie discovered prior to labor; the risks of this procedure are likely to outweigh possible benefits.

C. Transverse lie in association with a living, previable fetus warrants an attempt to arrest premature labor (p. 124). If successful, it may give the patient an opportunity to convert spontaneously to vertex presentation. Close follow-up is in order if the labor is successfully arrested. If it fails or is not feasible because labor is far advanced or conditions (such as amnionitis) dictate expeditious evacuation, vaginal delivery may be a possible option.

D. If the fetus is known to be dead or is nonviable, the feasibility of vaginal delivery should be weighed. The mechanisms of conduplicato corporis or spontaneous evolution may occur. One should always be aware that overdistention of the lower uterine segment is hazardous even if the fetus is relatively small. Under such circumstances, the risk of uterine rupture exists, especially if labor becomes arrested. Thus, patients have to be followed carefully and cesarean section done whenever indicated.

E. The choice of uterine incision for delivering a fetus in transverse lie by cesarean section will depend upon the position of the back relative to the pelvic inlet as well as consideration of concurrent conditions such as placenta previa or pelvic tumor. Lower uterine segment incision is feasible and acceptable only if the fetal back is up and the lower segment well formed. This will allow one to grasp the legs for purposes of breech extraction or manipulate the fetal head into the incision for delivery. If the back is down or the lower segment not well formed, classic incision is preferable.

REFERENCES

Hall JE, Kohl SG, Kavaler F: Transverse lie and perinatal mortality. NY J Med 62:2186, 1962

Johnson CE: Transverse presentation of the fetus. JAMA 187:642, 1964

Ranney B: The gentle art of external cephalic version. Am J Obstet Gynecol 116:239, 1973

Ylikorkala O, Hartikainen-Sorri A: Value of external version in fetal malpresentation in combination with use of ultrasound. Acta Obstet Gynecol Scand 56:63, 1977

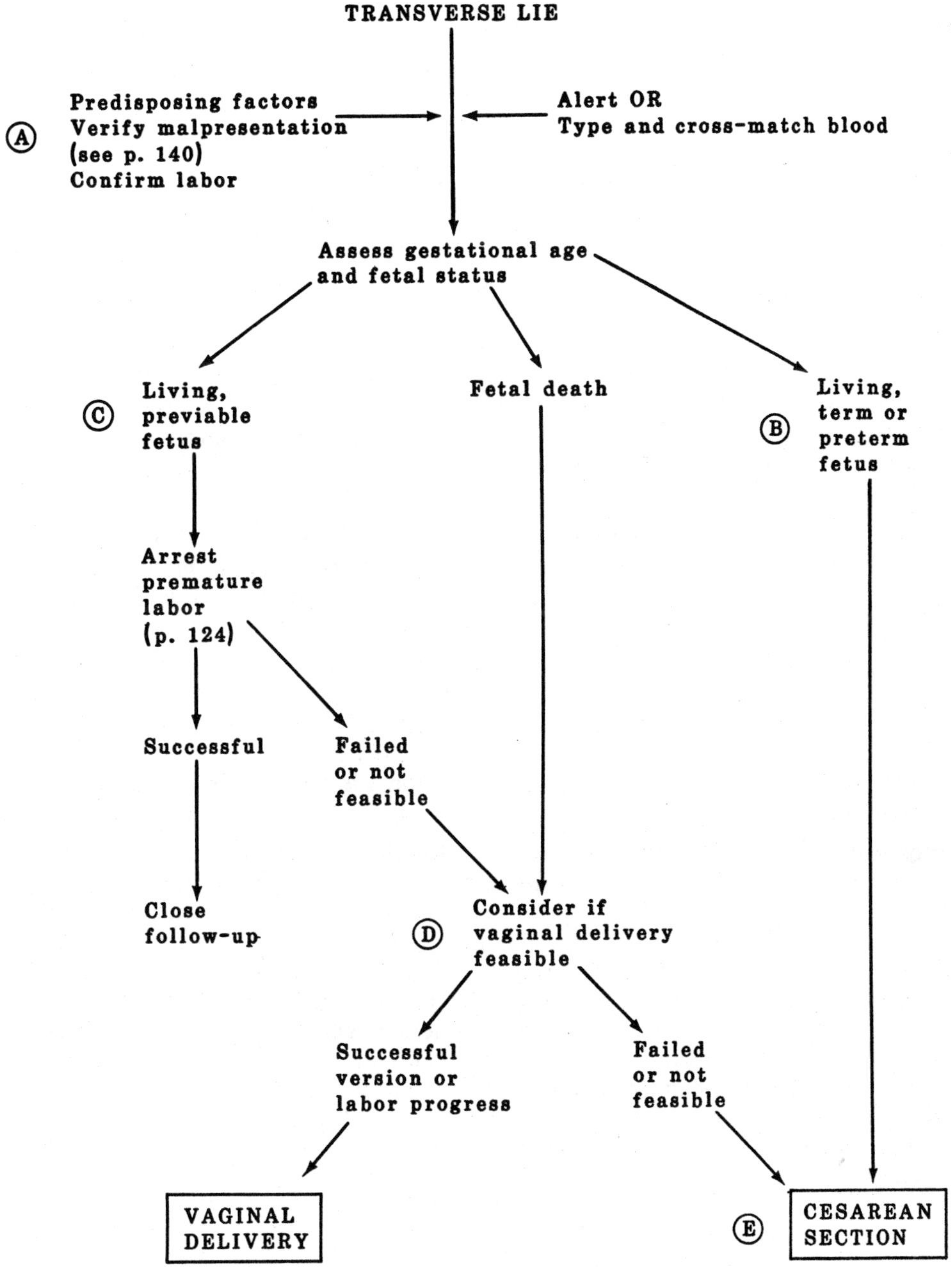
TRANSVERSE LIE
Ⓐ Predisposing factors
Verify malpresentation
(see p. 140)
Confirm labor
Alert OR
Type and cross-match blood
Assess gestational age
and fetal status
Ⓒ Living,
previable
fetus
Fetal death
Ⓑ Living,
term or
preterm
fetus
Arrest
premature
labor
(p. 124)
Successful
Failed
or not
feasible
Close
follow-up
Ⓓ Consider if
vaginal delivery
feasible
Successful
version or
labor progress
Failed
or not
feasible
VAGINAL
DELIVERY
Ⓔ CESAREAN
SECTION

PERSISTENT OCCIPUT POSTERIOR

Lenard Simon, M.D.

COMMENTS

A. The major predisposing factor is the type of pelvic architecture, especially anthropoid and android pelves. The position may also be seen in mixed types when there is an associated contracture of the forepelvis or midplane dimensions.

B. The diagnosis of fetal occiput posterior (OP) position is made primarily by vaginal examination, although one may be alerted by abdominal palpation. Since the fetal back is directed posteriorly, one may find it difficult to palpate the fetus transabdominally. Vaginal examination reveals the fetal head deflexion commonly seen with OP position. The sagittal suture is directed anteroposteriorly and both anterior and posterior fontanelles can usually be felt.

C. The abnormal labor pattern associated with OP positions is almost always the result of some degree of cephalopelvic disproportion and not directly related to the fetal position itself. Thus, protraction and arrest disorders are frequently seen. Conduction anesthesia or excessive sedation may also contribute.

D. Any patient who develops a major labor aberration with the fetus in OP position must be considered at high risk because of the probability that cephalopelvic disproportion is present. It is essential, therefore, to evaluate critically to determine if the pelvis can accommodate this fetus, using clinical means and, if necessary for confirmation, x-ray pelvimetry (p. 18). Confirmation of disproportion warrants cesarean section without further trial of labor.

E. In most cases in which the pelvis is adequate for the fetus, spontaneous internal rotation will occur to occiput anterior. With rare exceptions, an uneventful vaginal delivery can be expected. In some, the OP position will persist. Here, careful reassessment of the pelvic adequacy is essential. The fetus may have descended to a level at which obstruction can now be demonstrated objectively by dynamic assessment (p. 18). Even with the head well down in the pelvis, cesarean section is indicated for disproportion. In the absence of evidence of disproportion, one may gently attempt digital rotation to occiput anterior; if successful, vaginal delivery should occur in due course. In the case of a persistent OP that cannot be digitally rotated, allowing the fetus to deliver as an OP is preferable to forceps rotation, because the latter risks maternal and fetal damage. Attempts at forceps rotation or forceps delivery of the fetus from the midpelvis are generally unwarranted because of the high frequency of fetal damage associated with these procedures. They are contraindicated unless it can be shown that the risks of alternative actions are greater (p. 208).

REFERENCES

Phillips RD, Freeman M: The management of the persistent occiput posterior: A review of 552 consecutive cases. Obstet Gynecol 43:171, 1974

Pridmore BR, Hey EN, Aherne WA: Spinal cord injury of the fetus during delivery with Kielland's forceps. Brit J Obstet Gynaecol 81:168, 1974

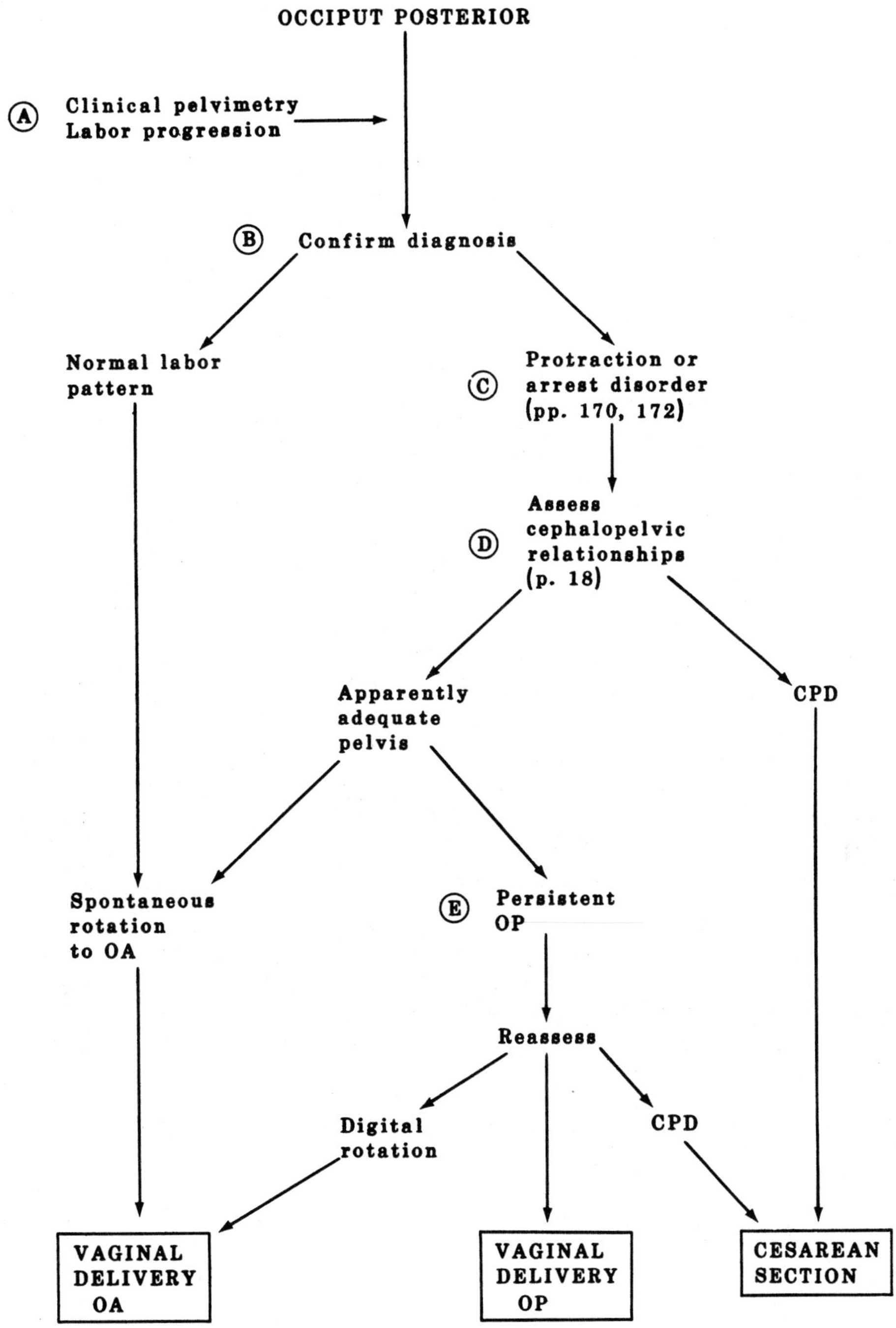
OCCIPUT POSTERIOR
Ⓐ Clinical pelvimetry
Labor progression
Ⓑ Confirm diagnosis
Normal labor pattern
Ⓒ Protraction or arrest disorder (pp. 170, 172)
Ⓓ Assess cephalopelvic relationships (p. 18)
Apparently adequate pelvis
CPD
Spontaneous rotation to OA
Ⓔ Persistent OP
Reassess
Digital rotation
CPD
VAGINAL DELIVERY OA
VAGINAL DELIVERY OP
CESAREAN SECTION

PROLAPSED CORD

Wayne R. Cohen, M.D.

COMMENTS

A. Factors that increase the risk of cord prolapse include breech presentation, transverse lie, unengaged fetal presenting part, rupture of membranes before term or in association with hydramnios, and delivery of the second twin.

B. The diagnosis is obvious in overt prolapse of the cord when a loop of the umbilical cord appears externally, is encountered in the vagina, or can be palpated by vaginal examination in front of or adjacent to the presenting part. Occult prolapse is a condition in which the cord lies adjacent to the presenting part and is not palpable on vaginal examination. Occult prolapse is a presumptive diagnosis made on the basis of an abnormal FHR pattern. Most often this consists of severe recurrent variable decelerations that do not respond to standard maneuvers of intrauterine resuscitation, including hydration, change in maternal position, and administration of oxygen.

C. Salutary maternal positions for patients with cord prolapse are Trendelenburg, elevated lateral Sims, and knee-chest positions. Appropriate help from nursing staff and anesthesia personnel is summoned; an intravenous line is inserted; the maternal abdomen is shaved and prepared with antiseptic solution. Operating room facilities are prepared in anticipation of an emergency cesarean section.

D. When possible, it is better to allow the fetus to recover from asphyxia in utero rather than to deliver an hypoxic fetus that will require considerable resuscitative efforts.

E. When the fetal heart rate pattern is normal, excessive haste is unnecessary and may be potentially harmful to mother and fetus.

F. In rare situations, when a cord prolapse is noted through intact membranes, elevating the presenting part without rupturing the membranes may allow the cord to be replaced (not by manually repositing it, but spontaneously), thus averting the need for surgical intervention.

G. A dead fetus can sometimes transmit maternal electrocardiographic voltages via the scalp electrode. This can be misinterpreted to represent the signal from a live fetus. If persistent fetal bradycardia is noted on the monitor, it should be confirmed using the DeLee stethoscope for auscultation.

REFERENCES

Cohen WR, Schifrin BS, Doctor G: Elevation of the fetal presenting part: A method of intrauterine resuscitation. Am J Obstet Gynecol 123:646, 1975

Myles TJM: Prolapse of the umbilical cord. J Obstet Gynaecol Brit Emp 66:301, 1959

Savage EW, Kohn SG, Wynn RM: Prolapse of the umbilical cord. Obstet Gynecol 36:502, 1970

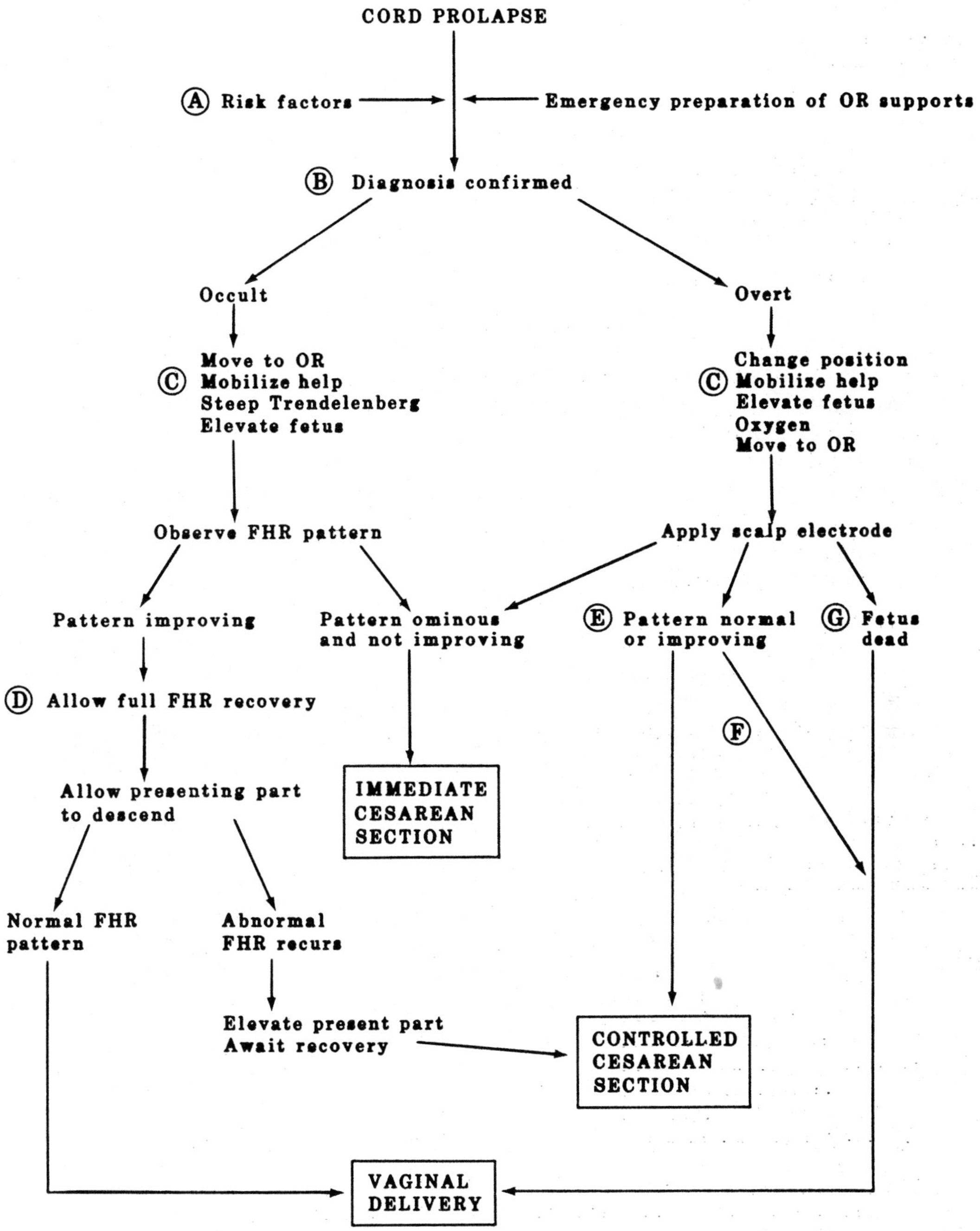
CORD PROLAPSE
(A) Risk factors
Emergency preparation of OR supports
(B) Diagnosis confirmed
Occult
Overt
Move to OR
(C) Mobilize help
Steep Trendelenberg
Elevate fetus
Change position
(C) Mobilize help
Elevate fetus
Oxygen
Move to OR
Observe FHR pattern
Apply scalp electrode
Pattern improving
Pattern ominous
and not improving
(E) Pattern normal
or improving
(G) Fetus
dead
(D) Allow full FHR recovery
(F)
IMMEDIATE
CESAREAN
SECTION
Allow presenting part
to descend
Normal FHR
pattern
Abnormal
FHR recurs
Elevate present part
Await recovery
CONTROLLED
CESAREAN
SECTION
VAGINAL
DELIVERY

HYDRAMNIOS

Henry Klapholz, M.D.

COMMENTS

A. Hydramnios refers to excessive accumulation of amniotic fluid, usually more than 2000 ml at term. Only about 1 in 1000 shows volumes greater than 3000 ml. It is characterized clinically by rapid weight gain accompanied by rapid increase in abdominal girth, usually with a tense, painful abdomen. Often there will be considerable stasis edema of the lower extremities. The fetal heart is difficult to hear because of the intervening fluid. The patient may experience nausea and vomiting.

B. B-scan ultrasonography is particularly useful in confirming the presence of a large volume of amniotic fluid relative to the fetal size. Volumetric determinations are available to help quantitate the amount. Ultrasound examination will also show concomitant multiple pregnancy (see p. 158) and reveal some fetal anomalies, such as anencephalus. If twins are found, suspect monozygous twins, because hydramnios, which is seen in about 10 percent of twins, is more common among them.

C. About half the anencephalic fetuses will have hydramnios. All cases of fetal esophageal atresia are associated with hydamnios, although the anomaly cannot be diagnosed by ultrasound. X-ray studies, with radiopaque material injected intra-amniotically, are needed for diagnosis. Overall, 29 percent of cases with hydramnios have anomalous fetuses. There is a 50 percent mortality rate associated with this condition.

D. It is important to assess these cases for fetal infection, maternal diabetes mellitus, and Rh isoimmunization. Infection may be uncovered by obtaining TORCH titers (an acronym referring to titers for toxoplasmosis, rubella, cytomegalovirus, and herpes virus, respectively). Although toxoplasmosis (see p. 104) may be treated with spiramycin, the prognosis for fetal survival or well-being is poor in cases associated with hydramnios.

E. Amniocentesis is done for therapeutic purposes only to relieve the intense pressure and respiratory compromise from impingement on the diaphragm. About 500 ml can be withdrawn per hour to a total of 1500 ml on each occasion. One can expect reaccumulation to be rapid. Labor often ensues. A technique for effecting permanent drainage has not yet been developed.

REFERENCES

Bates HR: Hydramnios and the fetal lung: A selective review. Am J Obstet Gynecol 135: 154, 1979

Harberg FJ, Pokorny WJ, Hahn H: Congenital duodenal obstruction: A review of 65 cases. Am J Surg 138:825, 1979

Phelas PD: Polyhydramnios, congenital malformations, and intrauterine detection. Pediatr 59:785, 1977

Pitkin RM: Acute polyhydramnios recurrent in successive pregnancies. Management with multiple amniocenteses. Obstet Gynecol 48(Suppl 1):42s, 1976

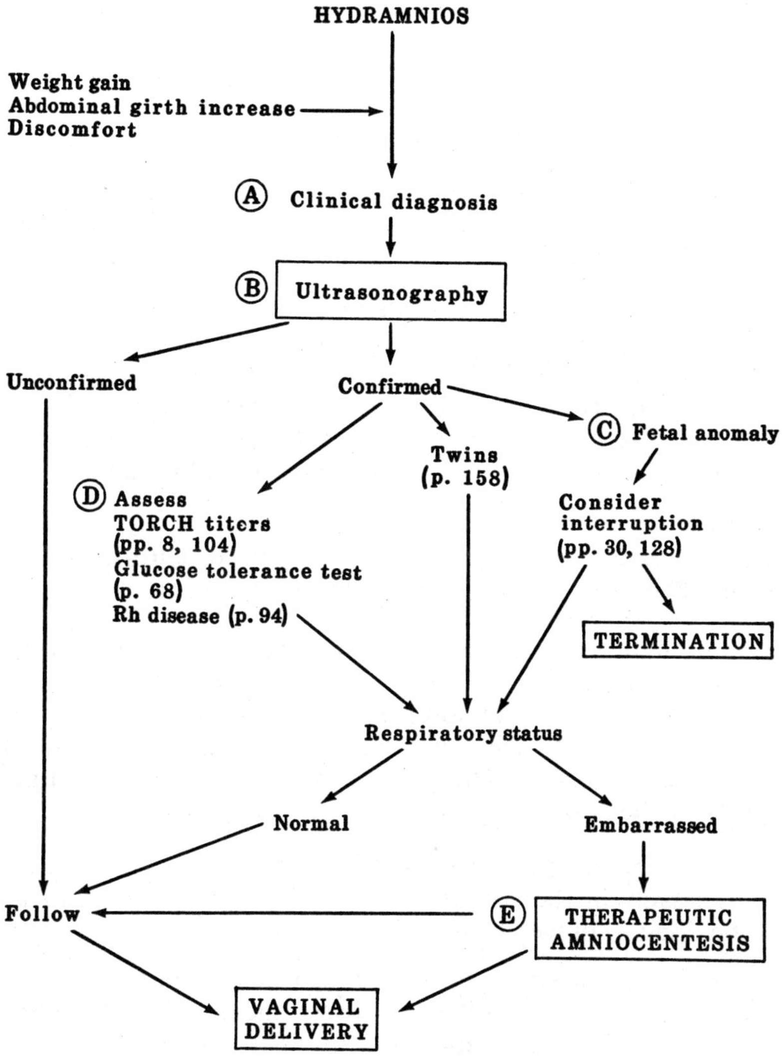
HYDRAMNIOS
Weight gain
Abdominal girth increase
Discomfort
(A) Clinical diagnosis
(B) Ultrasonography
Unconfirmed
Confirmed
(C) Fetal anomaly
Twins
(p. 158)
(D) Assess
TORCH titers
(pp. 8, 104)
Glucose tolerance test
(p. 68)
Rh disease (p. 94)
Consider
interruption
(pp. 30, 128)
TERMINATION
Respiratory status
Normal
Embarrassed
Follow
(E) THERAPEUTIC
AMNIOCENTESIS
VAGINAL
DELIVERY

HYDROCEPHALUS

Louis Burke, M.D.

COMMENTS

A. In vertex presentation, abdominal palpation may reveal a broad, hard mass presenting above the symphysis pubis. The lower abdomen may be rigid and the lower uterine segment tense. The cranial suture lines are widened and the fontanelles broad and distended; these are pathognomonic findings.

B. Ultrasonography is usually diagnostic, demonstrating enlargement of head size and dilated lateral ventricles. Amniography may reveal associated spina bifida or other anomaly. Alpha-fetoprotein may be helpful, especially if obtained in mid-trimester (p. 44). Erroneous x-ray diagnosis can occur, especially in breech presentation, owing to magnification of head dimensions. It may be helpful to note small facial bony features relative to head size and thinning of the cranial plates.

C. Ventricular tap is readily done if the fetal head is fixed. Ultrasound localization may be helpful. The technique is comparable to amniocentesis.

D. The diagnosis of hydrocephalus is often first made in labor. Ventricular tap can be done transcervically after the cervix is 2–3 cm dilated, provided the fetal head is fixed in the inlet. Transabdominal tap may have to be done to decrease head size and allow vaginal delivery; care must be taken to avoid puncturing the bladder. In breech presentation, if spina bifida is present, intrathecal tap is possible by way of the anomalous site.

E. The lower uterine segment may become quite overdistended if head size cannot be reduced effectively in the course of labor. If this occurs, cesarean section may have to be done to prevent uterine rupture.

F. Successful antepartum placement of an intraventricular shunt has been reported by way of amnioscopy. This will decompress the fetal cranium so that no further enlargement will occur and prevent progressive brain compression. Under these circumstances, cesarean section is favored for delivery to prevent possible dislodgement of the shunt during labor. Experience is limited with this experimental approach.

REFERENCES

Birnholz JC, Frigoletto FD: Antenatal treatment of hydrocephalus. New Engl J Med 304: 1021, 1981

Ferry PC, Pernoll ML: Rational management of perinatal hydrocephalus. Am J Obstet Gynecol 126:151, 1976

Freeman RK, McQuown DS, Secrist LJ, Larson EJ: The diagnosis of fetal hydrocephalus before viability. Obstet Gynecol 49:109, 1977

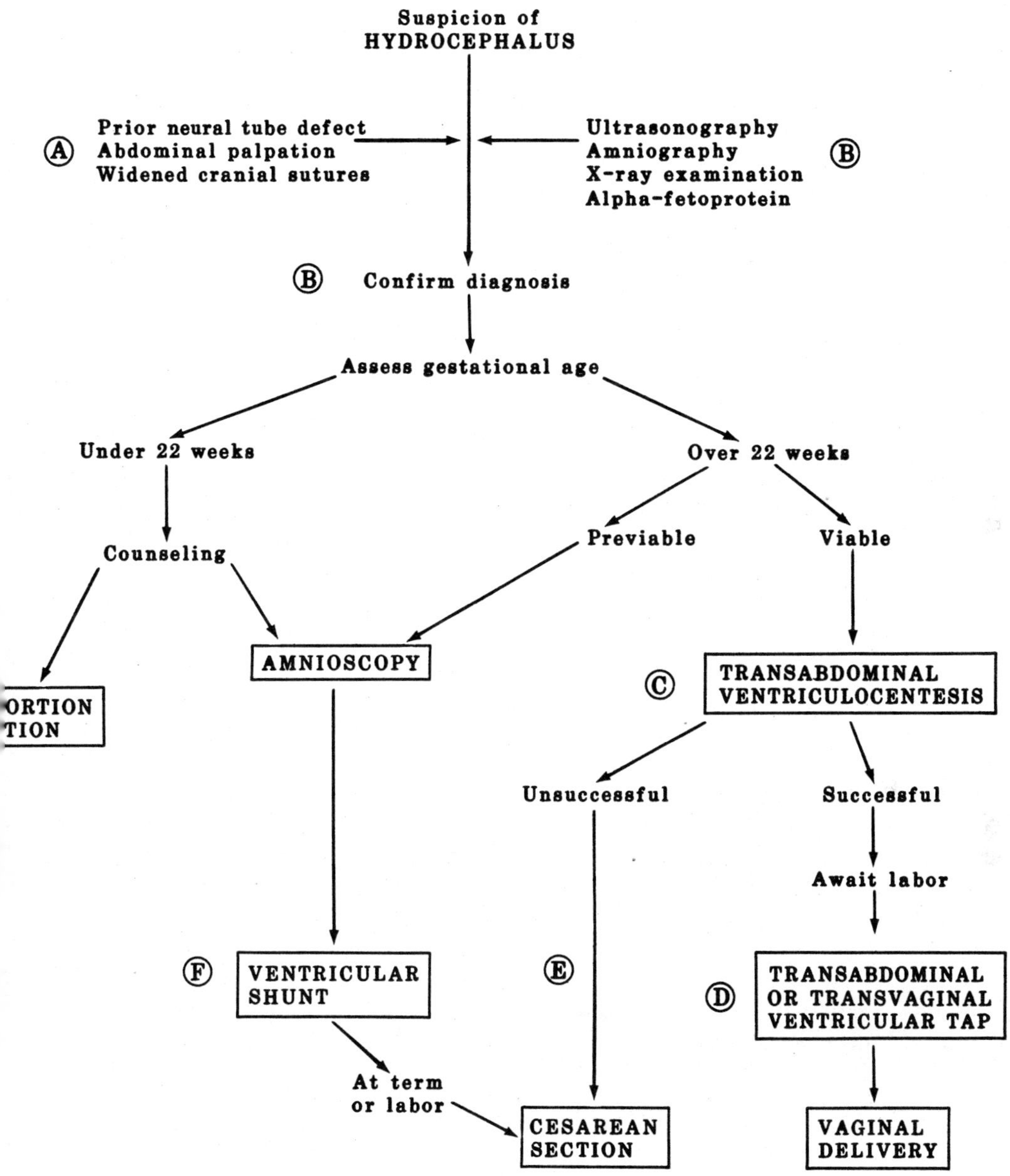
Suspicion of
HYDROCEPHALUS
Ⓐ
Prior neural tube defect
Abdominal palpation
Widened cranial sutures
Ultrasonography
Amniography
X-ray examination
Alpha-fetoprotein
Ⓑ
Ⓑ
Confirm diagnosis
Assess gestational age
Under 22 weeks
Over 22 weeks
Counseling
Previable
Viable
ORTION
TION
AMNIOSCOPY
Ⓒ
TRANSABDOMINAL
VENTRICULOCENTESIS
Unsuccessful
Successful
Await labor
Ⓕ
VENTRICULAR
SHUNT
Ⓔ
Ⓓ
TRANSABDOMINAL
OR TRANSVAGINAL
VENTRICULAR TAP
At term
or labor
CESAREAN
SECTION
VAGINAL
DELIVERY

MULTIPLE PREGNANCY

Louis Burke, M.D.

COMMENTS

A. The treatment of infertility by ovulation induction agents, such as Clomid and Pergonal, have increased the overall rate of multiple pregnancy. This applies particularly to triplets, quadruplets, and quintuplets; more than two-thirds of cases of these multiple births are now associated with these drugs. Suspect multiple pregnancy if the uterine size is excessive, if more than one fetal heart can be heard, or if the fetal presentation is difficult to assess.

B. Ultrasonography is usually definitive for diagnosis. Elevated levels of estriol, HCG, or HPL are suggestive.

C. The main fetal problem associated with multiple pregnancy is prematurity. Early diagnosis and prolonged bedrest may improve fetal salvage, especially if begun as early as 27 weeks and continued to 34 weeks. Tocolytic agents may be used if contractions occur, with or without cervical dilatation, to prolong the pregnancy.

D. Malpresentation is very common with three or more fetuses. Neonatal care is complex and requires team effort. Elective cesarean section at or beyond 36 weeks has been advocated to optimize outcome.

E. One or both twins may present in transverse presentation in about 10 percent of cases. While it is possible that the second twin will correct its malpresentation as the first twin is born, it is preferable to deliver by cesarean section so as to avoid the potential complications of an internal podalic version or a cesarean section under suboptimal emergency conditions.

F. Manage the delivery of the first twin as if it were a singleton, minimizing anesthesia for the delivery but preparing for general anesthesia in case it should become necessary for the second twin. Local or pudendal block is preferred at this point. If a nuchal cord is encountered, do not divide it, because it may prove to be the cord of the second twin.

G. As soon as the first twin is born, examine the patient internally to ascertain the presentation of the second twin. If it is a shoulder presentation, proceed with cesarean section. Otherwise, guide the presenting part into the pelvis, rupture the membranes (if they are not already ruptured), and apply a scalp electrode for FHR monitoring. Allow labor to evolve under close surveillance. Vaginal delivery can be expected, provided no cord or placental complications occur.

REFERENCES

Bieniarz J, Shah N, Dmowski WP, Rao R, Scommegna A: Premature labor treatment with ritodrine in multiple pregnancy with three or more fetuses. Acta Obstet Gynecol Scand 57:25, 1978

Duncan SL, Ginz B, Wahab H: Use of ultrasound and hormone assays in the diagnosis, management, and outcome of twin pregnancy. Obstet Gynecol 53:367, 1979

Powers WF, Miller TC: Bedrest in twin pregnancy: Identification of a critical period and its cost implications. Am J Obstet Gynecol 134:23, 1979

Ron-El R, Caspi E, Schreyer P, Weinraub Z, Arieli S, Goldberg M: Triplet and quadruplet pregnancies and management. Obstet Gynecol 57:458, 1981

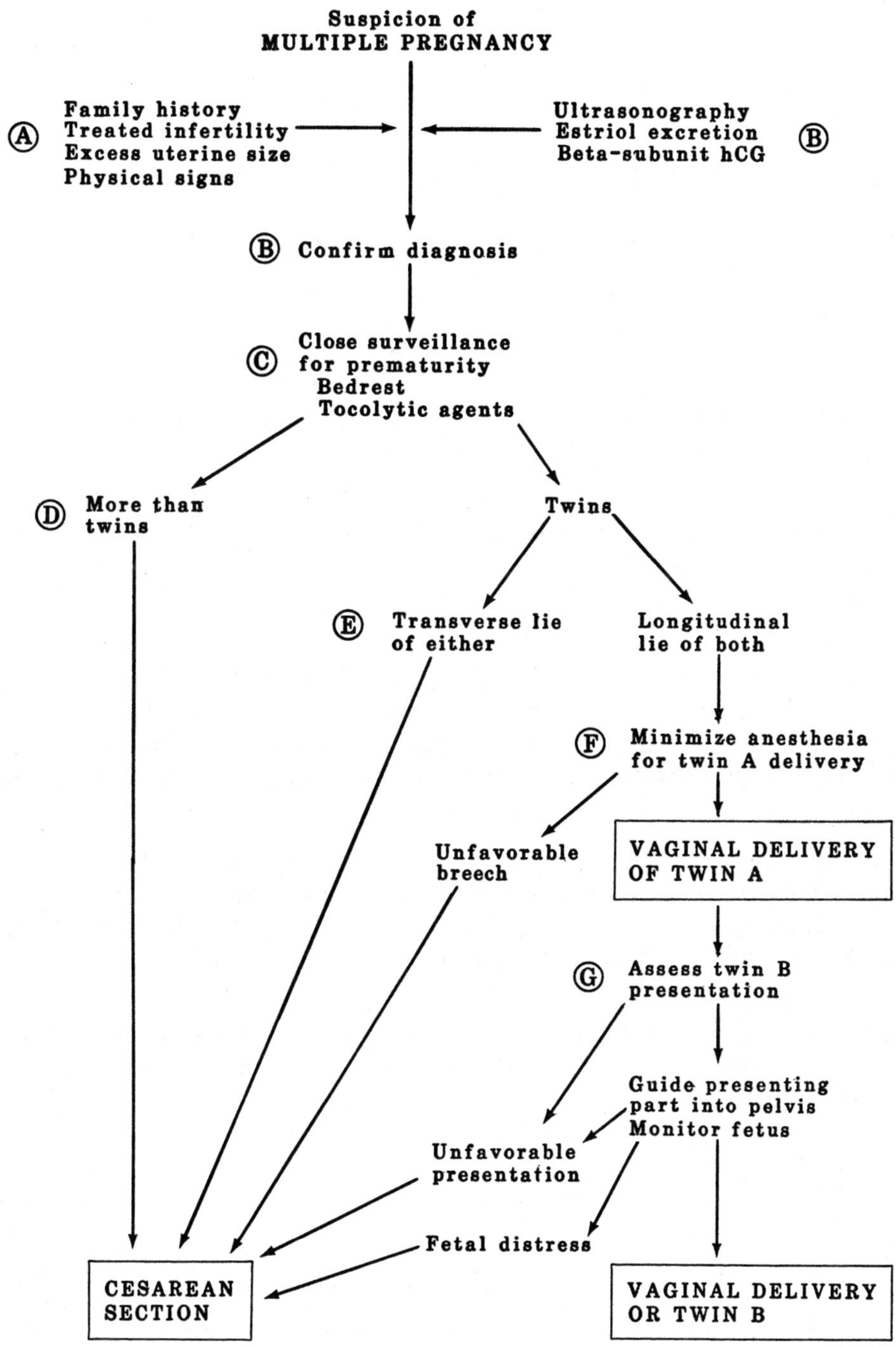
Suspicion of
MULTIPLE PREGNANCY
(A) Family history
Treated infertility
Excess uterine size
Physical signs
Ultrasonography
Estriol excretion
Beta-subunit hCG (B)
(B) Confirm diagnosis
(C) Close surveillance
for prematurity
Bedrest
Tocolytic agents
(D) More than
twins
Twins
(E) Transverse lie
of either
Longitudinal
lie of both
(F) Minimize anesthesia
for twin A delivery
Unfavorable
breech
VAGINAL DELIVERY
OF TWIN A
(G) Assess twin B
presentation
Guide presenting
part into pelvis
Monitor fetus
Unfavorable
presentation
Fetal distress
CESAREAN
SECTION
VAGINAL DELIVERY
OR TWIN B

LARGE FETUS

Selwyn P. Oskowitz, M.B.

COMMENTS

A. Be alert for fetal macrosomia if the gravida is diabetic or has a diabetic background (p. 68). Maternal obesity or excessive weight gain during pregnancy should raise one's index of suspicion. Post-term infants tend to be large as well.

B. Ultrasonography may show a large biparietal diameter, but fetal weight correlates better with abdominal circumference at the level of the ductus venosus. A head-to-abdomen ratio of less than one and an excessive rate of growth on serial measurements are very suggestive that the infant will be large.

C. Cephalopelvic disproportion is frequent in association with large fetuses. Moreover, failure of the fetal head to enter the pelvic inlet results in common occurrence of fetal malpresentation, including breech, brow, and transverse presentations.

D. When macrosomia is objectively diagnosed prior to delivery, a strong case can be made for elective cesarean section because of the high frequency of both maternal and fetal complications. Shoulder dystocia (p. 182), a serious complication frequently resulting in death or serious injury, can thereby be averted.

E. One must be prepared to mobilize appropriate supports in the event that shoulder dystocia develops. Rapid induction of general anesthesia as well as skilled ancillary obstetric and nursing personnel may be needed to manage this problem expeditiously and atraumatically.

F. Infants who are large for gestational age should be observed for hypoglycemia, hyperbilirubinemia, hyaline membrane disease, infections, and manifestations of birth injuries.

REFERENCES

Benedetti TJ, Gabbe SG: Shoulder dystocia: A complication of fetal macrosomia and prolonged second stage of labor with midpelvic delivery. Obstet Gynecol 52:526, 1978

Kearney K, Vigneron N, Frischman P, Johnson JWC: Fetal weight estimation by ultrasonic measurement of abdominal circumference. Obstet Gynecol 51:156, 1978

Parks DG, Ziel HK: Macrosomia: A proposed indication for primary cesarean section. Obstet Gynecol 52:407, 1978

Sack RA: The large infant: A study of maternal, obstetric, fetal and newborn characteristics, including a long term pediatric follow-up. Am J Obstet Gynecol 104:195, 1969

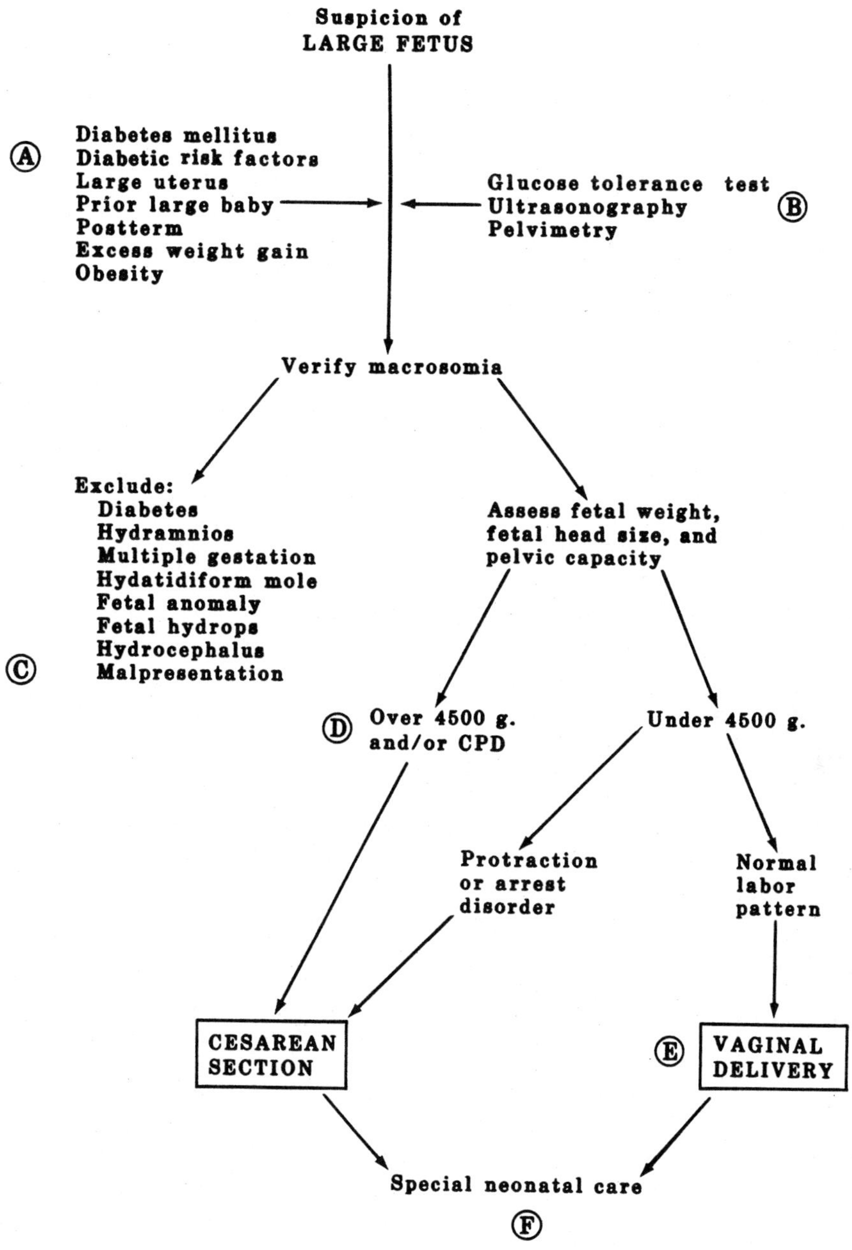
Suspicion of
LARGE FETUS
A
Diabetes mellitus
Diabetic risk factors
Large uterus
Prior large baby
Postterm
Excess weight gain
Obesity
Glucose tolerance test
Ultrasonography
Pelvimetry
B
Verify macrosomia
Exclude:
Diabetes
Hydramnios
Multiple gestation
Hydatidiform mole
Fetal anomaly
Fetal hydrops
Hydrocephalus
Malpresentation
C
Assess fetal weight,
fetal head size, and
pelvic capacity
D
Over 4500 g.
and/or CPD
Under 4500 g.
Protraction
or arrest
disorder
Normal
labor
pattern
CESAREAN
SECTION
E
VAGINAL
DELIVERY
Special neonatal care
F

RUPTURED UTERUS

Louis Burke, M.D.

COMMENTS

A. Uterine rupture can occur spontaneously, particularly if there has been prior uterine surgery (including cesarean section, myomectomy, metroplasty) or neglected obstructed labor. Excessive uterine contractions from uterotonic agents may be a precipitating factor as well. The clinical picture may vary from no symptoms at all (e.g., a window representing the dehisced scar of a prior cesarean section) to catastrophic shock with intraperitoneal hemorrhage. Acute pain is the most common presenting manifestation.

B. Laboratory data are of limited use for diagnosis. Even with considerable intraperitoneal bleeding, the fall in hematocrit may occur slowly. X-ray or ultrasound study may show abnormal fetal position with extremities extended and free intraperitoneal air. In most cases, the emergency nature of the condition will not permit such studies to be done.

C. It is usually possible to repair the thin or dehisced scar of a prior cesarean section incision at the time of the repeat cesarean by freshening the edges and resuturing. One should consider sterilization under these circumstances because of the risk of rupture in subsequent pregnancy.

D. When uterine rupture is discovered at the time of manual exploration following delivery of the placenta, immediate exploratory laparotomy is necessary. If the rupture site is smooth and not bleeding excessively, simple repair may be feasible; if not, hysterectomy may have to be done.

E. Severe hemorrhage usually requires hysterectomy. If the rupture is in the lower uterine segment, particularly if associated with broad ligament hematoma formation, hypogastric artery ligation should be done first; it may also be necessary to ligate the ovarian arteries (preferably at the site of the utero-ovarian ligaments to avoid compromising ovarian blood supply). Once the bleeding has been controlled, careful dissection can be done to avert injury to the ureters coursing under the uterine vessels.

REFERENCES

Golan A, Sandbank O, Rubin A: Rupture of pregnant uterus. Obstet Gynecol 56:549, 1980

Schrinsky DC, Benson RC: Rupture of pregnant uterus: A review. Obstet Gynecol Survey 33:217, 1978

Spaulding LB, Gallup DG: Current concepts of management of rupture of gravid uterus. Obstet Gynecol 54:437, 1979

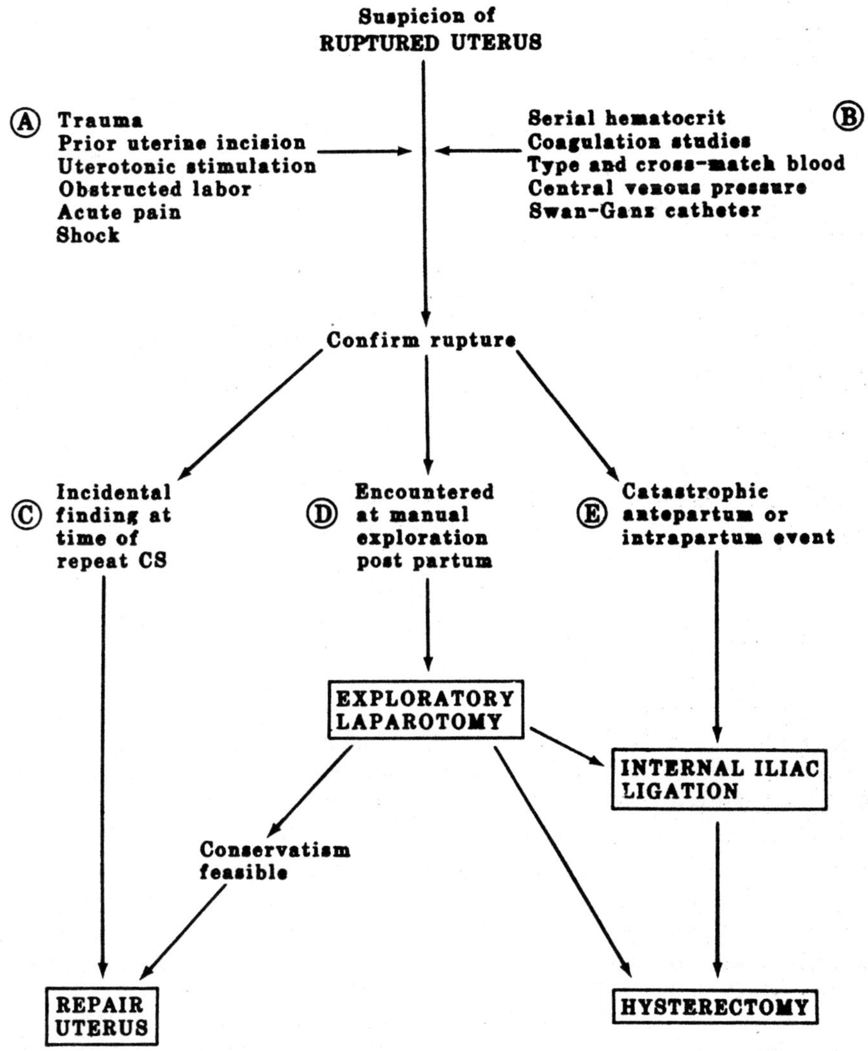
Suspicion of
RUPTURED UTERUS
Ⓐ Trauma
Prior uterine incision
Uterotonic stimulation
Obstructed labor
Acute pain
Shock
Serial hematocrit Ⓑ
Coagulation studies
Type and cross-match blood
Central venous pressure
Swan-Ganz catheter
Confirm rupture
Ⓒ Incidental finding at time of repeat CS
Ⓓ Encountered at manual exploration post partum
Ⓔ Catastrophic antepartum or intrapartum event
EXPLORATORY LAPAROTOMY
INTERNAL ILIAC LIGATION
Conservatism feasible
REPAIR UTERUS
HYSTERECTOMY

FEVER IN LABOR

Balmookoot Balgobin, M.D.

COMMENTS

A. Factors predisposing to infection in labor are poor socioeconomic status, anemia, diabetes, sickle cell disease, chronic renal and respiratory disease, and premature rupture of the membranes. Be alert to localizing symptoms that point to the source. Physical examination may help differentiate pre-existing infection or concurrent appendicitis, pyelonephritis, pneumonia, or other infection from chorioamnionitis.

B. The most common cause of temperature elevation in labor is dehydration, unless measures are routinely taken to ensure good fluid balance. Rapid intravenous infusion is useful as a therapeutic trial while diagnostic investigations are simultaneously pursued.

C. It is most important to rule out amnionitis by examining the amniotic fluid. A sample can be obtained transcervically or, if necessary, by amniocentesis. This is good practice even in the presence of signs suggesting an extrauterine source of infection. Gram stain is useful for demonstrating bacteria and polymorphonuclear leukocytes.

D. The choice of antibiotic therapy is guided by the results of the culture and the sensitivity tests; however, one cannot await such results before initiating treatment. Gram stain may help to decide initial therapy, which can later be modified when the laboratory results are available. One must take into account the undesirable side effects on mother and fetus. Because of the risk of kernicterus from hyperbilirubinemia, one must avoid sulfonamides. Tetracycline may cause dysplasia of bone and discoloration of the deciduous teeth; in large doses, tetracycline may precipitate jaundice, azotemia, and pancreatitis in the gravida who has impaired renal function. Streptomycin, kanamycin and gentamycin may be nephrotoxic and ototoxic. Chloramphenicol may produce serious fetal blood dyscrasia, and nitrofurantoin may cause hemolytic anemia in individuals with glucose-6-phosphate dehydrogenase deficiency.

E. Delivery guidelines include allowing spontaneous vaginal delivery whenever possible. Intervention is reserved for strict obstetric indications. In the presence of infection, one should be careful to avoid traumatizing maternal tissues. Thus, instrumentation by forceps, Crédé maneuver or forceful massage, and manual removal of the placenta should be avoided if possible. Check carefully for injuries of the genital tract and repair any lacerations encountered. At the time of delivery, appropriate cultures should be obtained (if they have not already been done) from mother, infant, and placenta. One should alert the pediatrician beforehand so that appropriate neonatal management can be instituted promptly. Needless to say, good aseptic technique is essential at all times.

REFERENCES

Charles D: *Infections in Obstetrics and Gynecology.* Philadelphia: WB Saunders, 1980

Friedman EA: Obstetric infections in labor. In Charles D, Finland M (eds): *Obstetric and Perinatal Infections.* Philadelphia: Lea & Febiger, 1973

Larsen JW, Goldkrand JW, Hanson TM, Miller CR: Intrauterine infection on an obstetrical service. Obstet Gynecol 43:838, 1974

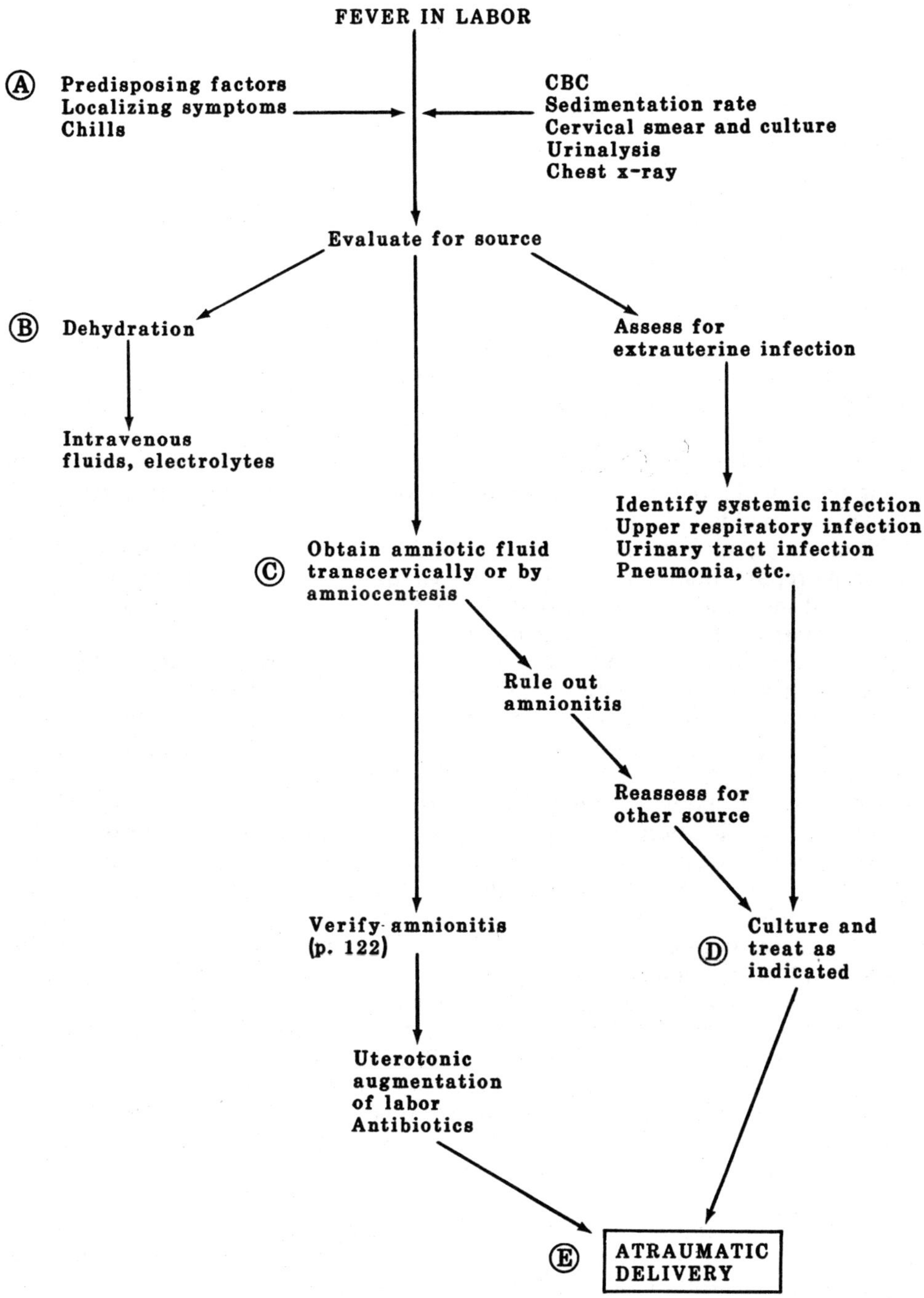
FEVER IN LABOR
(A) Predisposing factors
Localizing symptoms
Chills
CBC
Sedimentation rate
Cervical smear and culture
Urinalysis
Chest x-ray
Evaluate for source
(B) Dehydration
Intravenous
fluids, electrolytes
Assess for
extrauterine infection
Identify systemic infection
Upper respiratory infection
Urinary tract infection
Pneumonia, etc.
(C) Obtain amniotic fluid
transcervically or by
amniocentesis
Rule out
amnionitis
Reassess for
other source
Verify amnionitis
(p. 122)
(D) Culture and
treat as
indicated
Uterotonic
augmentation
of labor
Antibiotics
(E) ATRAUMATIC
DELIVERY

ASSESSING LABOR PROGRESSION

Emanuel A. Friedman, M.D.

COMMENTS

A. Whereas uterine contractions are essential for labor, their characteristics are not very helpful for judging the progress of labor. As a broad general (but not reliable) guide, the better the contractile pattern, the better the labor. The progression of the pain pattern may aid in differentiating a normal latent phase from an abnormally dilatory active phase (see *D*, below).

B. Periodic assessments of the cervix (via sterile vaginal examinations) are important for following the progress of labor. They should be done as often as is consistent with the progress being made, that is, more often (hourly) if progress is rapid and less frequently (at 2–4 hour intervals) if it is slow. Features to study objectively are dilatation, effacement, consistency, and cervical position relative to vaginal axis. At each examination, one should obtain updated information on membrane status, fetal position, asynclitism, molding, and caput formation.

C. For nulliparas, adequate active phase progress requires a rate of dilatation of 1.2 cm/hr or more; for multiparas, 1.5 cm/hr. Graphing the observations on square-ruled paper will show the expected upswing of dilatation when the active phase begins.

D. A particularly difficult diagnosis presents itself if a gravida is admitted with some degree of cervical dilatation (especially if >3 cm) and fails to advance. She could have begun labor with this dilatation and still be in the latent phase, or she could have advanced into the active phase earlier and is now secondarily arrested, a much more serious problem. The duration and pattern of contractions may help (e.g., if the contractions are unimpressive and of short duration, the patient is probably still in the latent phase). If in doubt, assume it is an arrest.

E. The normal deceleration phase, the last part of the dilatation curve prior to full cervical dilatation, should not exceed 3 hours in nulliparas or 1 hour in multiparas. Here, too, graphic display helps make the diagnosis easy.

F. The latent phase, the initial part of the dilatation pattern from onset of labor to the upswing at the beginning of the active phase, is normally less than 20 hours in nulliparas or 14 hours in multiparas.

G. Station can be readily determined by vaginal examination, relating the plane of the forward leading edge of the presenting part to the plane of the ischial spines (station zero). For each centimeter the fetus descends below the spines, it has advanced one station (+1) until it reaches and distends the perineum at station +5. Stations cephalad to the spines are designated by negative numbers (up to −5 at the true pelvic inlet). It is often important to verify that descent is really occurring (rather than molding) by suprapubic palpation of the fetal head.

H. Descent is expected to reach its maximum rate by the time the dilatation process reaches the deceleration phase and to continue uninterruptedly into second stage until the fetal presenting part reaches the perineum. The rate of descent is normally at least 1 cm/hr in nulliparas or 2 cm/hr in multiparas.

REFERENCE

Friedman EA: *Labor: Clinical Evaluation and Management*, 2nd ed. New York: Appleton-Century-Crofts, 1978

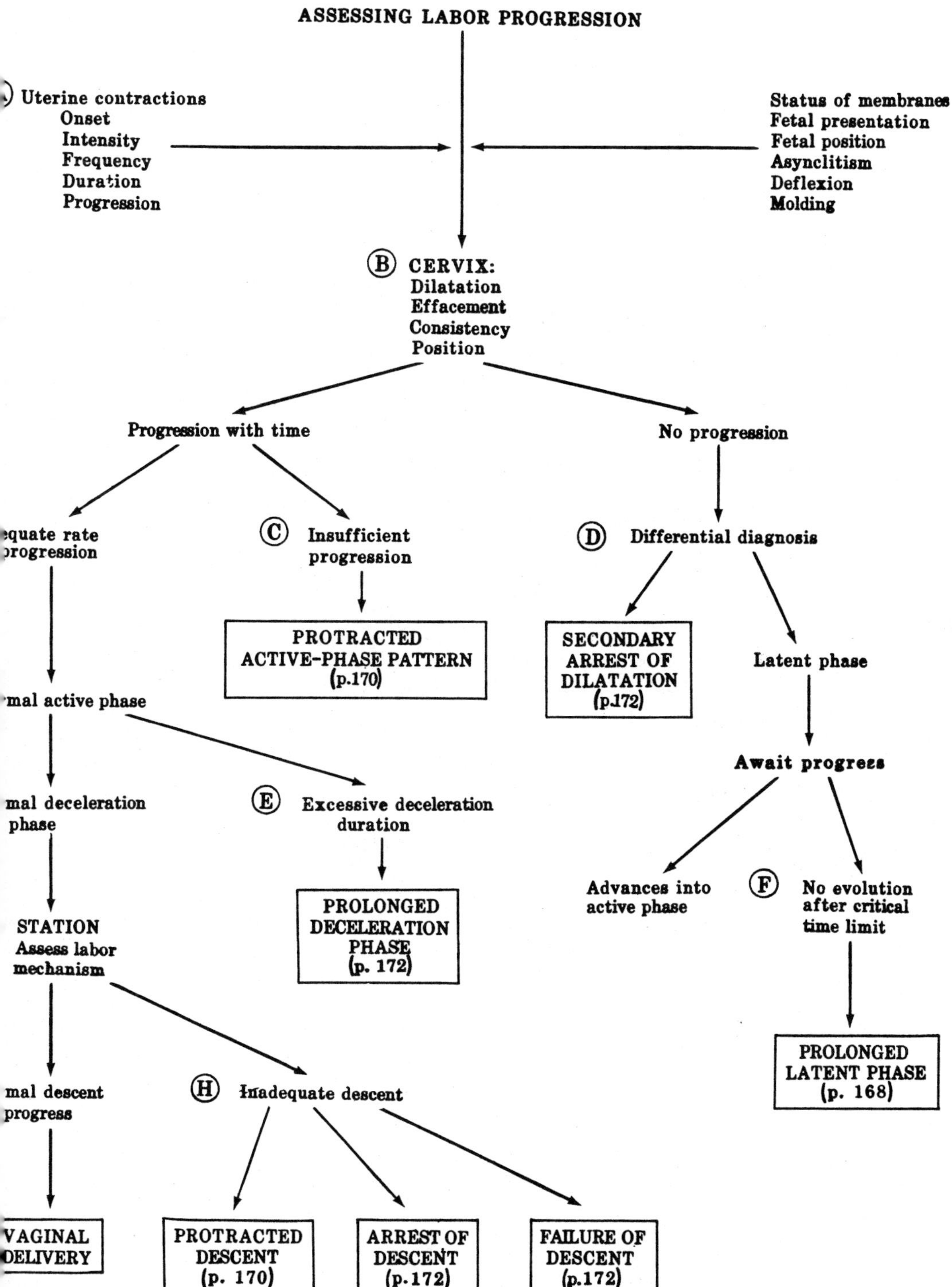
ASSESSING LABOR PROGRESSION
Uterine contractions
Onset
Intensity
Frequency
Duration
Progression
Status of membranes
Fetal presentation
Fetal position
Asynclitism
Deflexion
Molding
B CERVIX:
Dilatation
Effacement
Consistency
Position
Progression with time
No progression
equate rate
progression
C Insufficient progression
D Differential diagnosis
PROTRACTED ACTIVE-PHASE PATTERN (p.170)
SECONDARY ARREST OF DILATATION (p.172)
Latent phase
mal active phase
Await progress
mal deceleration phase
E Excessive deceleration duration
PROLONGED DECELERATION PHASE (p. 172)
Advances into active phase
F No evolution after critical time limit
STATION
Assess labor mechanism
PROLONGED LATENT PHASE (p. 168)
mal descent
progress
H Inadequate descent
VAGINAL
DELIVERY
PROTRACTED DESCENT (p. 170)
ARREST OF DESCENT (p.172)
FAILURE OF DESCENT (p.172)

PROLONGED LATENT PHASE

Emanuel A. Friedman, M.D.

COMMENTS

A. Most patients who lack progressive cervical dilatation when they first come under observation are in a perfectly normal latent phase. Those who began labor with some prelabor dilatation may mistakenly be thought to be in the active phase. The differential diagnosis is sometimes difficult (p. 166). Slow dilatation is sometimes seen in the latent phase, but it is usually less than 0.6 cm/hr. If more rapid but abnormal, consider protracted active-phase dilatation (p. 170).

B. The normal latent phase, from onset of regular contractions to the active phase upswing, should not exceed 20 hours in nulliparas or 14 hours in multiparas. If prolonged beyond these critical limits, diagnose prolonged latent phase.

C. Search for common causes, such as excessive narcotic-analgesic-sedative agents and inhalation or regional block anesthesia. The latent phase is particularly sensitive to the inhibitory effects of such agents; therefore, they should be avoided, minimized, or allowed to abate. False labor can only be diagnosed retrospectively.

D. The principal mode of managing gravidas with prolonged latent phase is a program of therapeutic rest. We use morphine sulfate, 15 mg subcutaneously or intramuscularly (20 mg for a large woman). After 20 minutes, the patient is reevaluated. Nothing more is given if the contractions have ceased or respirations are depressed. If contractions are continuing, check the cervix for any active phase change; if unchanged, an additional 10 mg morphine sulfate is given. Patients will usually sleep soundly for 6-10 hours. The time can be used profitably to correct fluid and electrolyte imbalance.

E. Rarely (2 percent incidence or less), overriding urgency prevails to try to conclude the labor as quickly as feasible (short of cesarean section). Careful uterotonic stimulation with oxytocin infusion is then used.

F. Those gravidas who awaken and are out of labor (10 percent) were in false labor. They can await onset of true labor.

G. Most (85 percent) will awaken with effective uterine contractions in the active phase of labor. Their subsequent management is no different from other parturients.

H. A few (5 percent) will wake up and resume ineffectual contractions. These failures have benefited from the rest and support. Oxytocin stimulation may now be invoked (p. 128) to effect active dilatation.

REFERENCE

Friedman EA: *Labor: Clinical Evaluation and Management*, 2nd ed. New York: Appleton-Century-Crofts, 1978

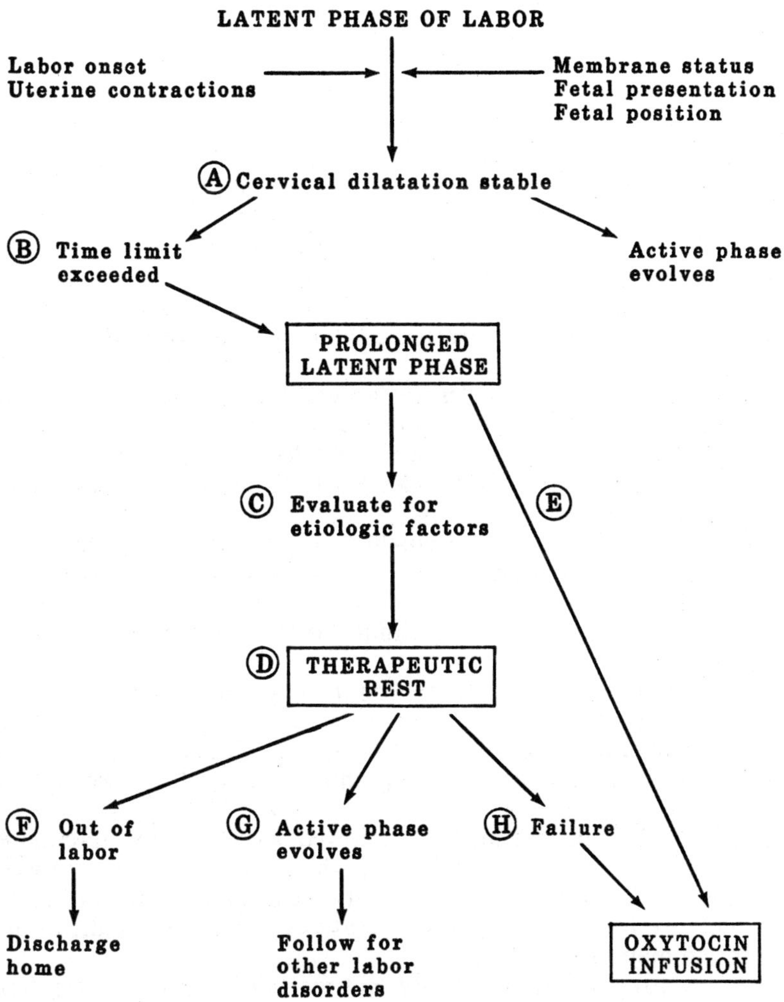
LATENT PHASE OF LABOR
Labor onset
Uterine contractions
Membrane status
Fetal presentation
Fetal position
A Cervical dilatation stable
B Time limit exceeded
Active phase evolves
PROLONGED LATENT PHASE
C Evaluate for etiologic factors
E
D THERAPEUTIC REST
F Out of labor
G Active phase evolves
H Failure
Discharge home
Follow for other labor disorders
OXYTOCIN INFUSION

PROTRACTION DISORDERS

Emanuel A. Friedman, M.D.

COMMENTS

A. Once the active phase of dilatation has begun, one should expect the cervix to dilate at least at a rate of 1.2 cm/hr in nulliparas or 1.5 cm/hr in multiparas. If less, diagnose protracted active-phase dilatation. Early in the active phase, one may discern the slow progression of the acceleration phase, representing a transition from the latent phase to the phase of maximum slope. Calculating the rate of dilatation at that time may thus result in a misdiagnosis of protracted dilatation. The error will be corrected as the true maximum slope develops.

B. After prelabor engagement, further descent generally does not begin until late in the active phase of dilatation. The descent process normally reaches its maximum slope about the time the dilatation process reaches the deceleration phase. Therefore, one cannot properly evaluate whether or not descent is occurring normally until after the deceleration phase of dilatation has begun.

C. The normal rate of descent is at least 1 cm/hr in nulliparas or 2 cm/hr in multiparas. Periodically assessing fetal station in centimeters above or below the plane of the ischial spines (station zero) will facilitate this calculation (see p. 83). Patients with rates of descent less than these critical limits are diagnosed as having protracted descent.

D. Since 30 percent of gravidas with a protraction disorder have insurmountable cephalopelvic disproportion, it is essential to evaluate the cephalopelvic relationships of every woman who develops this aberration (see p. 18). If disproportion is found to be present, safe vaginal delivery becomes very unlikely. Therefore, cesarean section is indicated.

E. Absent disproportion, the patient must be followed very carefully. Internal electronic fetal heart rate monitoring is essential. Because these labors are easily slowed or even stopped by analgesic and anesthetic agents, their use should be minimized. Arrest disorders (see p. 172) are frequent complicating features among these patients and should be watched for and managed accordingly.

F. There are high rates of perinatal morbidity and mortality as well as long-term neurologic and developmental problems associated with forceps delivery after a protraction disorder. If at all possible, therefore, one should try to deliver these babies spontaneously without instrumentation. This may require a second-stage duration of considerable length, but it is entirely acceptable provided descent is occurring (as opposed to molding) and the fetus and mother are in good condition.

REFERENCES

Friedman EA: *Labor: Clinical Evaluation and Management*, 2nd ed. New York: Appleton-Century-Crofts, 1978

Friedman EA, Sachtleben MR, Bresky PA: Dysfunctional labor: XII. Long-term effects on infant. Am J Obstet Gynecol 127:779, 1977

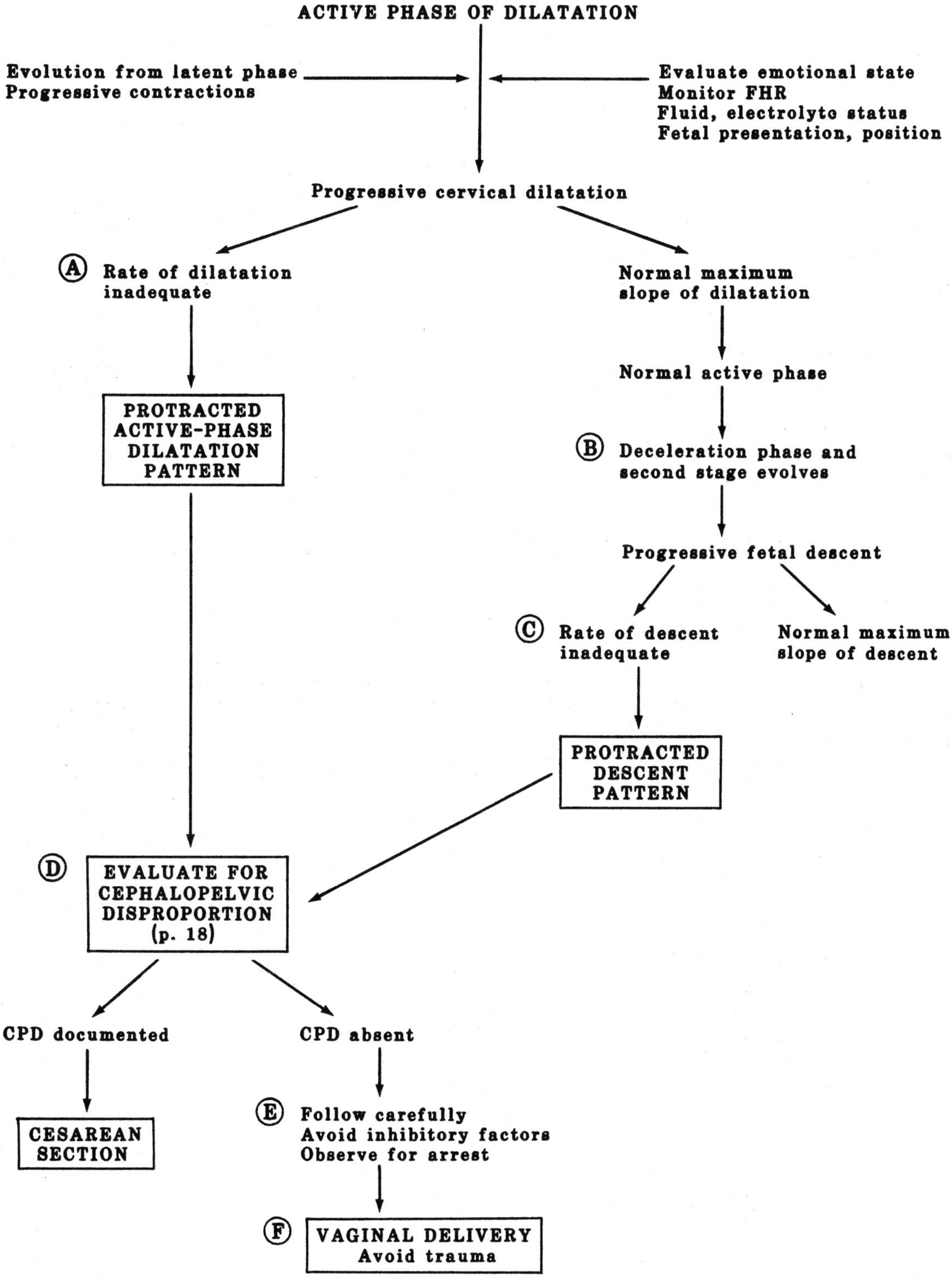
ACTIVE PHASE OF DILATATION
Evolution from latent phase
Progressive contractions
Evaluate emotional state
Monitor FHR
Fluid, electrolyte status
Fetal presentation, position
Progressive cervical dilatation
A Rate of dilatation inadequate
Normal maximum slope of dilatation
Normal active phase
B Deceleration phase and second stage evolves
Progressive fetal descent
C Rate of descent inadequate
Normal maximum slope of descent
PROTRACTED ACTIVE-PHASE DILATATION PATTERN
PROTRACTED DESCENT PATTERN
D EVALUATE FOR CEPHALOPELVIC DISPROPORTION (p. 18)
CPD documented
CPD absent
CESAREAN SECTION
E Follow carefully
Avoid inhibitory factors
Observe for arrest
F VAGINAL DELIVERY
Avoid trauma

ARREST DISORDERS

Emanuel A. Friedman, M.D.

COMMENTS

A. Once active dilatation begins, it should continue without interruption until the cervix is fully dilated and fully retracted. If dilatation stops — as documented by two vaginal examinations, preferably by the same person, spaced at least 2 hours apart — diagnose secondary arrest of dilatation. Without documented progression from latent phase to active, one has to differentiate a normal latent phase (p. 166).

B. About half the women with arrest disorders have obstructed labors based on cephalopelvic disproportion. It is imperative, therefore, to rule out disproportion before using any form of uterotonic stimulation (p. 18).

C. The risks of death and damage are great (for both mother and baby) if labor is allowed to proceed and vaginal delivery attempted in the presence of disproportion. If disproportion cannot be ruled out, one is obligated to conclude the arrested labor by cesarean section.

D. Those cases in which disproportion can be effectively ruled out will benefit from oxytocin infusion given in a carefully titrated manner. Additional dilatation and descent may occur, however, even in the presence of disproportion. Continuous electronic fetal heart rate monitoring must be done.

E. The degree of response to oxytocin may help signal that disproportion actually exists even though it is not suspected. Compare the postarrest slope of progressive dilatation or descent with the prearrest slope. If the postarrest slope is the same as or greater than the prearrest slope, the prognosis for vaginal delivery is excellent. A lower postarrest slope or nonprogression demands reevaluation of pelvic adequacy. Cesarean section should be done unless it is quite clear that the baby can be delivered vaginally. Outcome for babies born vaginally is poor unless disproportion is first clearly ruled out and the postarrest progression is optimal.

F. The terminal segment of the active phase, the deceleration phase, reflects cephalad retraction of the cervix around the fetal head. The same factors associated with other arrest disorders occur with prolonged deceleration phase, especially disproportion. A deceleration phase is abnormal if it lasts longer than 3 hours in nulliparas or 1 hour in multiparas.

G. Although active descent may begin before the deceleration phase, it is a serious disorder (failure of descent) if it does not occur at this time. If descent begins, but the fetal presenting part does not reach the perineum, arrest of descent is present. The diagnosis of arrest of descent is usually made in the second stage by two vaginal examinations spaced at least one hour apart.

REFERENCES

Friedman EA: *Labor: Clinical Evaluation and Management*, 2nd ed. New York: Appleton-Century-Crofts, 1978

Friedman EA, Sachtleben MR: Station of the fetal presenting part: VI. Arrest of descent in nulliparas. Obstet Gynecol 47:129, 1976

Friedman EA, Sachtleben MR, Bresky PA: Dysfunctional labor: XII. Long-term effects on infant. Am J Obstet Gynecol 127:779, 1977

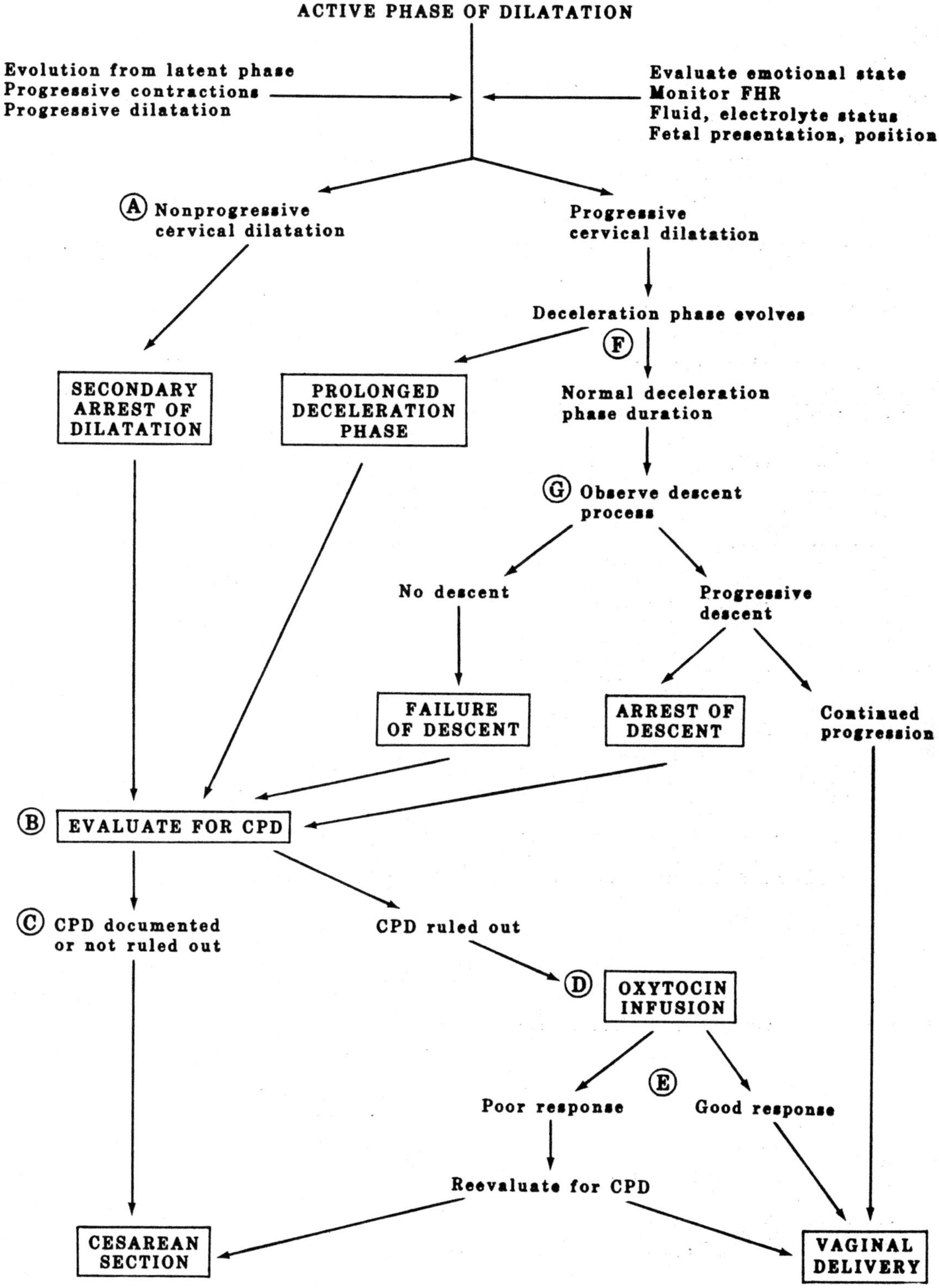
ACTIVE PHASE OF DILATATION
Evolution from latent phase
Progressive contractions
Progressive dilatation
Evaluate emotional state
Monitor FHR
Fluid, electrolyte status
Fetal presentation, position
(A) Nonprogressive cervical dilatation
Progressive cervical dilatation
Deceleration phase evolves
(F)
Normal deceleration phase duration
SECONDARY ARREST OF DILATATION
PROLONGED DECELERATION PHASE
(G) Observe descent process
No descent
Progressive descent
FAILURE OF DESCENT
ARREST OF DESCENT
Continued progression
(B) EVALUATE FOR CPD
(C) CPD documented or not ruled out
CPD ruled out
(D) OXYTOCIN INFUSION
(E)
Poor response
Good response
Reevaluate for CPD
CESAREAN SECTION
VAGINAL DELIVERY

FAILURE TO PROGRESS

Emanuel A. Friedman, M.D.

COMMENTS

A. Failure to progress is a "catch-basket" diagnosis encompassing a range of conditions, some serious and some benign. Since specific diagnosis enables one to provide specific, optimal therapy, it is important to differentiate.

B. Active phase of the first stage is readily recognized by the change in the slope of the dilation curve. The guideline of 0.6 cm/hr is sometimes helpful in differentiating between a normal latent phase (a slope less than this cut-point) and an abnormal active phase (more than this rate). One should note, however, that exceptions do occur.

C. The absence of any progress at advanced dilatation makes the differential diagnosis difficult. If prior dilatation is known (for example, if the patient had recently been examined in the office), this can be very helpful. Recent progress, even though unobserved, probably signifies active-phase dilatation, now arrested. If the differential diagnosis cannot be made, assume that the more serious problem (of arrest) exists.

D. Latent phase durations in excess of 20 hours in nulliparas or 14 hours in multiparas are abnormal (see p. 168). "Failure to progress" under these circumstances is a relatively minor problem, albeit common, with good prognosis.

E. Secondary arrest of dilatation and failure or arrest of descent (see p. 172) are readily diagnosed by following the labor pattern. They are far more serious forms of "failure to progress" than normal or prolonged latent phase. This is so because of the probable need for operative intervention in an arrest disorder which may have concomitant cephalopelvic disproportion.

F. Continuing dilatory progression in dilatation or in descent (see p. 170) is not actually a true arrest, but it is sometimes mistakenly included under the umbrella of "failure to progress." Such protraction disorders require astuteness for diagnosis and skill and patience for proper management.

REFERENCE

Friedman EA: *Labor: Clinical Evaluation and Management*, 2nd ed. New York: Appleton-Century-Crofts, 1978

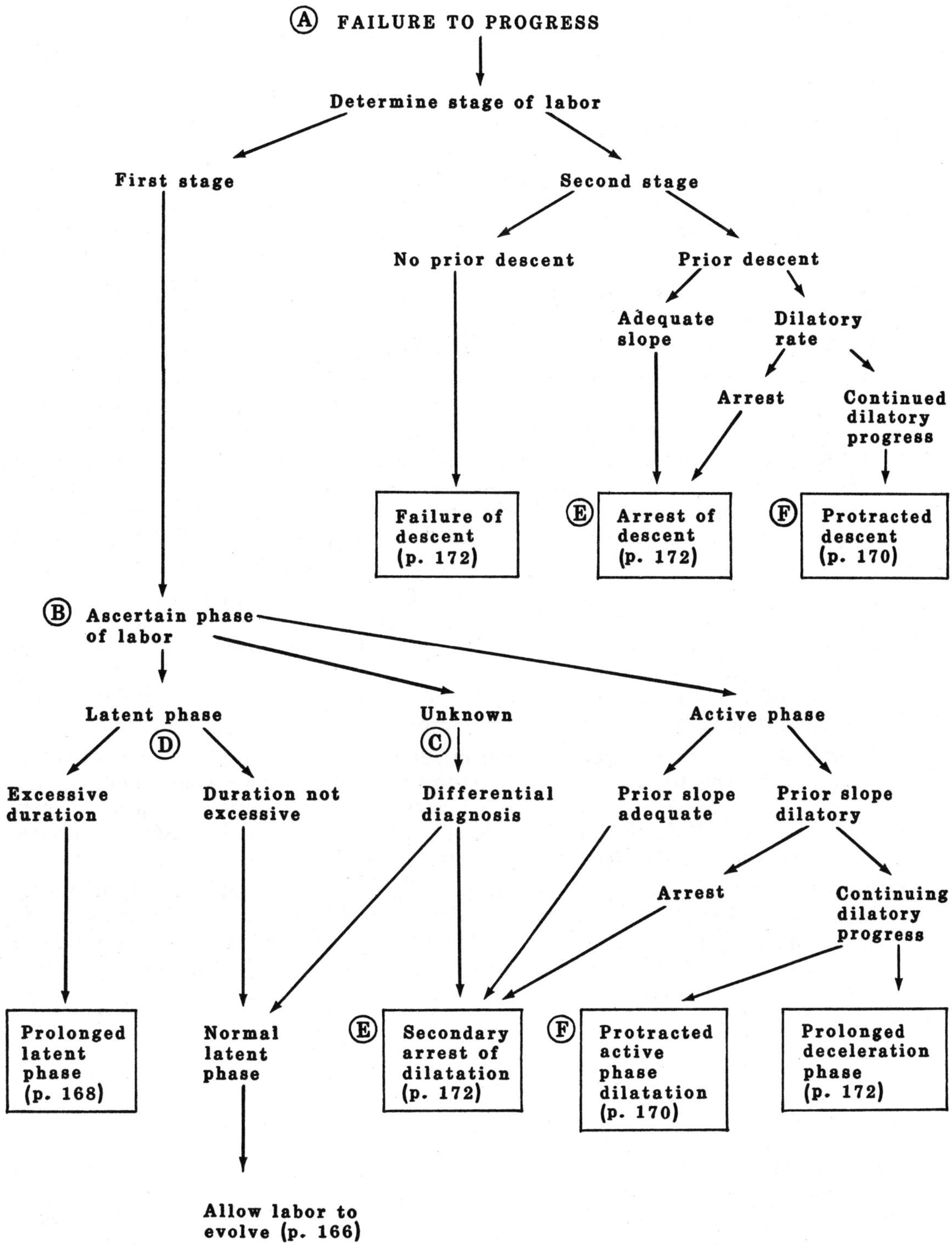
Ⓐ FAILURE TO PROGRESS
Determine stage of labor
First stage
Second stage
No prior descent
Prior descent
Adequate slope
Dilatory rate
Arrest
Continued dilatory progress
Failure of descent (p. 172)
Ⓔ Arrest of descent (p. 172)
Ⓕ Protracted descent (p. 170)
Ⓑ Ascertain phase of labor
Latent phase
Unknown
Active phase
Ⓓ
Ⓒ
Excessive duration
Duration not excessive
Differential diagnosis
Prior slope adequate
Prior slope dilatory
Arrest
Continuing dilatory progress
Prolonged latent phase (p. 168)
Normal latent phase
Ⓔ Secondary arrest of dilatation (p. 172)
Ⓕ Protracted active phase dilatation (p. 170)
Prolonged deceleration phase (p. 172)
Allow labor to evolve (p. 166)

MANAGEMENT OF SECOND STAGE

Wayne R. Cohen, M.D.

COMMENTS

A. One should be alert to malpresentation and cephalopelvic disproportion in order to ensure close surveillance. A second stage longer than 2 hours is not necessarily abnormal, but it is imperative that a gravida with a long second stage be evaluated very carefully.

B. Routine electronic fetal heart rate monitoring is recommended in all high-risk circumstances. If it is not being performed routinely, the fetal risk of abnormal descent with long second stage mandates such monitoring.

C. Periodic close assessment of the descent process is critical. Progress is noted by the rate of descent. If the rate of descent is at least 1 cm/hr in nulliparas or 2 cm/hr in multiparas, one can expect continued progress and uneventful vaginal delivery.

D. If there is no progression in fetal descent for 1 hour or more, diagnose arrest of descent and proceed with intensive evaluation for cephalopelvic disproportion. Unless one can rule out cephalopelvic disproportion, proceed with cesarean section. If there is adequate room for further fetal descent, expect uterotonic stimulation to yield good post-arrest response with adequate descent, leading to vaginal delivery (p. 172).

E. If descent is occurring but at an abnormally slow rate, diagnose protracted descent (p. 170) and rule out disproportion. Continued labor is permitted provided no disproportion exists. Periodically verify descent by confirming one's vaginal estimates of fetal station by means of suprapubic palpation. This will ensure that the head is actually descending and is not merely fixed in the inlet, elongating as a consequence of extreme molding. If descent is confirmed, manage expectantly.

F. During a long second stage, close patient support and encouragement are necessary. Allowing patients to assume the position in which they are most comfortable can aid in their bearing-down efforts. Upright postures, such as sitting and squatting, may enhance descent in some individuals. Avoid the supine position because of its adverse effect on venous cardiac return (supine hypotension syndrome).

G. Strive for a spontaneous vaginal delivery after a long second stage. Instrumental delivery, particularly a midforceps operation, increases the risk of perinatal morbidity after abnormal descent. Episiotomy is often helpful and desirable. Alternatively, one may soften and stretch the perineum by gradual massage. Delivery positions other than lithotomy may reduce the need for episiotomy.

REFERENCES

Cohen WR: Influence of the duration of second stage labor on perinatal outcome and puerperal morbidity. Obstet Gynecol 49:266, 1977

Friedman EA, Sachtleben MR: Station of the fetal presenting part: I. Pattern of descent. Am J Obstet Gynecol 93:522, 1965

Friedman EA, Sachtleben MR, Bresky P: Dysfunctionl labor: XII. Long-term effects on infant. Am J Obstet Gynecol 127:779, 1977

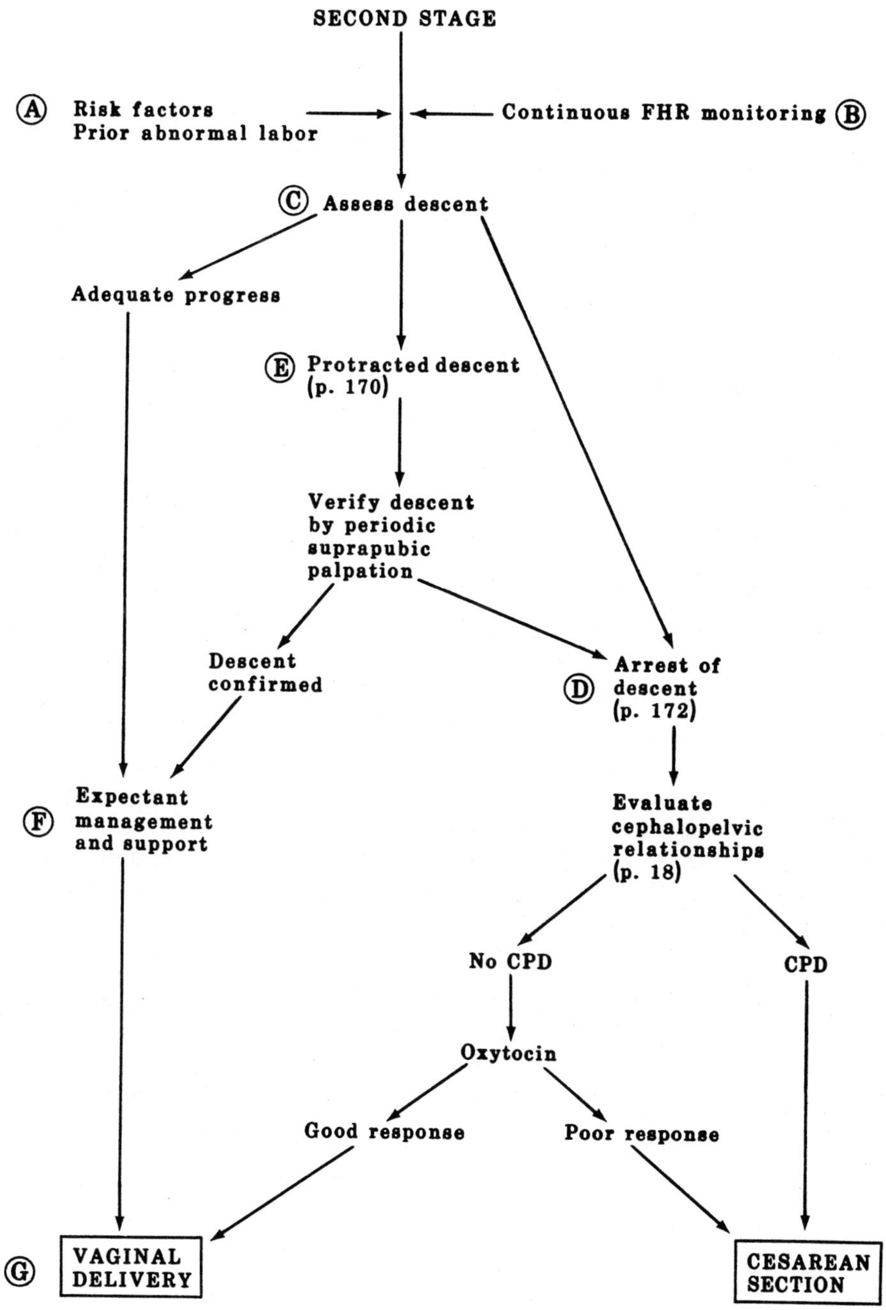
SECOND STAGE
Ⓐ Risk factors
Prior abnormal labor
Continuous FHR monitoring Ⓑ
Ⓒ Assess descent
Adequate progress
Ⓔ Protracted descent (p. 170)
Verify descent by periodic suprapubic palpation
Descent confirmed
Arrest of Ⓓ descent (p. 172)
Ⓕ Expectant management and support
Evaluate cephalopelvic relationships (p. 18)
No CPD
CPD
Oxytocin
Good response
Poor response
Ⓖ VAGINAL DELIVERY
CESAREAN SECTION

SOFT TISSUE DYSTOCIA

Emanuel A. Friedman, M.D.

COMMENTS

A. Whereas inadequate uterine contractions are more often the cause of labor aberrations than bony dystocia, it is rare for the soft tissues of the cervix to impede labor progression. A past history of cervical trauma, electrocautery, cryosurgery, conization, amputation or trachelorrhaphy should enhance one's suspicion, although most of these women have either a normal labor or a clinical picture of incompetent cervix (p. 40).

B. The unfavorable cervix (long, closed, tough, rigid, and posteriorly positioned in the vaginal axis) serves to suggest that the patient is not in true labor. If contractions do not subside spontaneously, an intensive regimen of therapeutic rest (p. 168) will usually stop the process.

C. Oxytocin infusion (p. 128) is an effective means for treating those few women who continue to have regular uterine contractions without perceptible change in the cervix after a suitable interval of therapeutic rest. Most will respond to uterotonic stimulation with active dilatation, leading ultimately to vaginal delivery (provided some other problem does not arise). The rare individual with true cervical dystocia may be distinguished at this time by failure to respond to oxytocin.

D. A foregoing interval of labor during which active cervical dilatation occurs is evidence to support the contention that the latent phase ended and that the current nonprogression probably represents secondary arrest of dilatation. An intensive program of evaluation and management is therefore in order (p. 172).

E. Cervical conglutination is an unusual condition in which the external os remains closed, but the labor process evolves nonetheless. The lower uterine segment is ballooned out as the fetal head descends. Effacement occurs, often to an extreme degree, as the internal os dilates and the cervix is then incorporated into the lower uterine segment. Insinuating a finger into the pinpoint cervical opening will often initiate rapid dilatation.

REFERENCES

Gibbs CE, Moore SF: The scarred cervix in pregnancy and labor. Gen Pract 37:85, 1968

Greenhill JP, Friedman EA: Soft-tissue dystocia. Hosp Med 4:73, 1968

Jones JM, Sweetnam P, Hibbard BM: Outcome of pregnancy after cone biopsy of the cervix: Case-control study. Brit J Obstet Gynaecol 186:913, 1979

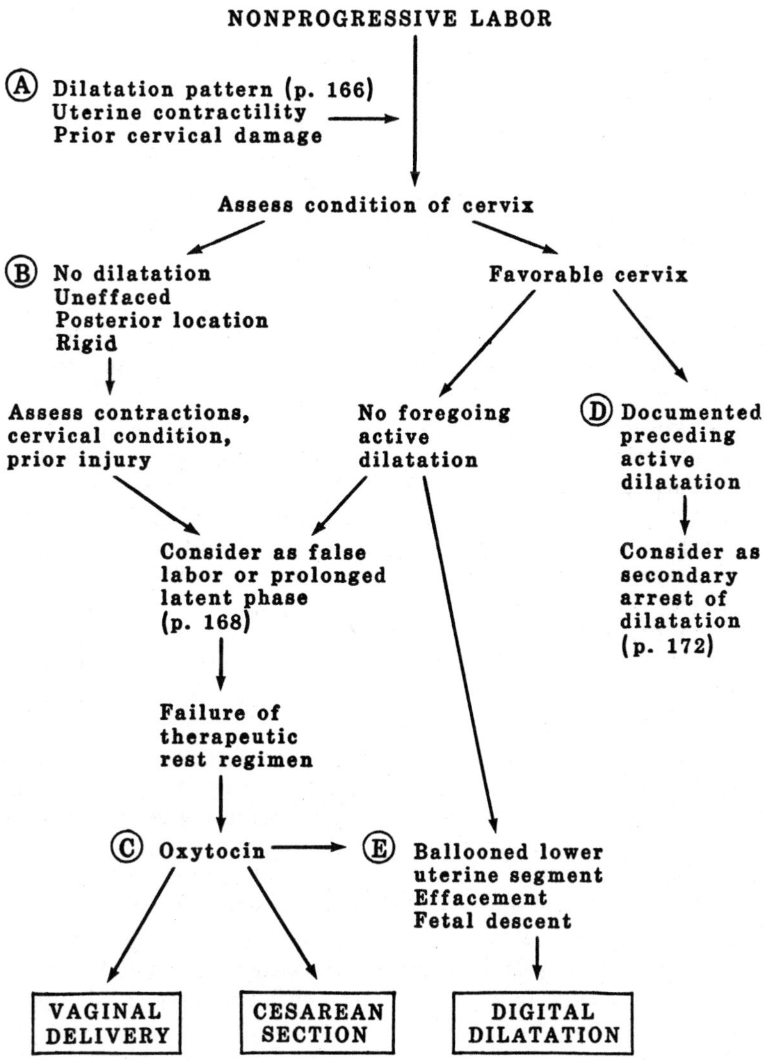
NONPROGRESSIVE LABOR
(A) Dilatation pattern (p. 166)
Uterine contractility
Prior cervical damage
Assess condition of cervix
(B) No dilatation
Uneffaced
Posterior location
Rigid
Favorable cervix
Assess contractions, cervical condition, prior injury
No foregoing active dilatation
(D) Documented preceding active dilatation
Consider as false labor or prolonged latent phase (p. 168)
Consider as secondary arrest of dilatation (p. 172)
Failure of therapeutic rest regimen
(C) Oxytocin
(E) Ballooned lower uterine segment
Effacement
Fetal descent
VAGINAL DELIVERY
CESAREAN SECTION
DIGITAL DILATATION

UTERINE TETANY

Emanuel A. Friedman, M.D.

COMMENTS

A. By convention, a contraction that lasts longer than 90 seconds is a tetanic contraction. Its importance stems from the fetal hypoxia that can result. Comarable hypoxia may result from uterine hypertonus (basal tonus increased above 12–15 mm Hg) or polysystole (frequent contractions with very short intervening resting intervals) that interferes with uterine blood flow and fetal oxygenation in the same way. Speed in evaluation and management is critical, because the longer the contraction lasts, the greater its potential for causing fetal death or irreversible brain damage. Thus, while assessing for cause, one should be actively pursuing measures for correcting the problem, determining both fetal and maternal status, and simultaneously preparing for emergency intervention if that should prove necessary.

B. Oxytocin use and abruptio placentae are the most common identifiable causes of tetanic uterine contractions. Uterine tetany can also occur spontaneously or result from the administration of drugs not ordinarily considered to be uterotonic. Aside from ergot preparations (such as those used for treating migraine) and prostaglandins, a wide variety of pharmacologic agents have uterine stimulating effects, including diphenhydramine (especially if given intravenously), vasopressor amines (such as methoxamine and mephentermine), histamine, digoxin (and related cardiotonic agents, ouabain and strophanthin G), acetylcholine, neostigmine, and pilocarpine. Tetanic contractions caused by these agents are rare and usually short-lived; nonetheless, they must be managed carefully and expeditiously to avoid fetal injury. The paradigm for oxytocin-induced tetany is applicable here as well.

C. The single most effective means for interrupting a tetanic contraction that occurs in response to oxytocin use is to stop administering the drug. As soon as the intravenous infusion of dilute oxytocin is discontinued, the circulating levels rapidly diminish (half-life about 3 minutes) and, in consequence, the contraction usually subsides promptly. Giving oxytocin by any other route can yield tetanic contractions that are not readily reversible; thus, these other routes of administration are not recommended.

D. Tocolysis by pharmacologic means (p. 124) generally takes too long to be very useful. Uterine-relaxing anesthesia is quickly effective, however, especially in the form of halogenated inhalation agents (e.g., halothane, enflurane, etc.), if appropriately trained and skilled personnel and suitable facilities are immediately available. Under most circumstances, by the time everything is in readiness to initiate the anesthesia, the oxytocin-induced tetanic contraction will have subsided spontaneously.

REFERENCES

Caldeyro-Barcia R, Pose SV, Poseiro JJ, Mendez-Bauer C, Escarcena L, Behrman R: Effects of several factors on fetal pO_2 recorded continuously in the fetal monkey. In Gluck L (ed): *Intrauterine Asphyxia and the Developing Fetal Brain.* Chicago: Year Book Medical Publishers, 1977

Odendaal HJ: Frequency of uterine contractions in abruptio placentae. S Afr Med J 50:2129, 1976

Ramsey EM, Donner MW: *Placental Vasculature and Circulation.* Philadelphia: WB Saunders Co, 1980

Schifrin BS: Fetal heart rate patterns following epidural anaesthesia and oxytocin infusion during labour. J Obstet Gynaecol Brit Comm 79:332, 1972

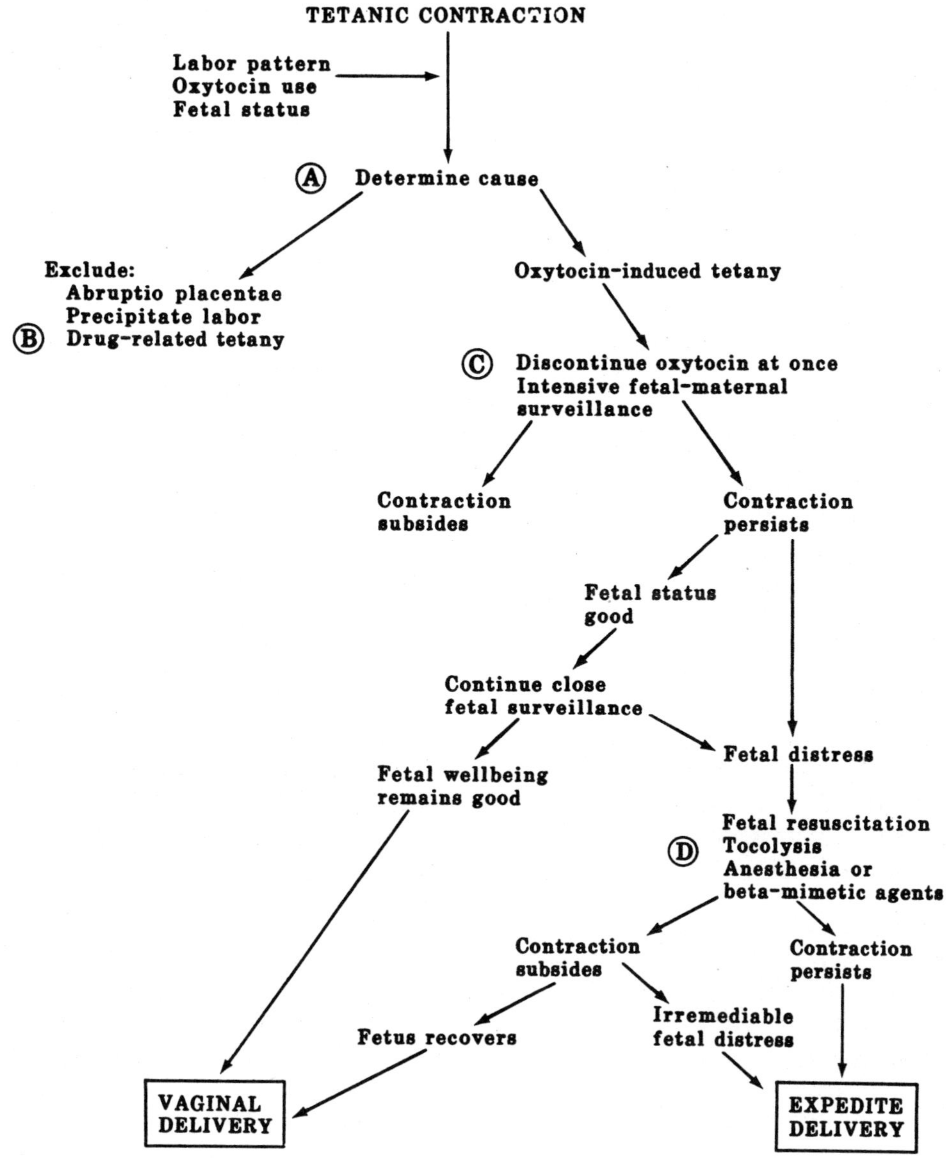
TETANIC CONTRACTION
Labor pattern
Oxytocin use
Fetal status
Ⓐ Determine cause
Exclude:
Abruptio placentae
Precipitate labor
Ⓑ Drug-related tetany
Oxytocin-induced tetany
Ⓒ Discontinue oxytocin at once
Intensive fetal-maternal surveillance
Contraction subsides
Contraction persists
Fetal status good
Continue close fetal surveillance
Fetal wellbeing remains good
Fetal distress
Fetal resuscitation
Ⓓ Tocolysis
Anesthesia or beta-mimetic agents
Contraction subsides
Contraction persists
Fetus recovers
Irremediable fetal distress
VAGINAL DELIVERY
EXPEDITE DELIVERY

SHOULDER DYSTOCIA

Wayne R. Cohen, M.D.

COMMENTS

A. Anticipate shoulder dystocia when there is a history of large babies, diabetes mellitus, obesity, contracted pelvis (especially at the outlet), or long second stage.

B. Characteristically, as the fetal head is being delivered, it will retract firmly back onto the perineum. Although shoulder dystocia requires efficient, forthright, and aggressive interventive action, undue haste and the temptation to use extreme traction or excessive fundal or suprapubic pressure must be avoided. Serious permanent or lethal damage to mother or fetus may result.

C. If an episiotomy has not yet been made, it is essential that a large mediolateral episiotomy, or preferably a complete median perineotomy, be done at once. Summon expert assistance to help in the delivery and mobilize expert anesthesia and pediatric consultants. Examine the patient internally to determine the degree of descent of the shoulders and the orientation of the bisacromial diameter (which is usually directed anteroposteriorly).

D. A combination of suprapubic pressure and gentle downward traction on the restituted fetal head should first be tried, taking special care not to damage the brachial plexus. Head traction must be gentle; do not persist if the anterior shoulder does not stem under the symphysis pubis.

E. Once the anterior shoulder is properly stemmed under the symphysis, gently elevating the fetal head should result in delivery of the posterior shoulder. If the posterior shoulder does not advance spontaneously, one may place a finger in the axilla and gently pull to dislodge the posterior shoulder from the sacral promontory or the hollow of the sacrum.

F. With the posterior shoulder well down in the pelvis, one may attempt to "corkscrew" the fetus by rotating the posterior shoulder 180° while simultaneously applying traction to deliver it under the pubic arch. If necessary, the shoulder now located posteriorly can be rotated 180° in the opposite direction. Kristellar pressure is useful during this maneuver.

G. In cases in which the posterior shoulder has not descended below the ischial spines, rotate the posterior shoulder so that the bisacromial diameter is obliquely oriented. Then dislodge the posterior shoulder and pull it below the midplane by axillary traction. The aforementioned corkscrew maneuver should then effect delivery.

H. The clavicle may be fractured or cut with heavy scissors. Both measures should be considered extreme, because they are hazardous to mother and fetus. Moreover, it is very difficult to fracture the clavicle, especially in a large, heavy-boned fetus. Nonetheless, it may be potentially lifesaving.

REFERENCES

Benedetti JJ, Gabbe SG: Shoulder dystocia: A complication of fetal macrosomia and prolonged second stage of labor with midpelvic delivery. Obstet Gynecol 52:526, 1978

Morris WIC: Shoulder dystocia. J Obstet Gynaecol Brit Emp 62:302, 1955

Woods CE: A principle of physics as applicable to shoulder delivery. Am J Obstet Gynecol 45:796, 1943

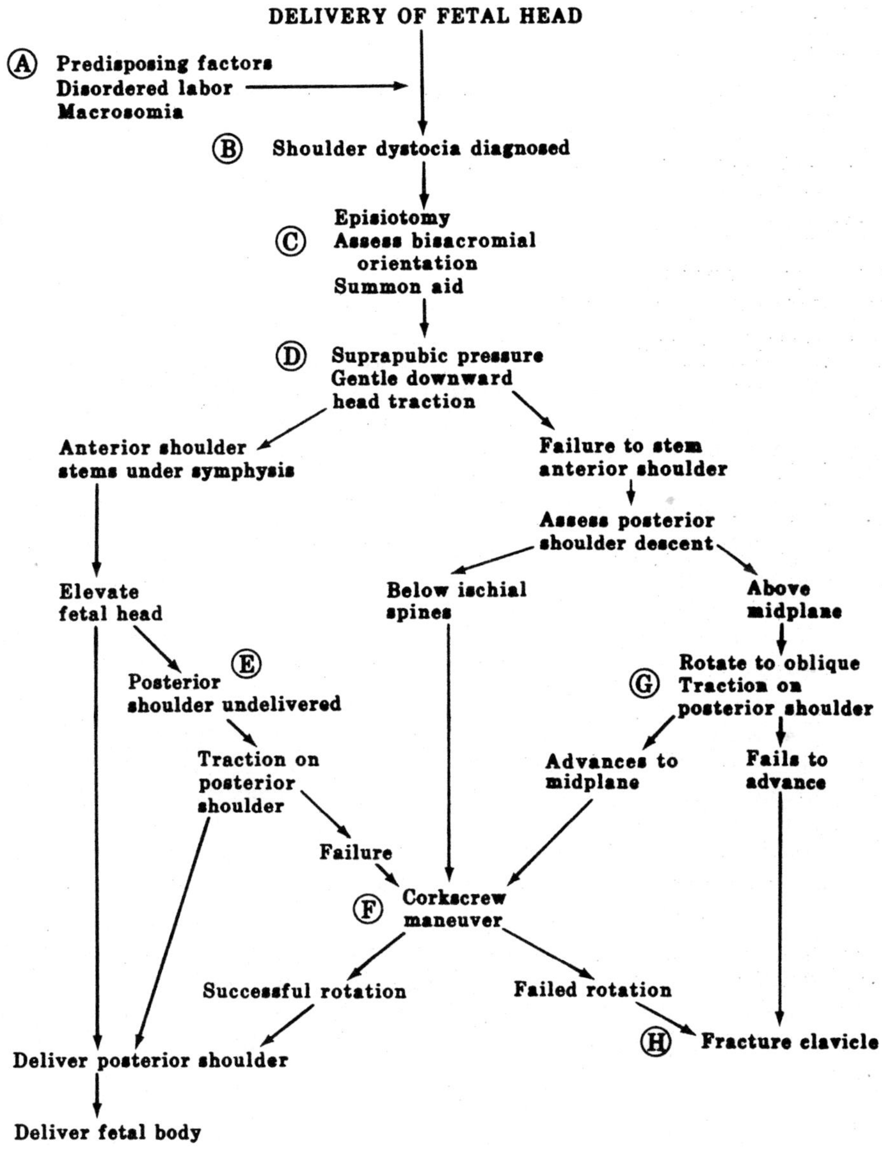
DELIVERY OF FETAL HEAD
A Predisposing factors
Disordered labor
Macrosomia
B Shoulder dystocia diagnosed
C Episiotomy
Assess bisacromial orientation
Summon aid
D Suprapubic pressure
Gentle downward head traction
Anterior shoulder stems under symphysis
Failure to stem anterior shoulder
Assess posterior shoulder descent
Elevate fetal head
Below ischial spines
Above midplane
E Posterior shoulder undelivered
G Rotate to oblique
Traction on posterior shoulder
Traction on posterior shoulder
Advances to midplane
Fails to advance
Failure
F Corkscrew maneuver
Successful rotation
Failed rotation
H Fracture clavicle
Deliver posterior shoulder
Deliver fetal body

DELIVERY TRAUMA

Selwyn P. Oskowitz, M.B.

COMMENTS

A. Risk factors for delivery trauma include a large fetus – especially in association with cephalopelvic disproportion – malpresentations, fetal anomalies, maternal obesity, grand multiparity, precipitate labor, obstructed labor, delivery manipulations and instrumentation, and shoulder dystocia.

B. In the interest of maternal welfare, it is important to replace lost blood by transfusion as quickly as possible; in the interim, blood volume can be maintained for purposes of ensuring cardiovascular stability and tissue perfusion by administering volume-expanding solutions. Since at minimum it will be necessary to explore the birth canal to ascertain the source of bleeding, one should mobilize anesthesia and operating room facilities (a fully equipped delivery room will usually suffice for this purpose).

C. Exploration of the birth canal will usually disclose the site of the bleeding. If no laceration or hematoma is encountered, consider uterine atony as the most likely cause (p. 186). Manual exploration of the uterus under anesthesia may reveal uterine rupture or uterine inversion. Second only to atony as a cause of postpartum hemorrhage are lacerations resulting from delivery trauma and subsurface disruptions leading to hematoma formation.

D. Lacerations in the lower vagina and perineum are readily repaired by careful hemostasis and suturing. Special attention should be paid to tears occurring in the vaginal fornices and lateral sulci, because damage to ureter or bladder may already exist or be incurred by suturing. Lacerations that enter the rectum require careful closure in layers with care taken to approximate the mucosa and anal sphincter. Lacerations near the ischial spine require special attention to avoid pudendal nerve damage.

E. Small, stable hematomas can be treated expectantly. If they are progressive with continued bleeding, expanding size, and increasing pain, they must be surgically evacuated with careful attention to hemostasis. Primary closure is sometimes possible but drainage is often necessary. Secondary infection demands evacuation and open drainage.

F. Hematoma in the broad ligament may be difficult to detect. Suspect it if the patient's cardiovascular instability or falling hematocrit cannot be accounted for by external blood loss. Internal iliac artery ligation is often necessary to stop the bleeding before evacuating and dissecting down to the bleeding source (usually a uterine artery or vein); special care must be taken to avoid ureteral injury.

REFERENCES

Lieberman BA: Repair to injuries of the genital tract. Clin Obstet Gynaecol 7:621, 1980
Massey WE, Cefalo RC: Neuropathies of pregnancy. Obstet Gynecol Survey 34:489, 1979
Pieri RJ: Pelvic hematomas associated with pregnancy. Obstet Gynecol 12:249, 1958

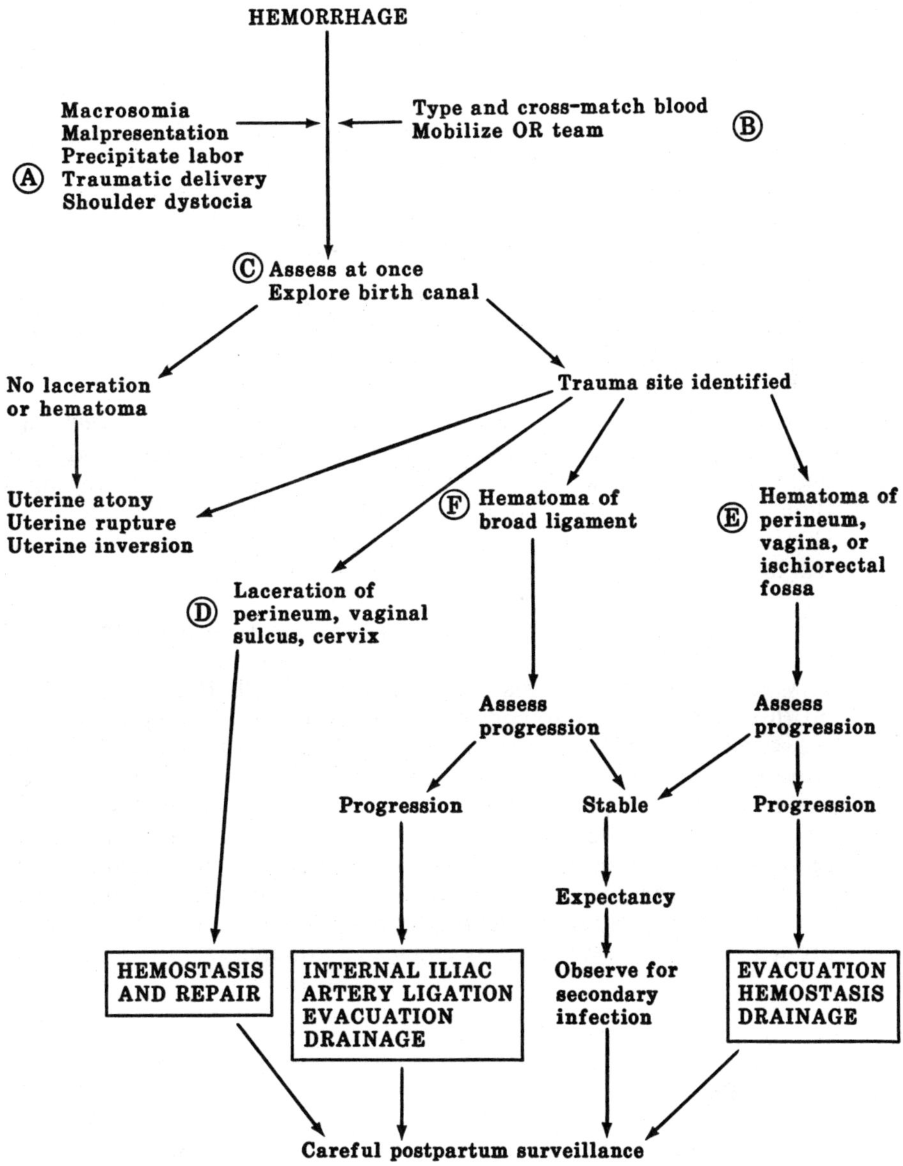
HEMORRHAGE
Macrosomia
Malpresentation
Precipitate labor
Ⓐ Traumatic delivery
Shoulder dystocia
Type and cross-match blood
Mobilize OR team Ⓑ
Ⓒ Assess at once
Explore birth canal
No laceration
or hematoma
Trauma site identified
Uterine atony
Uterine rupture
Uterine inversion
Ⓕ Hematoma of
broad ligament
Ⓔ Hematoma of
perineum,
vagina, or
ischiorectal
fossa
Ⓓ Laceration of
perineum, vaginal
sulcus, cervix
Assess
progression
Assess
progression
Progression
Stable
Progression
Expectancy
HEMOSTASIS
AND REPAIR
INTERNAL ILIAC
ARTERY LIGATION
EVACUATION
DRAINAGE
Observe for
secondary
infection
EVACUATION
HEMOSTASIS
DRAINAGE
Careful postpartum surveillance

UTERINE ATONY

Louis Burke, M.D.

COMMENTS

A. Anticipate uterine atony in grand multiparas and gravidas with uterine overdistention (e.g., large baby, multiple pregnancy, or hydramnios), prolonged labor (especially if stimulated with oxytocin), deep general anesthesia, abruptio placentae, and even placenta previa. Postpartum bleeding, particularly in association with the uterus that does not contract well, means uterine atony until proved otherwise.

B. The uterus should be elevated out of the pelvis and gently massaged. Uterotonic drugs are given, including rapid intravenous oxytocin drip or ergonovine in intravenous bolus. Prostaglandins may also be tried.

C. Exploration of the birth canal under sterile conditions in a well-equipped operating or delivery room is necessary to identify the bleeding site. Good lighting, assistance, and exposure are essential. Any lacerations encountered require immediate attention. Bimanual compression and massage of the noncontractile uterus should be done. Uterine packing is condemned because it is ineffective and wastes time; moreover, it will interfere with uterine contractility, which is desirable.

D. Uterine exploration will rule out retained fragments of placenta. If retained secundines are encountered, they must be evacuated by digital or instrumental means applied very gently to avoid traumatizing the uterine wall. If atony persists and bleeding is profuse, one may have to consider bilateral internal iliac ligation as a lifesaving measure. It must be undertaken before irreversible shock develops. Continued bleeding may require ovarian artery ligations as well at the uterovarian ligament site. If all else fails, hysterectomy may be necessary even in young women of low parity. For the patient who continues to bleed at a more moderate flow rate and in whom conservation of reproductive function is critical, one may consider newer techniques of arterial embolization by means of transvascular catheterization under radiographic control. These sophisticated angiographic techniques may be especially well suited for managing this problem, but they are not yet available everywhere.

REFERENCES

Brown BJ, Heaston DK, Poulson AM, Gabert HA, Mineau DE, Miller FJ Jr: Uncontrollable postpartum bleeding: A new approach to hemostasis through angiographic arterial embolization. Obstet Gynecol 54:361, 1979

Corson SL, Bolognese RJ: Postpartum uterine atony treated with prostaglandin. Am J Obstet Gynecol 129:918, 1977

Fribourg SR, Rothman LA, Rovinsky JJ: Intrauterine lavage for control of uterine atony. Obstet Gynecol 41:876, 1973

Lee CY, Madrazo B, Druker BH: Ultrasonic evaluation of the postpartum uterus in the management of postpartum bleeding. Obstet Gynecol 58:227, 1981

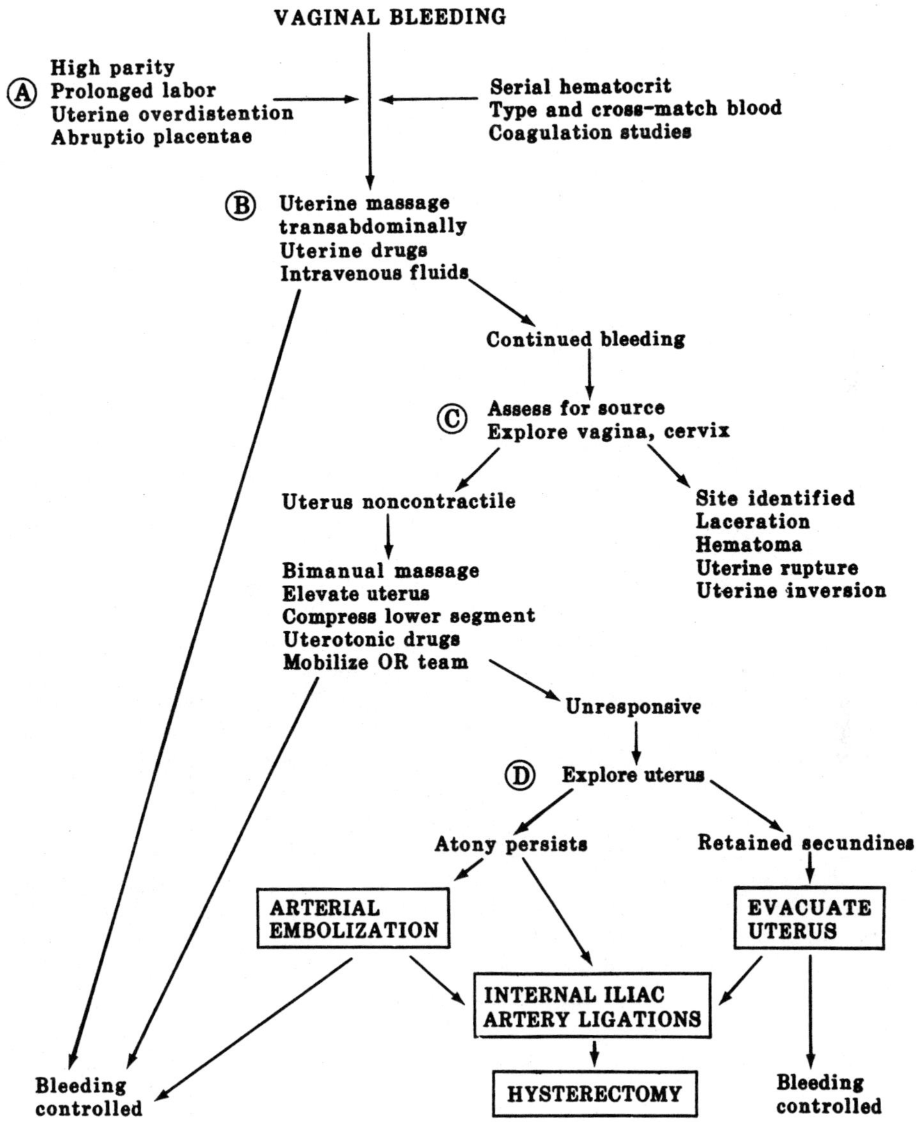
VAGINAL BLEEDING
A
High parity
Prolonged labor
Uterine overdistention
Abruptio placentae
Serial hematocrit
Type and cross-match blood
Coagulation studies
B
Uterine massage transabdominally
Uterine drugs
Intravenous fluids
Continued bleeding
C
Assess for source
Explore vagina, cervix
Uterus noncontractile
Site identified
Laceration
Hematoma
Uterine rupture
Uterine inversion
Bimanual massage
Elevate uterus
Compress lower segment
Uterotonic drugs
Mobilize OR team
Unresponsive
D
Explore uterus
Atony persists
Retained secundines
ARTERIAL EMBOLIZATION
EVACUATE UTERUS
INTERNAL ILIAC ARTERY LIGATIONS
HYSTERECTOMY
Bleeding controlled
Bleeding controlled

POSTPARTUM HEMORRHAGE

Harold Rubin, M.D.

COMMENTS

A. Postpartum hemorrhage during the first 24 hours after delivery requires that steps be taken immediately to identify the presence of uterine atony, retained placenta, trauma to the genital tract, or unsuspected coagulation defects.

B. Predisposing factors include high parity, uterine scars, tumors or anomalies, prolonged labor, augmented labor, prior postpartum hemorrhage, traumatic delivery, twins, and hydramnios.

C. Bleeding in the presence of a large, boggy, or difficult to delineate uterus indicates atony. Atony is frequently associated with retained placenta. Atony should respond to bimanual massage, oxytocin intramuscularly or intravenously (by rapid infusion, not bolus), and ergonovine intramuscularly.

D. Retained placenta is a frequent cause of bleeding. The uterus contracts poorly. A piece of unrecognized membrane, cotyledon or succenturiate lobe may be retained. Immediate manual exploration of the uterine cavity will confirm the diagnosis. Manual removal of the retained products followed by gentle exploration with placental forceps, curet or gauze-covered hand, in addition to the administration of oxytocin and ergonovine intramuscularly, should control the bleeding. If adherent, placenta accreta must be suspected (p. 62).

E. If excessive bleeding persists, management must become aggressive. Bilateral hypogastric artery ligation is performed and, if necessary, bilateral ovarian artery ligation at the level of the utero-ovarian ligaments. Hysterectomy is a last resort. Sometimes, acute bleeding can be stemmed by compressing the uterus firmly between the vaginal fist and the abdominal hand or by grasping the lower uterus through the abdominal wall.

F. If the uterus is well-contracted, bleeding is probably due to traumatic lacerations that can be located by inspection and manual exploration. Periurethral, vaginal and cervical lacerations are usually repaired without difficulty. Laceration of the uterus demands immediate laparotomy. If the laceration is linear and the bleeding is easily controlled, simple repair may suffice; otherwise, total hysterectomy is indicated.

G. Von Willebrand's (p. 80) disease is the most common clinically significant abnormality of blood coagulation in women. Postpartum hemorrhage may occur. The administration of fresh frozen plasma or cryoprecipitate in amounts adequate to increase Factor VIII will control the excessive bleeding.

REFERENCES

Dieckmann WS, Odell LD, Williger VM, Seski AG, Pottinger R: The placental stages and postpartum hemorrhage. Am J Obstet Gynecol 54:415, 1947

Melody GF: Primary postpartum hemorrhage. Calif Med 75:425, 1951

O'Leary JL, O'Leary JA: Uterine artery ligation for control of postcesarean section hemorrhage. Obstet Gynecol 43:849, 1974

Thomas WO Jr: Manual removal of the placenta. Am J Obstet Gynecol 86:600, 1963

Van Gelderen CJ: Internal iliac artery ligation in obstetrics and gynecology. S Afr Med J 49:1997, 1975

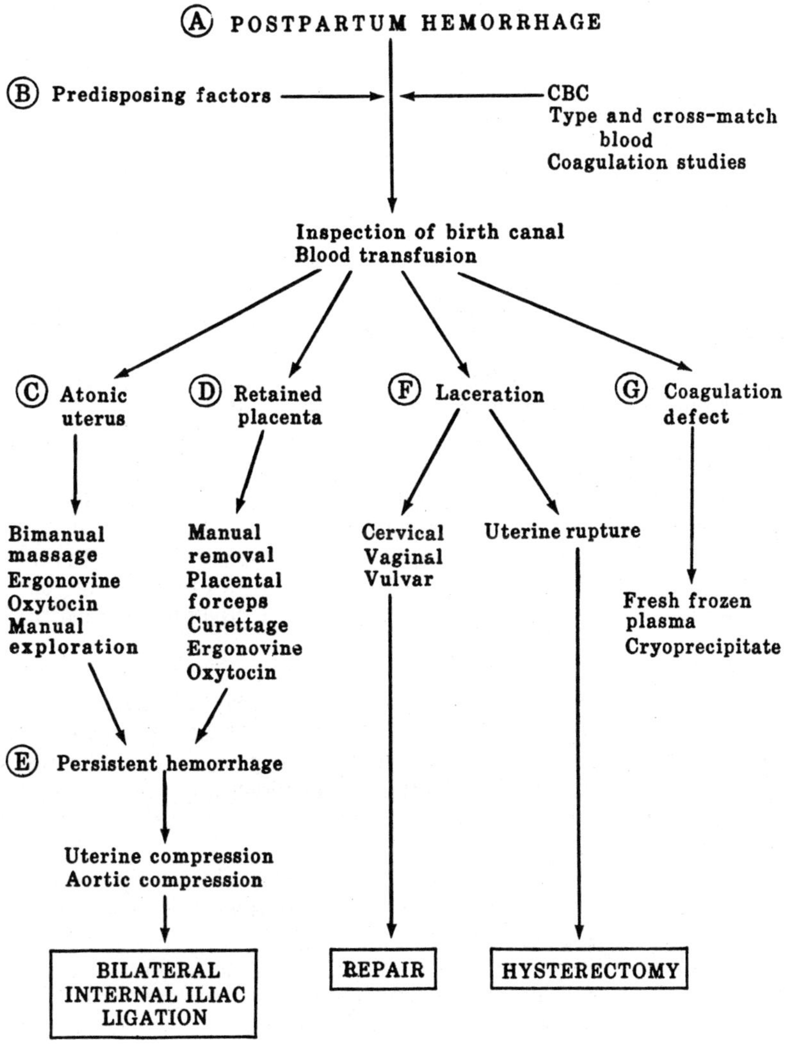

(A) POSTPARTUM HEMORRHAGE
(B) Predisposing factors
CBC
Type and cross-match blood
Coagulation studies
Inspection of birth canal
Blood transfusion
(C) Atonic uterus
(D) Retained placenta
(F) Laceration
(G) Coagulation defect
Bimanual massage
Ergonovine
Oxytocin
Manual exploration
Manual removal
Placental forceps
Curettage
Ergonovine
Oxytocin
Cervical
Vaginal
Vulvar
Uterine rupture
Fresh frozen plasma
Cryoprecipitate
(E) Persistent hemorrhage
Uterine compression
Aortic compression
BILATERAL INTERNAL ILIAC LIGATION
REPAIR
HYSTERECTOMY

PUERPERAL INFECTION

Harold Rubin, M.D.

COMMENTS

A. Febrile morbidity is defined as peak temperature elevation to 38°C (100.4°F) or more on any two of the first ten postpartum days except the first 24 hours.

B. Predisposing factors include prolonged labor, premature rupture of the membranes, traumatic delivery, manual removal of the placenta, cesarean section (especially if done after labor and if internal fetal heart rate monitoring was done during the labor), intrapartum fever, bladder catheterization, and atonic bladder.

C. Both aerobic and anaerobic organisms should be searched for in bacteriologic studies of cultures obtained from the endocervical and intrauterine areas as well as blood, urine and throat.

D. Coagulation parameters should be monitored so that impending disseminated intravascular coagulation can be recognized as early as possible.

E. Ultrasonography is especially useful for identifying an abscess in cases in which its presence is suspected.

F. Antibiotics for use against aerobic and anaerobic bacteria are given at once, as needed. The types and dosages are adjusted, if appropriate, on the basis of culture reports. Pelvic infections are best treated initially with broad-spectrum combinations of agents —such as (1) penicillin and streptomycin, (2) clindamycin and kanamycin, or (3) clindamycin, gentamycin, and ampicillin—so as to ensure coverage against both anaerobic and enterococcal pathogens.

G. If there has been no improvement in 72 hours, one must consider the possibilities of pelvic thrombophlebitis, abscess formation, and septic embolization.

H. All abscesses must be drained or excised. If the pelvic abscess points into the posterior vaginal fornix, it should be drained through the vagina; if not, the transabdominal approach is in order. If the uterus is involved, hysterectomy may be indicated, especially if the condition arose following cesarean section and the uterine incision has dehisced or is the seat of the infection.

I. Septic embolization is a rare but potentially life-threatening complication of puerperal sepsis, and it must be considered when the patient does not respond to appropriate antibiotics in adequate amounts.

J. Septic shock, diagnosed by the presence of high fever, unstable cardiovascular status, and falling WBC, demands intensive management with oxygen, volume replacement, blood transfusion, antibiotics, corticosteroids, vasomotor agents, digitalis, and anticoagulants, as needed.

REFERENCES

Gassner CB, Ledger WJ: The relationship of hospital acquired maternal infection to invasive intrapartum monitoring techniques. Am J Obstet Gynecol 126:33, 1976

Gibbs RS: Clinical risk factor for puerperal infection. Obstet Gynecol 55(Suppl):178s, 1980

Jewett JF, Reid DC, Safon LE, Easterday CL: Childbed fever: A continuing entity. JAMA 206: 344, 1968

Kitzmiller JL: Septic shock: An eclectic view. Obstet Gynecol Survey 26:105, 1971

Ledger WJ: Infections in obstetrics and gynecology. Surg Clin North Am 52:1447, 1972

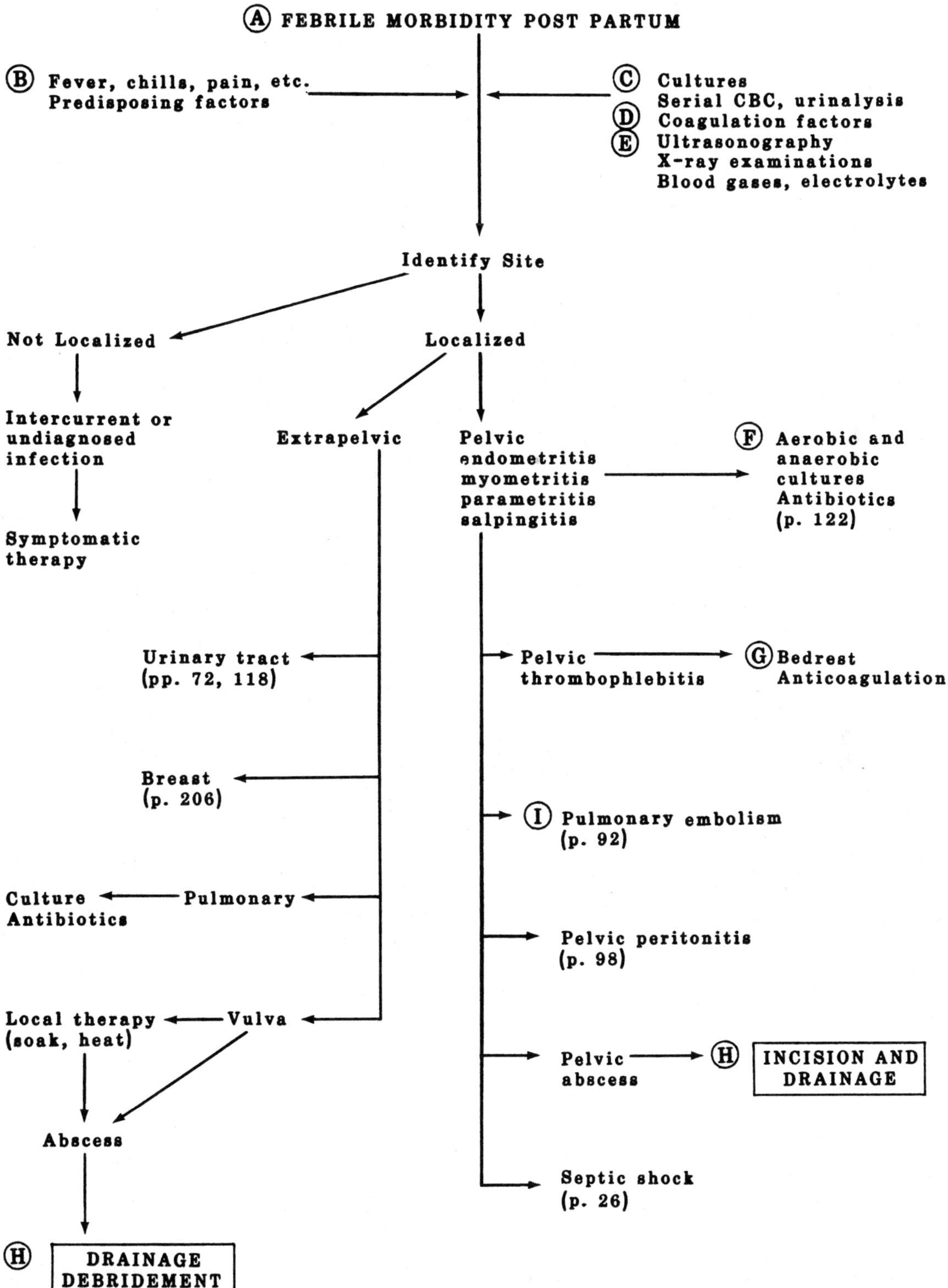
(A) FEBRILE MORBIDITY POST PARTUM
(B) Fever, chills, pain, etc.
Predisposing factors
(C) Cultures
Serial CBC, urinalysis
(D) Coagulation factors
(E) Ultrasonography
X-ray examinations
Blood gases, electrolytes
Identify Site
Not Localized
Localized
Intercurrent or undiagnosed infection
Symptomatic therapy
Extrapelvic
Pelvic
endometritis
myometritis
parametritis
salpingitis
(F) Aerobic and anaerobic cultures
Antibiotics
(p. 122)
Urinary tract
(pp. 72, 118)
Pelvic thrombophlebitis
(G) Bedrest
Anticoagulation
Breast
(p. 206)
(I) Pulmonary embolism
(p. 92)
Culture
Antibiotics
Pulmonary
Pelvic peritonitis
(p. 98)
Local therapy
(soak, heat)
Vulva
Pelvic abscess
(H) INCISION AND DRAINAGE
Abscess
Septic shock
(p. 26)
(H) DRAINAGE
DEBRIDEMENT

EVALUATING THE NEWBORN INFANT

William D. Cochran, M.D.

COMMENTS

A. Prenatal and intrapartum involvement of the pediatrician in cases in which high-risk infants may be delivered is strongly recommended. One must be especially alert to cases involving serious maternal illnesses, prematurity, abnormal labor patterns, difficult delivery processes, meconium staining of the amniotic fluid, and other evidences of fetal distress.

B. The Apgar score will provide an immediate assessment of the newborn infant. The 1-minute score helps direct the intensity of the resuscitative efforts (p. 194), but the 5-minute score tends to be a more valuable indicator of prognosis and the need for subsequent special neonatal care.

C. A modified Dubowitz examination, coupled with information obtained from the history and available laboratory data pertaining to fetal lung maturity, will help determine gestational age and functional maturity.

D. Premature infants and those with documented or suspected immature organ system function should be observed and cared for, as indicated, in a special care nursery setting. Similarly, those with recognizable high-risk conditions, including hemolytic disease (p. 94), congenital anomaly, intrauterine growth retardation (p. 52), or with possible meconium aspiration deserve comparable surveillance.

E. The otherwise normal term infant who develops any manifestation suggesting an underlying disorder or deterioration of his or her condition warrants pediatric consultation and special care. If such mature infants improve or stabilize on the basis of evaluation and management, they can be returned to the regular nursery for continued care and observation. Be especially attentive to the following: respiratory manifestations (grunting, tachypnea, nasal flaring, chest retraction, cyanosis), central nervous system abnormalities (lethargy, seizures, hyperactivity, tremors), abdominal signs (distention, propulsive vomiting, or vomiting bile-colored material), metabolic changes (particularly hypothermia and hypoglycemia), hemolytic effects (positive Coombs, hepatosplenomegaly, petechiae, and unusual bleeding), infection (manifested by anemia, hepatosplenomegaly, or petechiae), and any anomalies that may compromise the infant's well-being.

REFERENCES

Dubowitz LMS, Dobowitz V: *Gestational Age of the Newborn.* Menlo Park, Calif: Addison-Wesley Publishing Co, 1977

Parkin JM, Hey EN, Clowes JS: Rapid assessment of gestational age at birth. Arch Dis Child 51:259, 1976

Scanlon JW, Nelson T, Grylack L, Smith Y: *A System of Newborn Physical Examination.* Baltimore: University Park Press, 1979

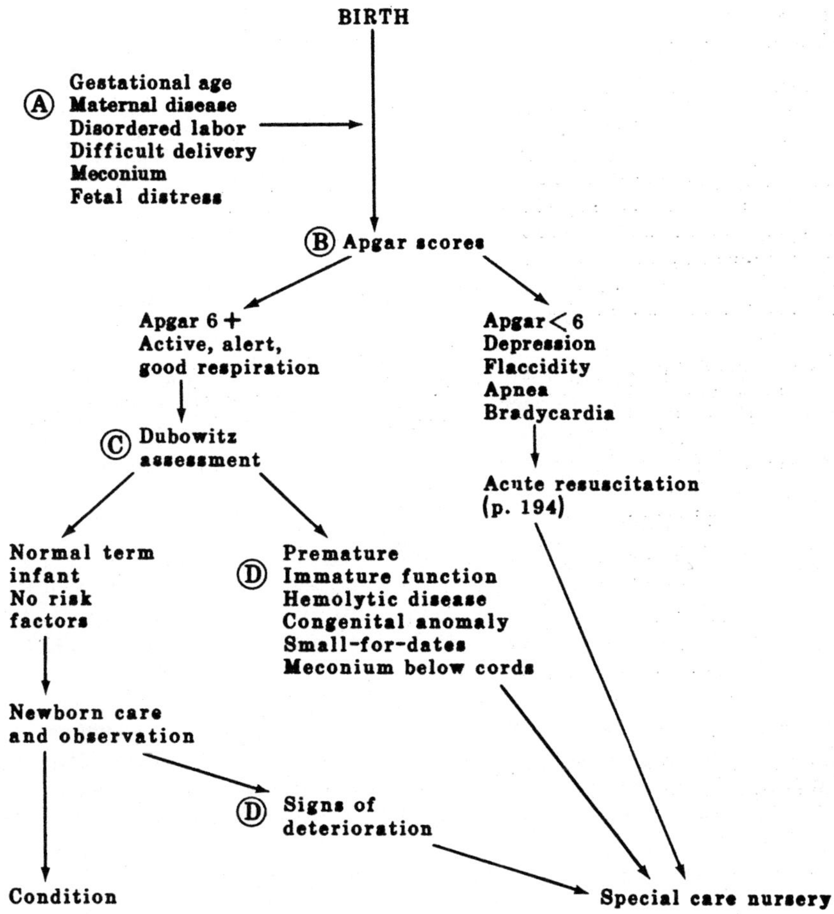
BIRTH
(A) Gestational age
Maternal disease
Disordered labor
Difficult delivery
Meconium
Fetal distress
(B) Apgar scores
Apgar 6 +
Active, alert,
good respiration
Apgar < 6
Depression
Flaccidity
Apnea
Bradycardia
(C) Dubowitz
assessment
Acute resuscitation
(p. 194)
Normal term
infant
No risk
factors
(D) Premature
Immature function
Hemolytic disease
Congenital anomaly
Small-for-dates
Meconium below cords
Newborn care
and observation
(D) Signs of
deterioration
Condition
Special care nursery

NEONATAL RESUSCITATION

William B. Cochran, M.D.

COMMENTS

A. Anticipate problems so as to alert specialists for resuscitating the newborn infant and mobilize full team supports. Each member of the team should know his or her position and review and coordinate specific tasks ahead of time.

B. The obstetric attendant must take special pains to clear the infant's oropharnyx as the baby's mouth appears over the perineum, preferably before the first breath and particularly if meconium is present.

C. In the presence of meconium, the first requisite of resuscitation should be to ascertain whether any meconium has been aspirated below the level of the vocal cords. Endotracheal suctioning is mandatory under such circumstances. Laryngoscopic visualization must precede the administration of oxygen under positive pressure to avert pushing the meconium down into the bronchial tree and alveoli.

D. The moderately depressed infant is resuscitated initially with a flow-through bag fitted with a pop-off valve device and a manometer for proper pressure control. Until assured that the chest wall is moving in response to ventilation, use pressures up to 60 cm of water. Thereafter, 40 cm generally suffices. The rate of ventilation should be between 40 and 80 per minute. Listen for air entry by stethoscope.

E. Whereas endotracheal intubation is clearly preferable, orotracheal or nasotracheal intubation may be effective (especially in emergency circumstances in which expert help may not be immediately available) as long as it is done correctly — that is, the tube must not be placed in the esophagus. The minimum amount of pressure necessary to move the chest should suffice; listen for air entry. Apply closed chest cardiac massage with 2 fingers on the midsternum at 60–80 per minute.

F. By 3 min, the unresponsive infant requires umbilical vein catheterization for correcting its rapidly developing acidosis. Measure the distance from the umbilicus to the right nipple, subtract 1 cm, and insert the catheter to that distance. If it cannot be inserted that far, it may be in the hepatic or portal vein; if so, inject drugs with extreme caution. Give an equal mixture of 1 M sodium bicarbonate and 10 percent dextrose in water (5–8 ml/kg). If there is no improvement in 1–2 min, inject epinephrine (1 ml 1:10,000). This may be given by direct intracardiac injection in babies with an Apgar score of zero. If there is still no improvement, consider giving Narcan (0.02 mg/ml, injecting 1–2 ml) as a narcotic antagonist, if indicated, and, calcium gluconate (10 percent, injecting 2 ml slowly), rechecking the airway and the chest for air entry. Subsequently, one may give whole blood (preferably the infant's own placental blood, 10–15 ml/kg) or 5 percent albumin. One generally terminates efforts after about 30 min if there is no response.

REFERENCES

Cloherty JP, Stark AR: *Manual of Neonatal Care.* Boston: Little, Brown & Co, 1980

Schreiner RL: *Care of the Newborn.* New York: Raven Press, 1981

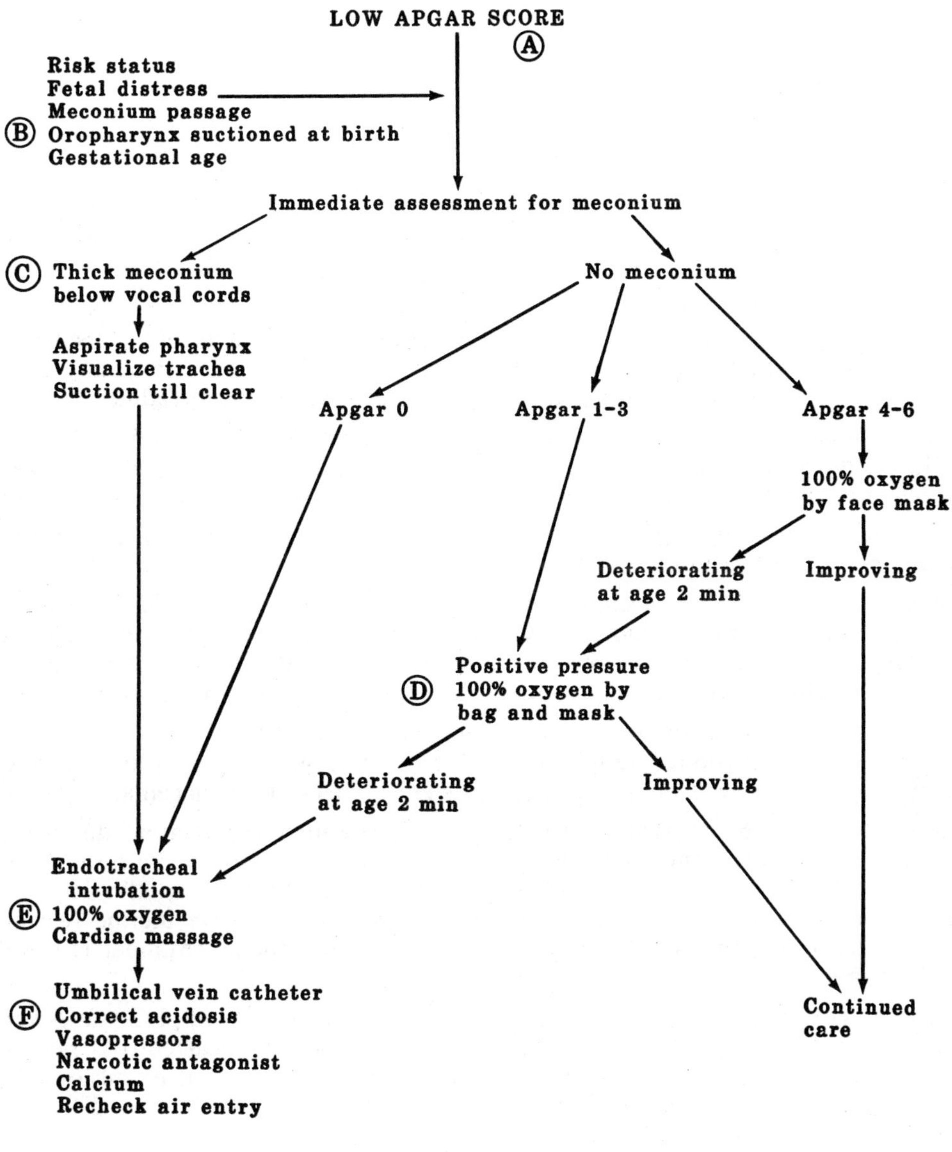
LOW APGAR SCORE
Ⓐ
Risk status
Fetal distress
Meconium passage
Ⓑ Oropharynx suctioned at birth
Gestational age
Immediate assessment for meconium
Ⓒ Thick meconium below vocal cords
Aspirate pharynx
Visualize trachea
Suction till clear
No meconium
Apgar 0
Apgar 1-3
Apgar 4-6
100% oxygen by face mask
Deteriorating at age 2 min
Improving
Positive pressure
Ⓓ 100% oxygen by bag and mask
Deteriorating at age 2 min
Improving
Endotracheal intubation
Ⓔ 100% oxygen
Cardiac massage
Umbilical vein catheter
Ⓕ Correct acidosis
Vasopressors
Narcotic antagonist
Calcium
Recheck air entry
Continued care

RETAINED PLACENTA

Selwyn P. Oskowitz, M.B.

COMMENTS

A. Predisposing factors include abnormal labor, uterotonic stimulation, uterine atony from general anesthesia, uterine overdistention (hydramnios or twins), prior curettage or myomectomy, and uterine anomalies.

B. Because hemorrhage is common and intrauterine exploration is often needed, one should prepare the patient beforehand with an open intravenous line (using a large-bore catheter), blood typing and cross-matching, and anesthesia in readiness.

C. Abdominopelvic examination (under sterile conditions) quickly determines if the placenta has descended into the vagina. Elevating the uterus out of the pelvis while applying slight countertension on the cord will show whether total separation has occurred.

D. Active uterine bleeding signifies separation, usually incomplete; it requires expeditious management to effect manual delivery of the placenta.

E. Manual removal of the placenta requires anesthesia. Blood should be available for transfusion but volume expanders may temporarily substitute to maintain cardiovascular stability (p. 198). Manual removal is carried out under sterile conditions in an operating theater. If cleavage plane cannot be found, one must not persist (p. 62).

F. Failure of the placenta to separate for 30 minutes or more after delivery warrants a trial of oxytocin infusion. Intermittent uterine contractions aid separation. Tonic contraction from excessive stimulation may cause entrapment of the placenta.

G. The placenta may be trapped in the uterine cavity by tonic contractions due to inappropriate use of uterotonic agents (e.g., giving oxytocin or ergotrate with the anterior shoulder, a common practice with little merit and some risk). One can allow the uterotonic effect to subside. If bleeding becomes a problem, effective uterine relaxation may be accomplished quickly with anesthesia (e.g., halothane). Manual removal is then feasible.

H. The Brandt-Andrews maneuver safely aids delivery of the separated placenta. A suprapubically placed hand gently lifts the uterus while the umbilical cord is held (not pulled) tautly at the vulva. This moves the placenta into the vagina. Expulsion efforts by the patient, enhanced by pressure on the uterus, if needed, then delivers the placenta.

REFERENCES

Taylor ES: Intrapartum and postpartum hemorrhage. Am J Obstet Gynecol 83:37, 1962

Verhoge JC: Retained placenta. Nederl T Verlosk 59:224, 1959

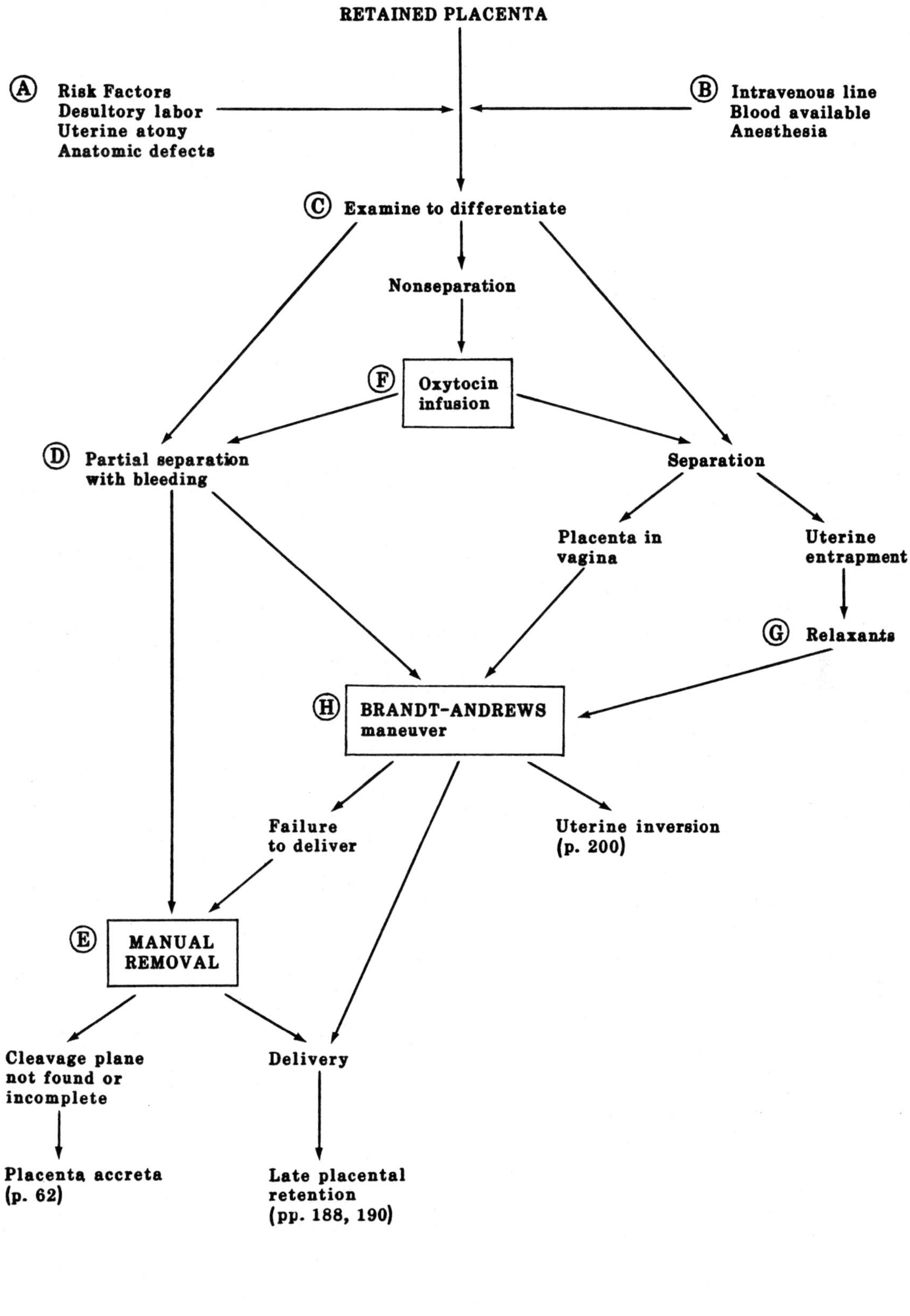
RETAINED PLACENTA
(A) Risk Factors
Desultory labor
Uterine atony
Anatomic defects
(B) Intravenous line
Blood available
Anesthesia
(C) Examine to differentiate
Nonseparation
(F) Oxytocin infusion
(D) Partial separation with bleeding
Separation
Placenta in vagina
Uterine entrapment
(G) Relaxants
(H) BRANDT-ANDREWS maneuver
Failure to deliver
Uterine inversion (p. 200)
(E) MANUAL REMOVAL
Cleavage plane not found or incomplete
Delivery
Placenta accreta (p. 62)
Late placental retention (pp. 188, 190)

SHOCK

Henry Klapholz, M.D.

COMMENTS

A. One should suspect that shock is present or imminent if there is hypotension. However, the blood pressure may not be a very sensitive indicator. Therefore, be alert to such early manifestations as peripheral or circumoral cyanosis or pallor indicative of peripheral vasoconstriction, oliguria, mental confusion, dyspnea, or chest pain. A patient who has had excessive blood loss or a recent infection is at special risk.

B. Aggressive, expeditious evaluation is essential. The pulse and blood pressure should be constantly monitored. Periodic auscultation of the lungs is also important. Check the extremities to assess peripheral circulation, edema, and reflexes, and to determine if warm or cold. Urinary output should be measured hourly by means of catheter drainage. A central venous pressure catheter (CVP) is invaluable as well. A large-bore (No. 14 gauge, for example) intravenous catheter will aid in the rapid administration of drugs and fluids, as indicated. Blood cultures should be obtained. Blood should be obtained for investigation of coagulation parameters (minimally, prothrombin time, partial thromboplastin time, fibrinogen level, and platelet count), hematocrit and electrolytes, and for cross-matching whole blood or packed red blood cells (at least 4 units) for later rapid transfusion, if needed. Chest x-ray may be helpful, too. Electrocardiographic monitoring is useful. Where available, a Swan-Ganz catheter can be very beneficial.

C. Patients with septic shock require large volumes of electrolytic solutions to help bring the CVP up to 8–10 cm water. They should be given gentamycin and penicillin in large doses and hydrocortisone, 1 gm intravenously. Pressor agents may be needed.

D. One should be alert to the possibility of the potentially fatal complication of amniotic fluid embolism (p. 92) in patients with tumultuous labors, especially grand multiparas and gravidas with polyhydramnios. Oxytocin administration is often a concomitant feature. Forceps procedures may also be associated. Characteristically, there is sudden hypotension, usually at the time of delivery or immediately post partum, accompanied by acute dyspnea.

E. Cardiogenic shock is managed with effective diuresis, using furosemide, 80 mg intravenously, in combination with pressor agents such as dopamine. Digitalis should be administered as well.

F. Hypovolemia demands circulatory volume replacement. Until blood is available, one can give electrolyte-containing solution with cystalloids or colloids, such as Ringer's lactate, normal saline, or 5 percent albumen in saline. Whole blood or packed red blood cells with fresh frozen plasma may be given. Consider giving fresh plasma to prevent losing coagulation factors.

G. Vagal syncope is readily reversed by placing the patient supine. Atropine is effective in 0.4- to 0.6-mg doses intravenously along with electrolyte-containing fluids.

REFERENCES

O'Donnell TF Jr, Belkin SC: The pathophysiology, monitoring, and treatment of shock. Orthop Clin North Am 9:589, 1978

Goldberg LI, Hsieh YY, Resnekov L: Newer catecholamines for treatment of heart failure and shock: An update on dopamine and a first look at dobutamine. Progr Cardiovasc Dis 19:327, 1977

Campbell CD, Carey LC: Shock: Differential diagnosis and immediate treatment. Postgrad Med 55: 85, 1974

Ledingham JM: Shock. Ann Roy Coll Surg 60:237, 1978

Watson P: Postpartum hemorrhage and shock. Clin Obstet Gynecol 23:985, 1980

Duff P: Pathophysiology and management of septic shock. J Reprod Med 24:109, 1980

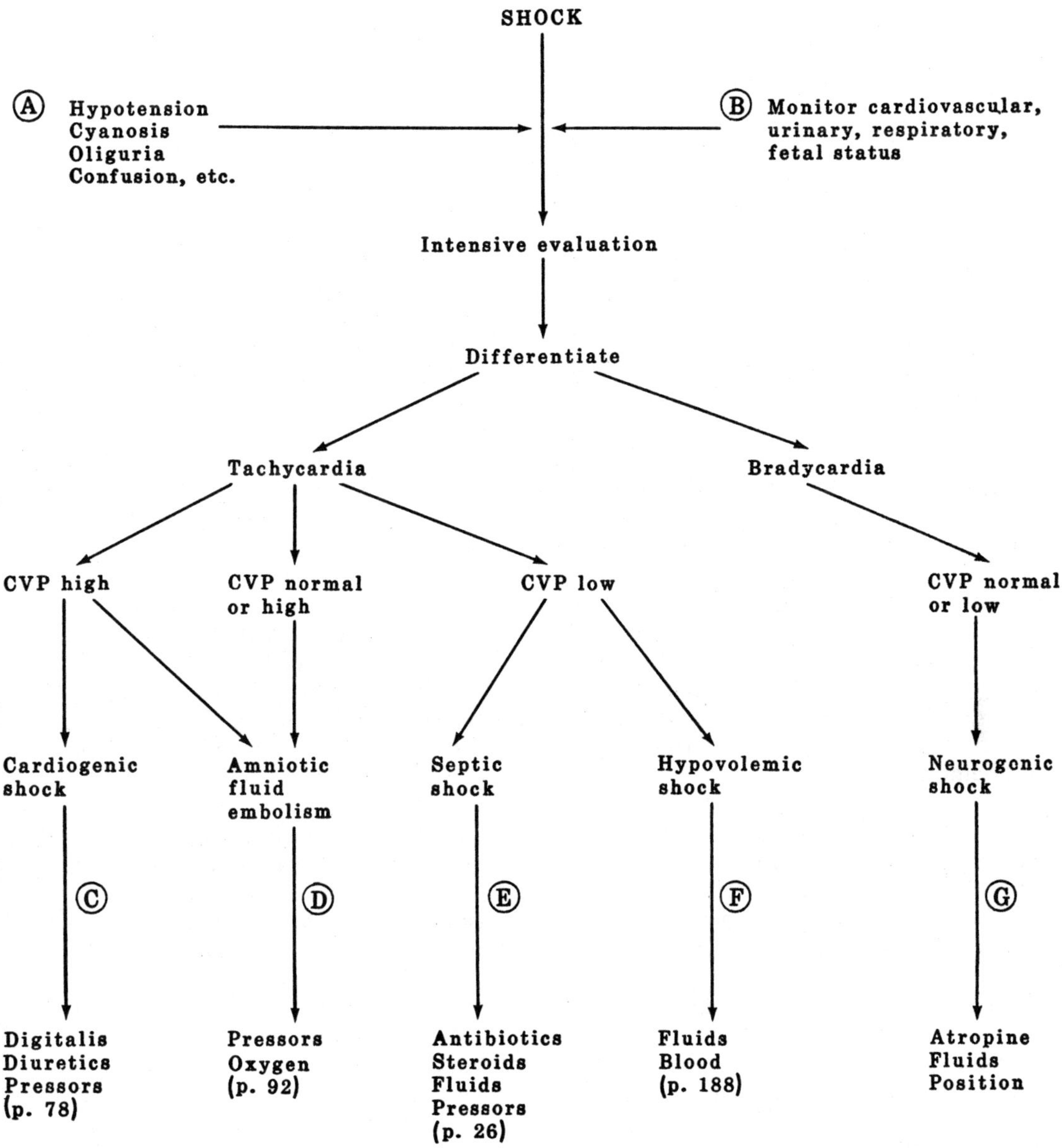
SHOCK
(A) Hypotension
Cyanosis
Oliguria
Confusion, etc.
(B) Monitor cardiovascular,
urinary, respiratory,
fetal status
Intensive evaluation
Differentiate
Tachycardia
Bradycardia
CVP high
CVP normal
or high
CVP low
CVP normal
or low
Cardiogenic
shock
Amniotic
fluid
embolism
Septic
shock
Hypovolemic
shock
Neurogenic
shock
(C)
(D)
(E)
(F)
(G)
Digitalis
Diuretics
Pressors
(p. 78)
Pressors
Oxygen
(p. 92)
Antibiotics
Steroids
Fluids
Pressors
(p. 26)
Fluids
Blood
(p. 188)
Atropine
Fluids
Position

UTERINE INVERSION

Lenard Simon, M.D.

COMMENTS

A. By far the most common cause of uterine inversion is excessive force placed upon the uterine fundus during the third stage of labor in attempts to extract the placenta using the Crédé maneuver. Alternatively, inversion may result from excessive traction on the umbilical cord in ill-advised attempts to deliver a placenta that is still attached, especially if a placental implantation site is in the uterine fundus. Inexplicably, nulliparas are more commonly affected by this condition than multiparas.

B. Diagnosis is usually made by means of vaginal examination, although abdominal palpation may reveal a defect in the uterine fundus. Partial inversion, which is easiest to treat, is most difficult to diagnose. Patients who do not have the usual symptoms of profound shock out of proportion to the amount of blood lost, severe lower abdominal pain, or uncontrolled hemorrhage may not be diagnosed early. Undue delay in the diagnosis means increased morbidity and mortality rates.

C. The earlier the diagnosis is made and the more expeditious and aggressive the management, the easier it will be to reposit the inverted uterus. Replacement should be done under sterile conditions in an operating room (or well-equipped delivery room) with appropriate resources available for anesthesia and cardiovascular support.

D. Patients who are in shock as a consequence of uterine inversion must be treated at once with vasopressors, fluid or blood replacement for reactive hypovolemia, and internal examination to determine the cervical status. If the cervix is sufficiently opened to allow manual replacement, this procedure is preferable. If not (and this is the usual state, especially if diagnosis has been delayed), surgical management will be required. The latter applies particularly if the patient is suffering acute intense pain and hemorrhage.

E. If the diagnosis is made at once, before the uterus has had a chance to contract down and the cervix to constrict, manual replacement of the inverted uterine corpus can generally be done easily. If more than several minutes' time has elapsed, however, it may be difficult. General anesthesia will be necessary to relax the uterus and to provide sufficient pain relief to permit the procedure to be accomplished.

F. Surgical intervention may require splitting the cervical ring to permit the inverted uterus corpus to be replaced. It can sometimes be accomplished vaginally (Spinelli procedure) but more often has to be done transabdominally (Huntington or Haultain operations). While attempting to reposit the corpus transvaginally, one may try to dilate the cervix manually, taking special care to avoid perforating the uterine wall with the fingers.

REFERENCES

Kitchin JD, Thiagarajh S, May HV, Thornton WJ: Puerperal inversion of the uterus. Am J Obstet Gynecol 123:51, 1975

Watson P, Besch N, Bowes WA: Management of acute and subacute puerperal inversion of the uterus. Obstet Gynecol 55:12, 1980

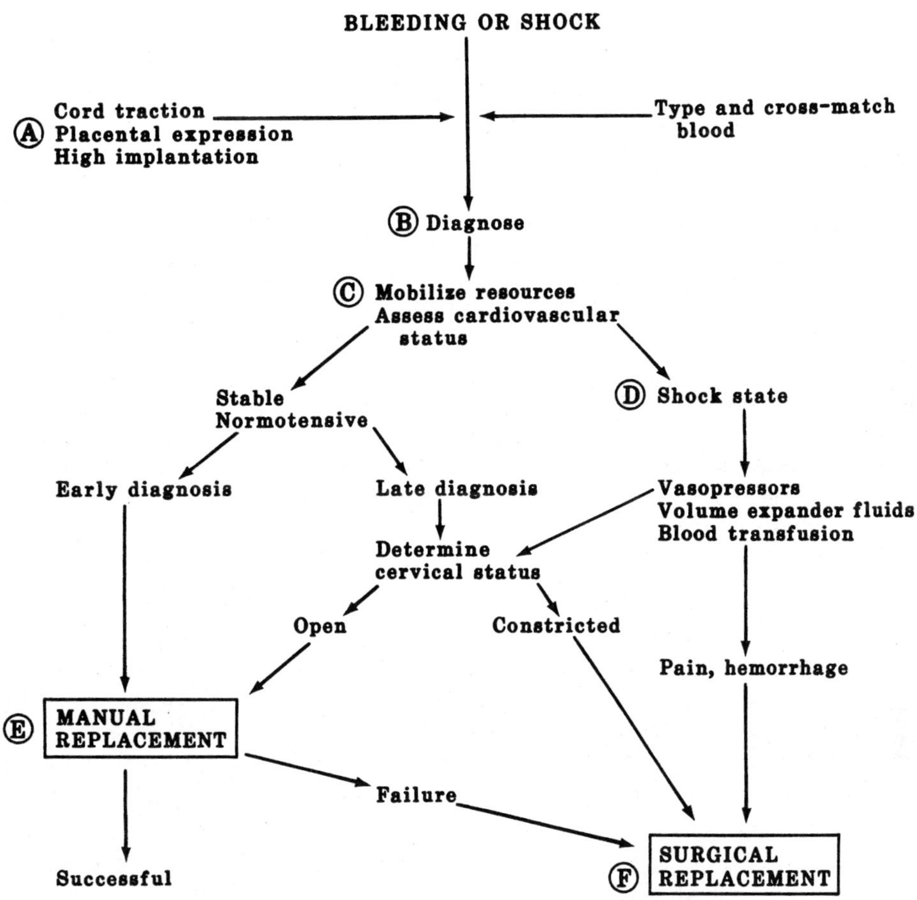
BLEEDING OR SHOCK
Ⓐ Cord traction
Placental expression
High implantation
Type and cross-match blood
Ⓑ Diagnose
Ⓒ Mobilize resources
Assess cardiovascular status
Stable
Normotensive
Ⓓ Shock state
Early diagnosis
Late diagnosis
Vasopressors
Volume expander fluids
Blood transfusion
Determine cervical status
Open
Constricted
Pain, hemorrhage
Ⓔ MANUAL REPLACEMENT
Failure
Successful
Ⓕ SURGICAL REPLACEMENT

LATE POSTPARTUM HEMORRHAGE

Harold Rubin, M.D.

COMMENTS

A. Bleeding from the genital tract which begins 24 hours or more post partum is called late postpartum hemorrhage. It may occur as late as 3–5 months following delivery. Even though it may be severe, it is rarely fatal.

B. Immediate hospitalization is mandatory; only in this environment can the patient be accurately and safely evaluated, observed, and treated.

C. Uterine inversion is a rare postpartum complication. When it occurs in the third stage of labor, it is usually complete and the placenta remains totally or partially attached in about 75 percent of patients. Shock is often present if the inversion is sudden and tends to be disproportionate to the amount of blood loss. Unrecognized incomplete inversion may be one source of late postpartum hemorrhage. Vaginal examination reveals the complication. It may be corrected vaginally by manual replacement or the Spinelli operation. The inversion may also be corrected by laparotomy utilizing the Huntington operation if the vaginal procedures fail (see p. 200).

D. Hematoma formation is a result of injury to blood vessels, spontaneous or traumatic, without laceration of the superficial tissue. Intense pain, swelling, and bluish discoloration are the characteristic symptom and signs. Hematomas tend to enlarge progressively and to follow the fascial planes. Large hematomas are very rare. Treatment consists of evacuating the hematoma and ligating the bleeding vessels. All dead space must be eliminated by suturing. If this cannot be accomplished, the vagina is firmly packed; the pack is removed in 12 hours.

E. The most common causes of late postpartum hemorrhage are thrombosed vessels at the placental site and subinvolution of the placental site. Rarely is placental tissue found on curettage. If bleeding is profuse, curettage must be performed at once. If bleeding is moderate it probably will be controlled by ergonovine, 0.2 mg given orally 3–4 times daily. Curettage is performed only if the bleeding does not abate after the ergonovine is given.

F. Degenerated fibroids usually require hysterectomy. For malignancy, appropriate radical surgery or radiation therapy must be carried out.

REFERENCES

Anderson WR, Davis J: Placental site involution. Am J Obstet Gynecol 102:23, 1968

Dewhurst CJ: Secondary post-partum haemorrhage. J Obstet Gynaecol Brit Cwlth 73:53, 1966

Fliegner JRH: Postpartum broad ligament haematomas. J Obstet Gynaecol Brit Cwlth 78: 184, 1971

Melody GF: An inquiry into late postpartum hemorrhage. Am J Surg 78:821, 1949

Rome RM: Secondary postpartum haemorrhage. Brit J Obstet Gynaecol 82:289, 1975

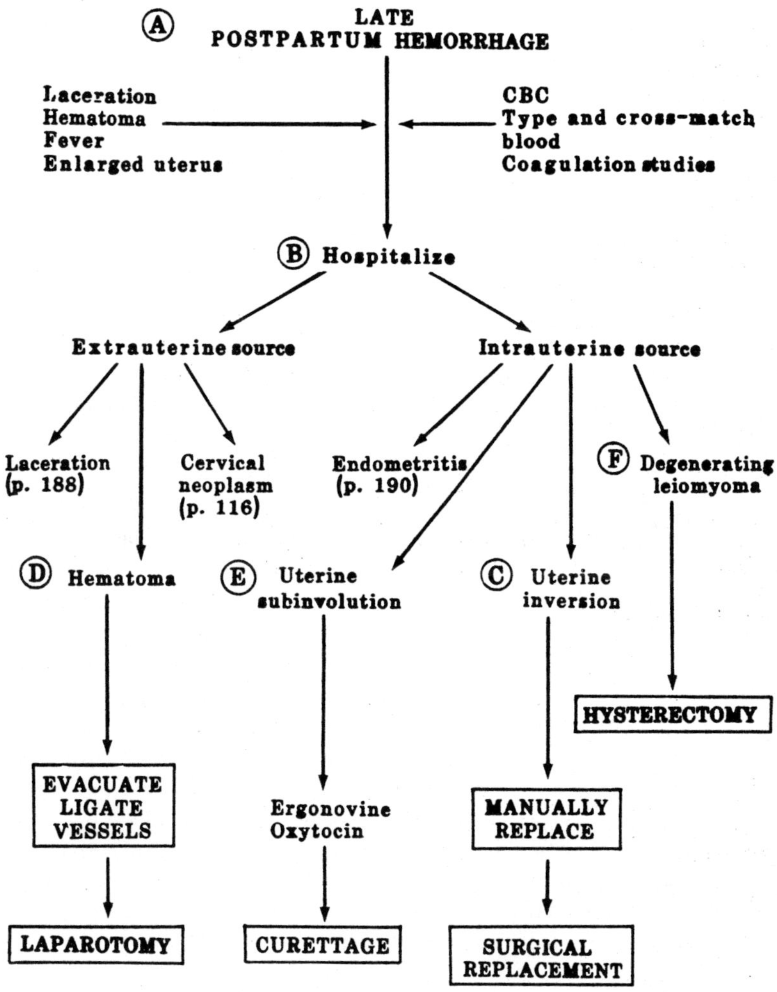
Ⓐ LATE POSTPARTUM HEMORRHAGE
Laceration
Hematoma
Fever
Enlarged uterus
CBC
Type and cross-match blood
Coagulation studies
Ⓑ Hospitalize
Extrauterine source
Intrauterine source
Laceration (p. 188)
Cervical neoplasm (p. 116)
Endometritis (p. 190)
Ⓕ Degenerating leiomyoma
Ⓓ Hematoma
Ⓔ Uterine subinvolution
Ⓒ Uterine inversion
HYSTERECTOMY
EVACUATE LIGATE VESSELS
Ergonovine Oxytocin
MANUALLY REPLACE
LAPAROTOMY
CURETTAGE
SURGICAL REPLACEMENT

LACTATION

Max Borten, M.D.

COMMENTS

A. One should discuss breast feeding at length during pregnancy. Deal with psychologic, social, and economic factors affecting breast feeding. Leave the final decision to the gravida, who should not feel pressured to make an unwanted or hurried choice. The disadvantages of breast feeding, such as constraints in work or social life, should not be interpreted as contraindications.

B. The size of the mammary glands is no indicator of their ability to produce milk. During pregnancy, adipose tissue is replaced by proliferating acini. Small breasts are usually quite capable of providing adequate infant nourishment. The psychologic support of positive feedback may be extremely beneficial to the self-image of a woman with small breasts.

C. The discomfort of tender or cracked nipples can be minimized by preparing the breast with lanolin rubbed in twice a day and by periodically placing gentle traction on the nipples. Flat or inverted nipples do not preclude breast feeding. Flat nipples respond to a program of stretching 2–3 times a day during the last 6–8 weeks of pregnancy. Inverted nipples respond well to massage during the last 2 months of pregnancy, although they may require nipple shields for nursing.

D. There are relatively few contraindications to breast feeding. Maternal breast cancer interdicts lactation and breast feeding because it could dangerously delay radiation or chemotherapy in the interest of the infant. Drugs given to the mother, such as chemotherapy or narcotic agents, may be secreted in breast milk and thereby adversely affect the infant.

E. When a delay in lactation is indicated — as for premature infants or those with congenital abnormalities, particularly if tracheoesophageal fistula is suspected — mechanical pumping of the breast is an excellent method for accumulating breast milk as well as for sustaining the gland secretion. For working mothers, the use of a mechanical pump can produce sufficient milk to feed the infant for those intervals when the mother is not available.

F. Suppression of lactation can be accomplished when desired or indicated within 72–96 hours of delivery merely by avoiding stimulation of the breast and providing good support of the mammary glands by use of a sturdy brassiere or binder. The routine use of lactation suppression agents is, therefore, considered unnecessary in most cases. Commonly used agents for lactation suppression include estrogenic hormones (Deladumone and Tace) and bromocryptine (Parlodel); the latter has proved especially effective for this purpose, if it should be necessary.

REFERENCES

Beer AE, Billingham RE: Immunologic benefits and hazards of milk in maternal-perinatal relationships. Ann Intern Med 83:865, 1975

Countryman BA: Breast care in the early puerperium. J Obstet Gynecol Nurs 2:36, 1973

Tyson JE: Mechanism of puerperal lactation. Med Clin North Am 61:153, 1977

Wing JP: Human versus cow's milk in infant nutrition and health: Update 1977. Curr Prob Pediatr 8:1, 1977

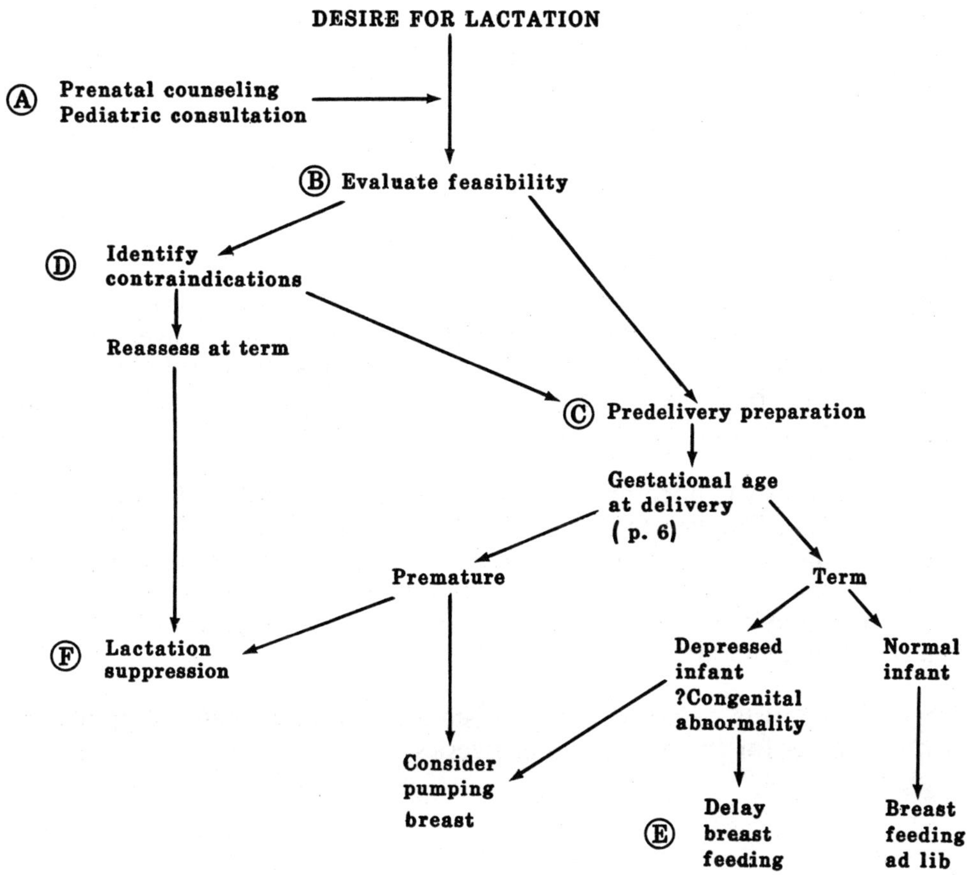
DESIRE FOR LACTATION
Ⓐ Prenatal counseling
Pediatric consultation
Ⓑ Evaluate feasibility
Ⓓ Identify contraindications
Reassess at term
Ⓒ Predelivery preparation
Gestational age at delivery
(p. 6)
Premature
Term
Ⓕ Lactation suppression
Depressed infant
?Congenital abnormality
Normal infant
Consider pumping breast
Ⓔ Delay breast feeding
Breast feeding ad lib

PUERPERAL MASTITIS

Austin Wertheimer, M.D. and Harold Rubin, M.D.

COMMENTS

A. The isolated case is a common occurrence. Usually, the clinical picture arises abruptly one to several weeks after delivery. Infection involves interlobular tissue and results in a wedge-shaped area of cellulitis. It is probably associated with milk stasis or cracked nipple. Pus is not seen in the milk. If staphylococci are cultured, they tend to be nonvirulent.

B. Epidemic mastitis is uncommon. It generally begins insidiously within 2 weeks of the delivery. The lactiferous apparatus (glands and ducts) are affected with virulent strains of staphylococci. Both breasts or several nonadjacent lobes of one breast may be involved. Pus can often be expressed from the nipple. Outbreaks of staphylococcal infections are seen in the nursery. They can be related to a carrier individual.

C. Treatment consists of penicillinase-resistant antibiotics, plus a supporting garment or binder for the breast and analgesics.

REFERENCES

Devereux WP: Acute puerperal mastitis: Evaluation of its management. Am J Obstet Gynecol 108:78, 1970

Gibbard GF: Sporadic and epidemic puerperal breast infections. Am J Obstet Gynecol 65: 1038, 1953

Marshall BR, Hepper JK, Zirbel CC: Sporadic puerperal mastitis: An infection that need not interrupt lactation. JAMA 233:1377, 1975

Niebyl JR, Spence MR, Parmley TH: Sporadic (nonepidemic) puerperal mastitis. J Reprod Med 20:97, 1978

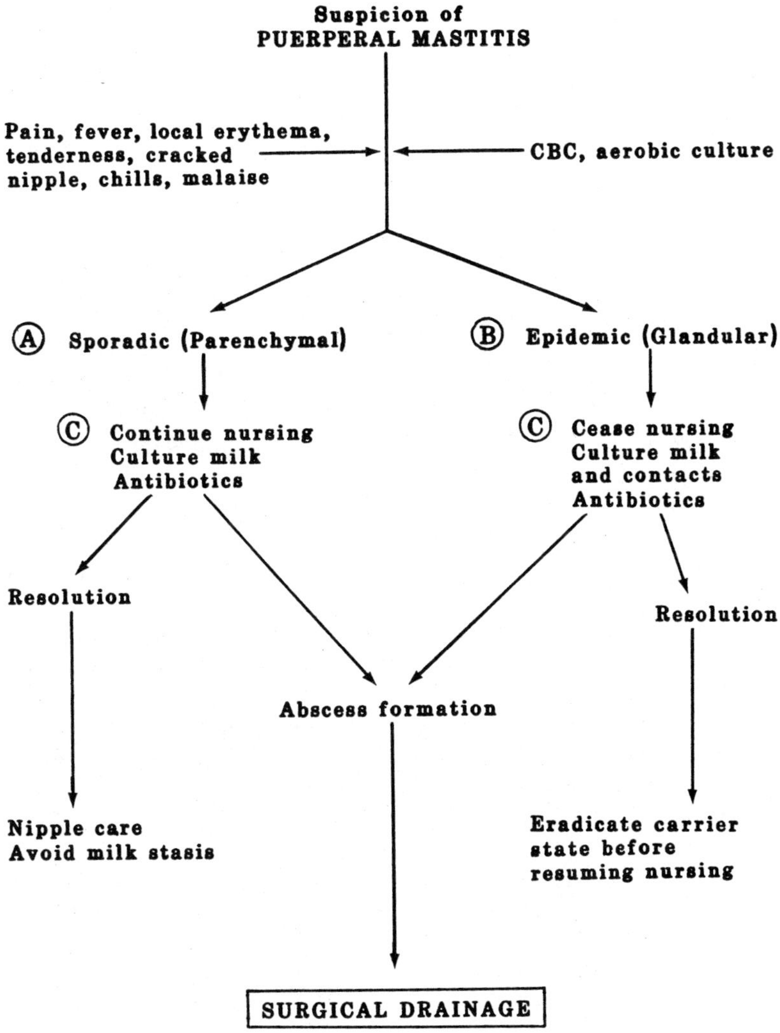
Suspicion of
PUERPERAL MASTITIS
Pain, fever, local erythema, tenderness, cracked nipple, chills, malaise
CBC, aerobic culture
(A) Sporadic (Parenchymal)
(B) Epidemic (Glandular)
(C) Continue nursing
Culture milk
Antibiotics
(C) Cease nursing
Culture milk
and contacts
Antibiotics
Resolution
Resolution
Abscess formation
Nipple care
Avoid milk stasis
Eradicate carrier
state before
resuming nursing
SURGICAL DRAINAGE

CHOICE OF FORCEPS

Emanuel A. Friedman, M.D.

COMMENTS

A. Before using forceps, assess the preceding labor, cephalopelvic relationship, type and capacity of pelvis, fetal position, station, flexion, synclitism, and molding, as well as fetal status based on the fetal heart rate pattern.

B. Weigh the risks of the procedure against its benefits, vis-à-vis the risks of allowing labor to continue or delivering by an alternative method. Documenting those benefits is good practice for justifying the operation, especially if prevailing conditions are suboptimal.

C. Conditions in which forceps risk fetal and maternal damage include midpelvic fetal station, malposition (occiput transverse or posterior), deflexion, marked molding, possible cephalopelvic disproportion, and a major labor abnormality.

D. The degree of urgency for delivery depends on maternal and fetal status. A strong indication for delivery may counterbalance the risk of the delivery procedure, although passage of time may make less hazardous options acceptable. Thus, indications for intervention have to be carefully assessed to determine if delivery is required and, if so, whether urgency dictates delivery at once or will permit one to prepare for abdominal delivery.

E. Strong indication for delivery and low risk with forceps justify delivery. With suboptimal conditions, the decision is not easy. Do not traumatize a baby by a difficult midforceps operation in an effort to prevent it from being damaged by an hypoxic insult. Cesarean section is a preferable alternative, if feasible. Even where there are strong indications and urgency dictates rapid intervention, there is often enough time for cesarean section.

F. With weak indications (e.g., maternal exhaustion, poor expulsive efforts), the risks of traumatic delivery cannot be justified. One should seriously entertain temporizing options. Merely allowing the labor to continue under close surveillance will often resolve the problem. Heavy sedation or regional block anesthesia can be permitted to abate. If indicated, oxytocin infusion may help.

G. Selecting the proper instrument can reduce risks. Use Elliott type forceps (with overlapping shank and rounded cephalic curve) for an unmolded fetal head and Simpson type (separated shanks and tapered curve) for a molded head. Special forceps are applicable for special purposes, including Kielland (occiput posterior or transverse in a deep anthropoid pelvis) and Barton forceps (occiput transverse in a flat pelvis). If unexpected difficulty is encountered, one must never persist.

REFERENCES

Chiswick ML, James DK: Kielland forceps: Association with neonatal morbidity and mortality. Brit Med J 1:7, 1979

Friedman EA: Patterns of labor as indicators of risk. Clin Obstet Gynecol 16:172, 1973

Friedman EA, Sachtleben MR, Bresky PA: Dysfunctional labor: XII. Long-term effects on infant. Am J Obstet Gynecol 127:79, 1977

Hughey MJ, McElin TW, Lussky R: Forceps operations in perspective: I. Midforceps rotation operations. J Reprod Med 20:253, 1978

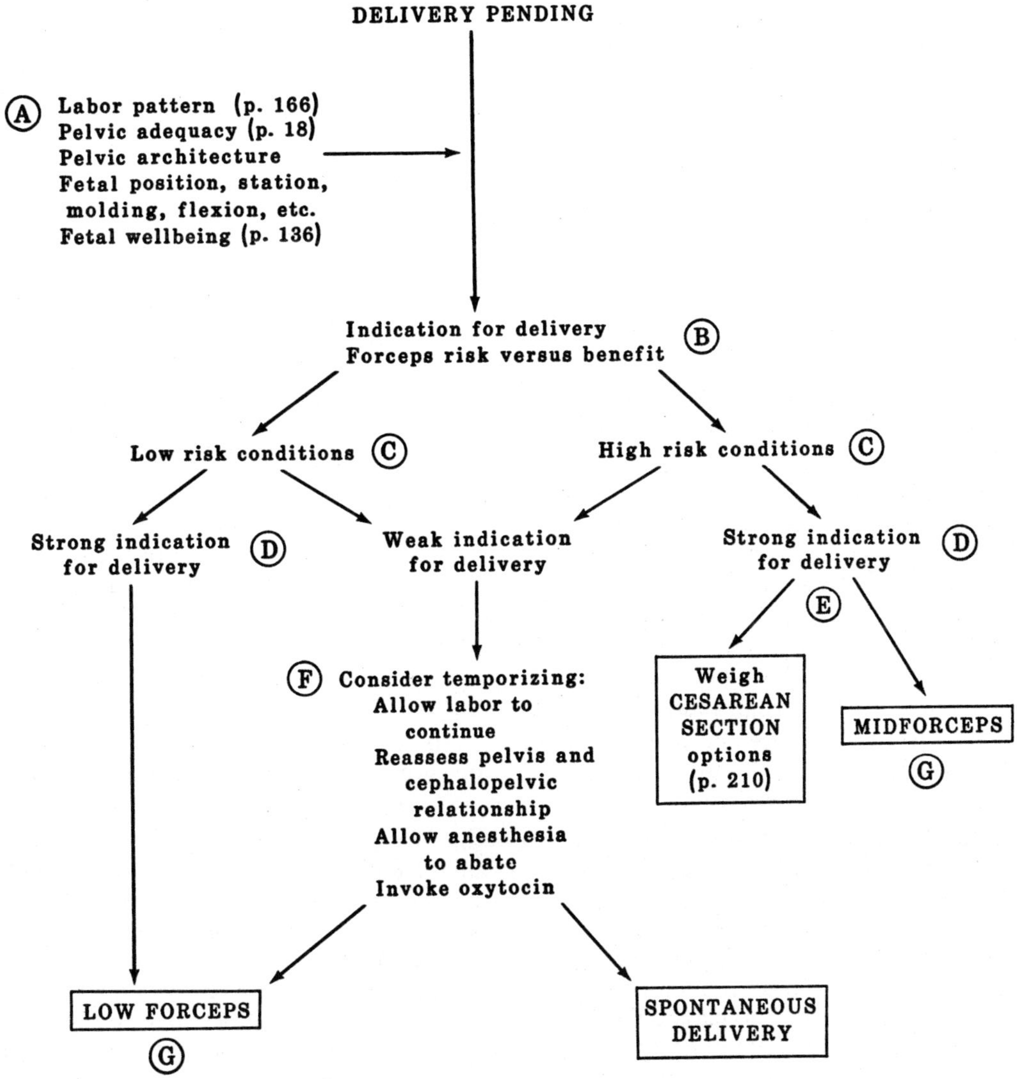
DELIVERY PENDING
A
Labor pattern (p. 166)
Pelvic adequacy (p. 18)
Pelvic architecture
Fetal position, station, molding, flexion, etc.
Fetal wellbeing (p. 136)
Indication for delivery
Forceps risk versus benefit
B
Low risk conditions
C
High risk conditions
C
Strong indication for delivery
D
Weak indication for delivery
Strong indication for delivery
D
E
F
Consider temporizing:
Allow labor to continue
Reassess pelvis and cephalopelvic relationship
Allow anesthesia to abate
Invoke oxytocin
Weigh CESAREAN SECTION options (p. 210)
MIDFORCEPS
G
LOW FORCEPS
G
SPONTANEOUS DELIVERY

CESAREAN OPTIONS

Louis Burke, M.D.

COMMENTS

A. Because cesarean section is a major surgical procedure carrying significant risk, one must try to ensure that the gravida is in optimal condition before proceeding. Optimally, full preoperative evaluation involves surveillance of blood, electrolyte, renal, cardiac, and pulmonary function status.

B. No matter how urgent the situation, it is imperative that the patient be counseled and reassured so that she is able to give some degree of informed consent. This can be accomplished in most cases while the operating room team is being mobilized and the preanesthetic evaluation is being done.

C. About half the elective repeat cesarean section patients can be delivered vaginally. Observe strict criteria for selection to ensure safety: facilities and personnel for immediate operative intervention, vertex presentation with adequate pelvis and good labor progression, a prior low cervical transverse incision, and the patient's desire and consent, of course. Labor can be interrupted any time problems arise in order to perform a cesarean section. Such trials of labor should not be undertaken in outlying areas or hospitals that cannot meet the criteria of immediately available on-site surgical facilities and personnel.

D. Prophylactic use of antibiotics, especially if instituted several hours prior to surgery, can effectively reduce the maternal morbidity so commonly associated with cesarean section in patients who are in labor. Antibiotics are not comparably effective for elective repeat cesarean section.

E. The choice of abdominal incision depends on the need for speed (vertical midline suprapubic incision is quicker), for room (transverse incision may give limited access), and for cosmetic consideration (transverse incision preferred). As to uterine incisions, the common transverse elliptical incision in the lower uterine segment (Kerr-Phaneuf) has many advantages (reduced bleeding, ease of repair, fewer postoperative adhesions or subsequent rupture), although lateral extension into uterine vessels and bladder injury may occur. The classic incision, made vertically in the upper uterine segment, has the single advantage of speed but is associated with more hemorrhage, poorer healing, and more frequent subsequent catastrophic rupture. Classic incisions are also used for transverse lie (especially with undeveloped lower uterine segment or when the fetal back is down), brech presentation with hyperextended head (to avoid transection of the cervical spinal cord), placenta previa (especially with anterior wall involvement), and severe fetal distress. Extraperitoneal cesarean for a grossly infected uterus is rarely done today.

REFERENCES

Amerikia H, Zarewych B, Evans TN: Cesarean section: A 15 year review of changing incidence, indications, and risks. Am J Obstet Gynecol 140:81, 1981

Farrell SJ, Andersen HF, Work BA Jr: Cesarean section: Indications and postoperative morbidity. Obstet Gynecol 56:696, 1980

Mann LI, Gallant J: Modern indications for cesarean section. Am J Obstet Gynecol 135:437, 1979

Pauerstein CJ: Labor after cesarean section: From precept to practice. J Reprod Med 26:409, 1981

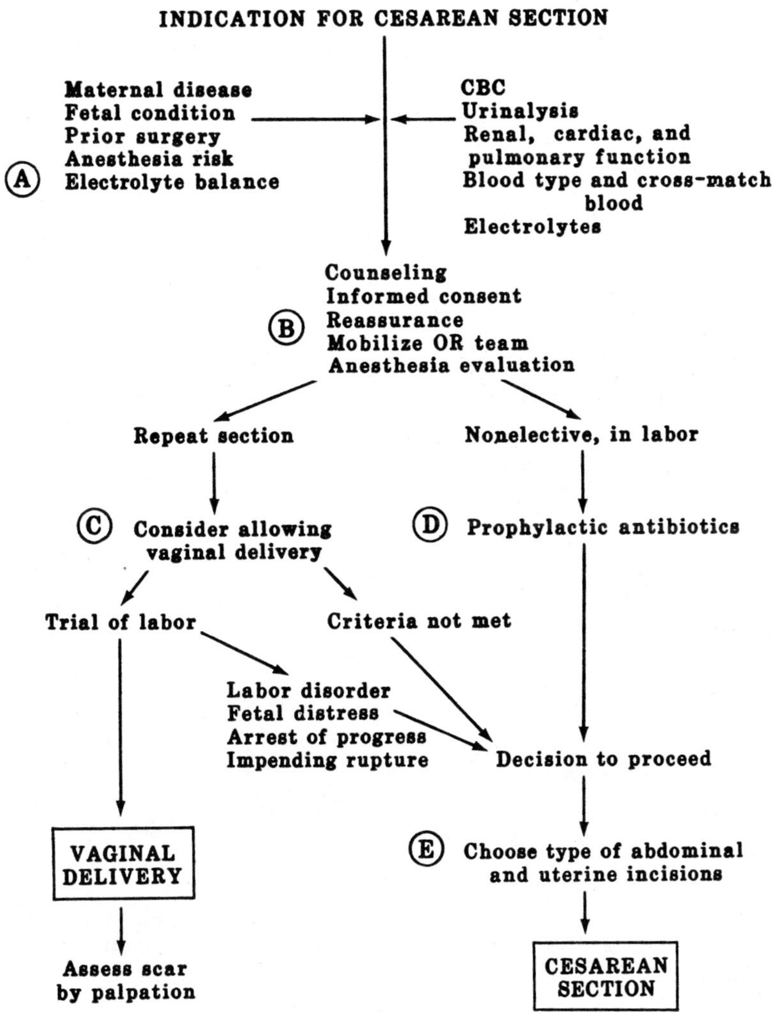
INDICATION FOR CESAREAN SECTION
Maternal disease
Fetal condition
Prior surgery
Anesthesia risk
Electrolyte balance
(A)
CBC
Urinalysis
Renal, cardiac, and pulmonary function
Blood type and cross-match blood
Electrolytes
(B)
Counseling
Informed consent
Reassurance
Mobilize OR team
Anesthesia evaluation
Repeat section
Nonelective, in labor
(C) Consider allowing vaginal delivery
(D) Prophylactic antibiotics
Trial of labor
Criteria not met
Labor disorder
Fetal distress
Arrest of progress
Impending rupture
Decision to proceed
VAGINAL DELIVERY
(E) Choose type of abdominal and uterine incisions
Assess scar by palpation
CESAREAN SECTION

PREVIOUS CESAREAN SECTION

Austin Wertheimer, M.D.

COMMENTS

A. The criteria to be applied in preselecting a patient for trial of labor and vaginal delivery include adequate institutional facilities and personnel for 24-hour blood bank, anesthesia, fetal monitoring, and emergency cesarean section without delay, plus the patient's willingness to accept a trial of labor and her understanding of the risks, as well as verification that the prior cesarean was done through a low transverse uterine incision. The patient should not have had more than one cesarean; if she has had more than one, a lateral hysterogram should be done in the nonpregnant state to confirm that the lower uterine segment scar is intact.

B. Gestational age assessment is based on information derived from the date of the last menstrual period, date of quickening (expected at about 18 weeks), date that nonamplified fetal heart sounds were first heard (20 weeks), biparietal diameter by ultrasonography between 20 and 30, weeks early crown-rump measurements, and uterine size.

C. Any discrepancy warrants objective verification of fetal lung maturity before proceeding with elective repeat cesarean section. The same applies if the dating is unsure or unknown or if the patient first presents for antepartum care late in pregnancy.

D. Labor management requires one to avoid anesthesia, such as epidural or caudal block, to minimize analgesia, and to eschew oxytocin for uterotonic stimulation. Constant attendance of trained personnel and continuous electronic fetal monitoring are essential.

E. The kinds of abnormalities that should serve to interrupt the trial of labor in favor of cesarean section include fetal distress, intensifying focal uterine or generalized abdominal pain or tenderness between contractions, deterioration of vital signs, irregular uterine outline, heavy vaginal bleeding, ascent of the fetal presenting part, regression of cervical dilatation, hematuria, protraction or arrest disorder of labor unresponsive to conservative measures, and sudden cessation of uterine contractions.

REFERENCES

Brudenell M, Chakravarti S: Uterine rupture in labour. Brit Med J 2:122, 1975

Merrill BS, Gibbs CE: Planned vaginal delivery following cesarean section. Obstet Gynecol 52:50, 1978

Saldana LR, Schulman H, Reuss L: Management of pregnancy after cesarean section. Am J Obstet Gynecol 135:555, 1979

Spaulding LB, Gallup DG: Current concepts of management of rupture of the gravid uterus. Obstet Gynecol 54:437, 1979

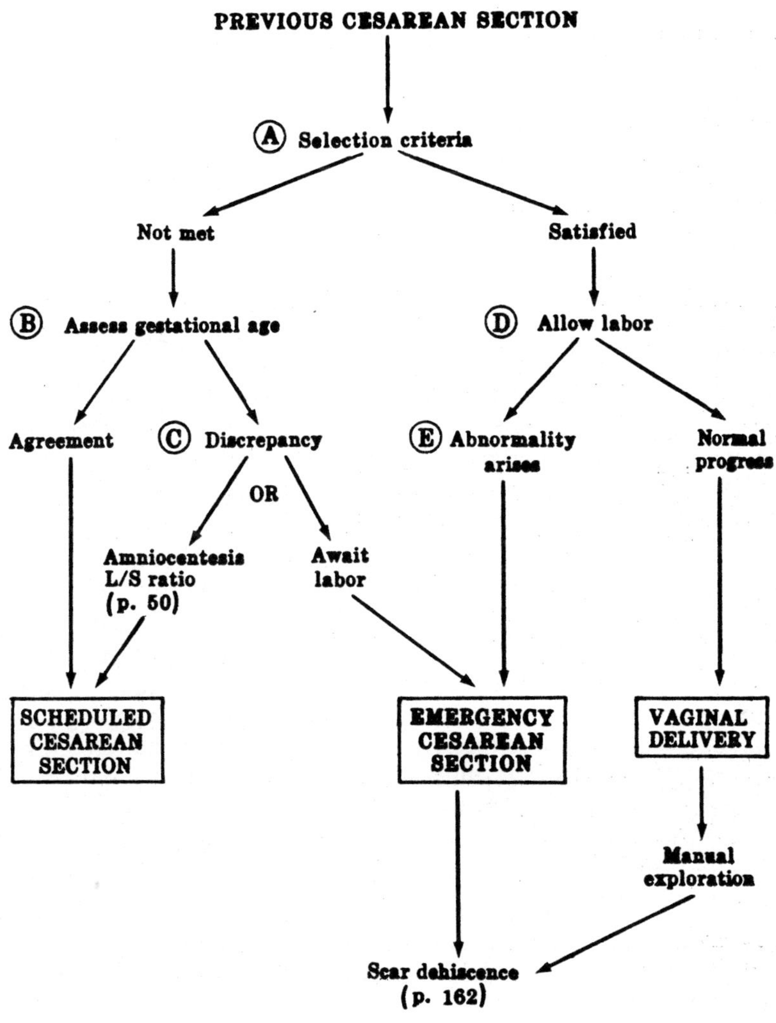
PREVIOUS CESAREAN SECTION
(A) Selection criteria
Not met
Satisfied
(B) Assess gestational age
(D) Allow labor
Agreement
(C) Discrepancy
OR
(E) Abnormality arises
Normal progress
Amniocentesis L/S ratio (p. 50)
Await labor
SCHEDULED CESAREAN SECTION
EMERGENCY CESAREAN SECTION
VAGINAL DELIVERY
Manual exploration
Scar dehiscence (p. 162)

CONTRACEPTION

Johanna F. Perlmutter, M.D.

COMMENTS

A. Birth control pills are inappropriate for lactating women because they may reduce milk production. Natural methods are least effective when menstruation is erratic.

B. Lactation will produce amenorrhea, but resumption of ovulation is unpredictable. For complete protection against pregnancy an alternative method of contraception should always be utilized.

C. Resumption of menstruation is highly variable, usually occurring 6 to 8 weeks post partum; with lactation, it may not occur for 3–4 months. If intercourse is begun prior to the 6-week visit, condoms are recommended.

D. Birth control pills can be initiated as early as 5 days post partum. They can mask manifestations of Sheehan's syndrome and make it difficult to differentiate breakthrough bleeding from pregnancy-related problems. Rule out early pregnancy before starting pills. If pills are begun before the first menstrual bleeding, contraceptive protection is unreliable.

E. Common postpartum problems include retained secundines, subinvolution of the uterus, and endometritis. Heavy bleeding and persistent spotting and bleeding may necessitate curettage.

F. An intrauterine device (IUD) may be inserted at any time after complete uterine involution. With subinvolution or endometritis it is advisable to wait for complete resolution, because poor IUD placement, sepsis, heavy vaginal bleeding, and perforation are more apt to occur. Uterine hyperinvolution with lactation may make the uterine cavity too small for an IUD and risk expulsion, pregnancy, and perforation.

G. Spontaneous IUD expulsion occurs mostly in the first 24 hours or at the first menstrual period. A check-up is done at 6 weeks or after the first menstrual period. Watch for bleeding and infection.

H. Even under the most ideal circumstances, natural methods yield frequent pregnancies. They are even less effective before normal menstrual rhythmicity is re-established. Study of basal body temperature and cervical mucus together give better results but may require long periods of abstention.

I. Spatial relationships of cervix and vagina, vaginal tone, and perineal muscle integrity must be restored for a proper diaphragm fit. Anatomic distortions preclude good diaphragm placement.

REFERENCES

Mackenzie P: Postpartum family planning in private practice. Obstet Gynecol 44:762, 1974

Van Praagh IGL, Munsick GW, Murdoch DE: Perforation of a puerperal uterus with two Lippes loops. Am J Obstet Gynecol 105:1286, 1969

Wade ME, McCarthy P, Braunstein GD, Abernathy JR, Suchindran CM, Harris GS, Danzer HC, Uricchio WA: A randomized prospective study of the use-effectiveness of two methods of natural family planning. Am J Obstet Gynecol 141:368, 1981

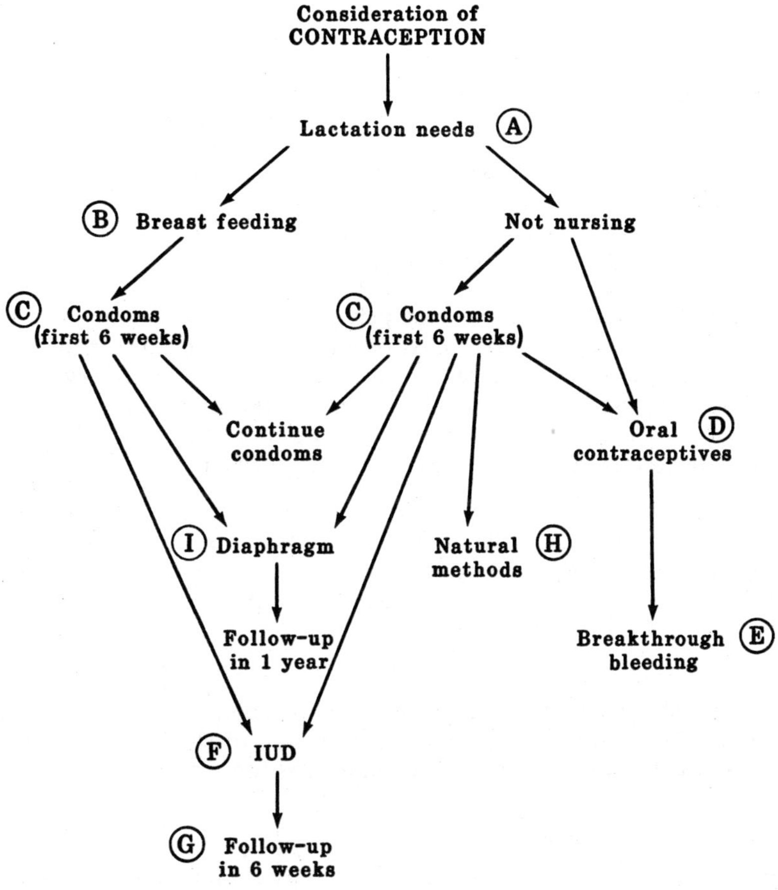
Consideration of CONTRACEPTION
Lactation needs (A)
(B) Breast feeding
Not nursing
(C) Condoms (first 6 weeks)
(C) Condoms (first 6 weeks)
Continue condoms
Oral contraceptives (D)
(I) Diaphragm
Natural methods (H)
Follow-up in 1 year
Breakthrough bleeding (E)
(F) IUD
(G) Follow-up in 6 weeks

STERILIZATION

Max Borten, M.D.

COMMENTS

A. Before performing permanent sterilization, be alert to potential problems in the patient's emotional and social background. Counseling should stress the irreversibility of the surgery. Discuss contraceptive alternatives, especially in younger women of low parity. Review the relative risks of sterilization options so that the patient can make an intelligent, informed decision. At least 72 hours should be given to all patients to weigh their decision before the operation is actually done.

B. Severe or recurrent pelvic infection, prior pelvic surgery, or abdominal surgery complicated by postoperative infection may produce adhesions distorting the adnexal anatomy and making the tubes inaccessible for transendoscopic surgery. Adherence of the intestines to the anterior abdominal wall places the bowel at risk of perforation during laparoscopy. These features in the past history constitute relative contraindications to endoscopic techniques for sterilization (except open laparoscopic techniques).

C. Whereas sterilization is commonly done during the immediate postpartum period, interval procedures are technically easier and have lower failure rates. For convenience, however, the patient who has just delivered and desires sterilization is a good candidate for the procedure.

D. Operative endoscopic techniques are usually applicable for sterilizing the recently pregnant woman. Hysteroscopic transuterine occlusion of the tubal ostia has not been shown to be as effective and cannot be recommended for general use yet.

E. Closed laparoscopy is the commonest surgical procedure in use. Puerperal sterilization is approached by the abdominal route. If laparotomy is chosen, a small elliptical subumbilical incision should be surgically satisfactory and cosmetically acceptable. Open laparoscopy is mainly indicated in cases with prior abdominal or pelvic surgery or history of intraperitoneal infection. Bipolar coagulation of the tube is done in 3 adjacent sites. Unipolar coagulation risks sparking across to the adjacent structures; serious bowel burn may occur. Division and resection of a segment of the tube, when done in conjunction with coagulation, inexplicably results in high failure and complication rates.

REFERENCES

Chi IC, Laufe LE, Gardner SD, Tolbert MA: An epidemiologic study of risk factors associated with pregnancy following female sterilization. Am J Obstet Gynecol 136:768, 1980

Fishburne JI: Anesthesia for laparoscopy: Considerations, complications and techniques. J Reprod Med 21:37, 1978

Neufeld R: Principles and hazards of electrosurgery including laparoscopy. Surg Gynecol Obstet 147:205, 1978

Penfield AJ: Minilaparotomy for female sterilization. Obstet Gynecol 54:184, 1979

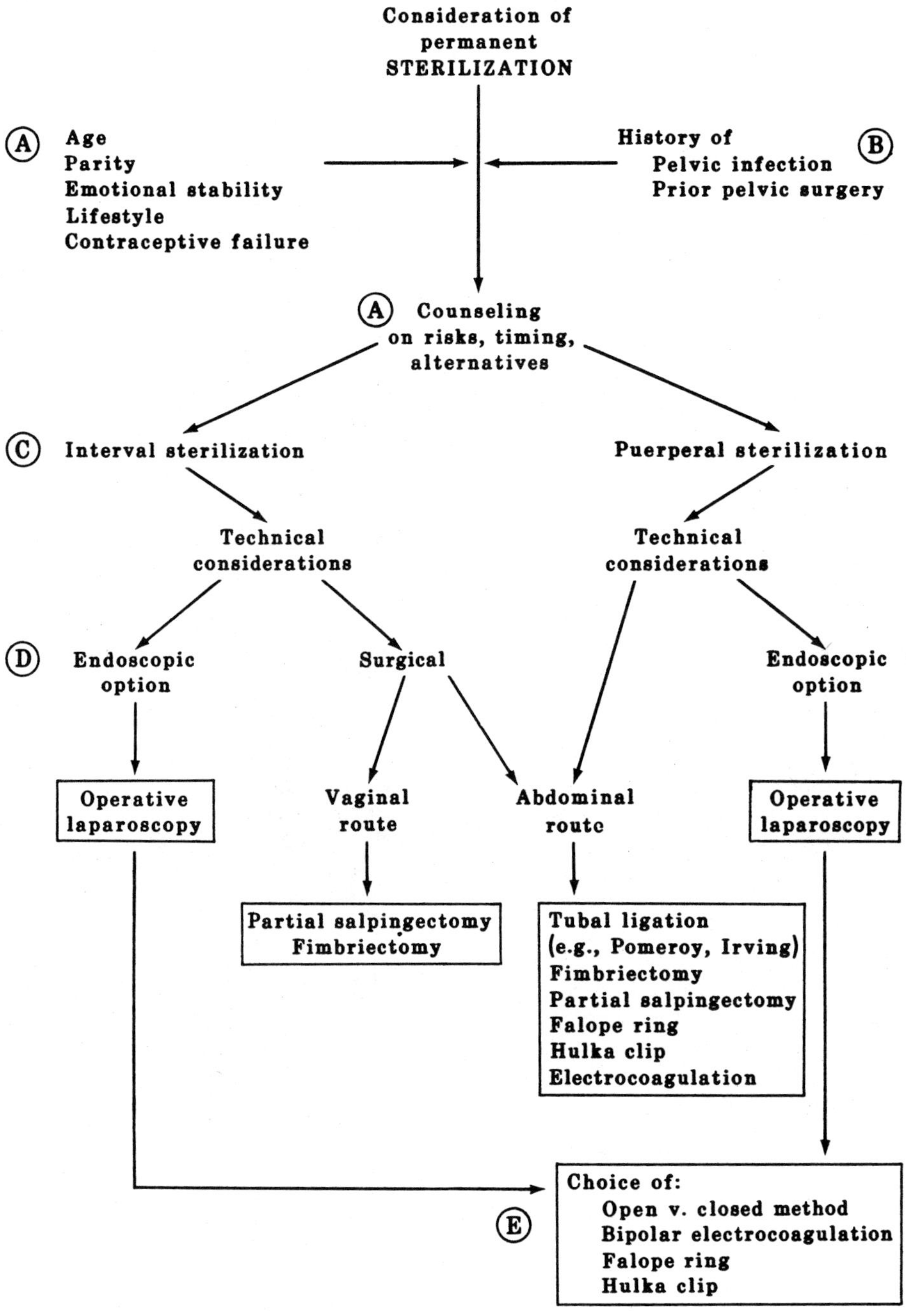
Consideration of permanent STERILIZATION
A
Age
Parity
Emotional stability
Lifestyle
Contraceptive failure
History of
Pelvic infection
Prior pelvic surgery
B
A Counseling on risks, timing, alternatives
C Interval sterilization
Puerperal sterilization
Technical considerations
Technical considerations
D Endoscopic option
Surgical
Endoscopic option D
Operative laparoscopy
Vaginal route
Abdominal route
Operative laparoscopy
Partial salpingectomy
Fimbriectomy
Tubal ligation
(e.g., Pomeroy, Irving)
Fimbriectomy
Partial salpingectomy
Falope ring
Hulka clip
Electrocoagulation
E
Choice of:
Open v. closed method
Bipolar electrocoagulation
Falope ring
Hulka clip

INDEX